NEUROLOGIC CRITICAL CARE

NEUROLOGIC CRITICAL CARE

Joan E. Davis/Celestine B. Mason

Critical Care Clinician
Manpower Health Services
Seattle, Washington

Assistant Professor
Pacific Luthern University
Tacoma, Washington

VNR VAN NOSTRAND REINHOLD COMPANY

NEW YORK   CINCINNATI   ATLANTA   DALLAS   SAN FRANCISCO
LONDON   TORONTO   MELBOURNE

Van Nostrand Reinhold Company Regional Offices:
New York Cincinnati Atlanta Dallas San Francisco

Van Nostrand Reinhold Company International Offices:
London Toronto Melbourne

Library of Congress Catalog Card Number: 79-4379
ISBN: 0-442-22004-9

Manufactured in the United States of America

Published by Van Nostrand Reinhold Company
135 West 50th Street, New York, N. Y. 10020

Published simultaneously in Canada by Van Nostrand Reinhold Ltd.

15 14 13 12 11 10 9 8 7 6 5 4 3 2 1

Library of Congress Cataloging in Publication Data

Davis, Joan, 1945–
  Neurologic critical care.

  Includes index.
  1. Neurological nursing. 2. Critical care medicine.
I. Mason, Celestine, joint author. II. Title.
[DNLM: 1. Critical care. 2. Nervous system diseases—
Nursing. WY160.3 D262n]
RC350.5.D38   610.73′6   79-4379
ISBN 0-442-22004-9

This book is dedicated to:

Those nurses who stimulated us to write by their insistance to grasp information which would enable them to improve their nursing care.

BUT ESPECIALLY TO OUR FAMILIES

William J. Davis and Ben and June Edmiston
Frank L. Mason, Kimberly, Michael, Daleen, Christel, and Michelle.

ACKNOWLEDGMENTS

We wish to express our sincere gratitude to:

Naomi Ruth Edmiston, B.S., M.A., Vancouver, Washington, who taught us the art of the English language.

Elke Tercier and Bill Davis, Seattle, Washington, for their expert art work. We commend them for their patience in drawing to our unique specifications.

The engineers and draftsmen of the Air Launch Cruise Missile (ALCM), Boeing Company, Seattle, Washington, for their consultation on the physics of trauma.

Special recognition is due the following people for their review of selected chapters:

Vicki Stockton, R.N., C.N.R.N., Neuro Nurse Specialist, Baylor College of Medicine, Houston, Texas.

Susan R. Richey, R.N., A.D.S., Intensive Care, Valley General Hospital, Renton, Washington.

Many people have influenced our writing in various ways. We would like to thank the following nurses for their continued interest, enthusiastic support, and invaluable motivation:

Joyce Zerweckh, R.N., B.S.N., M.A., Home Health Coordinator, Group Health Cooperative, Seattle, Washington.

Mat Acuff, R.N., B.S.N., M.S., Assistant Professor Psychiatric-Mental Health Nursing, Pacific Lutheran University, Tacoma, Washington.

Shirley Aikin, R.N., B.S.N., M.A., Instructor Medical-Surgical Nursing, Pacific Lutheran University, Tacoma, Washington.

The quality of the nursing profession has always been promoted by two interested friends:

Robert J. McHardy, M.S., Director Browne McHardy Clinic, Metairie, Louisiana.

George Yang, M.D., Neurosurgeon, Seattle, Washington.

Our book would not be possible without the conscientious, diligent, and expert work of our typist:

Bonnie Melander, Tacoma, Washington.

PREFACE

The incidence, frequency, and mortality of neurologic disorders demand the attention of the intensive care nurse. Many of the conditions presented in intensive care units are devastating in nature, not only in terms of the loss to the patient and family, but the loss to the community as well. These diseases are hideous in appearance and often incurable by man. The nurse involved in the care of the neurologic patient may become frustrated, disappointed, and even disheartened. The area, the conditions, and the patient become a challenge for nursing practice, as well as a framework that offers a personal growth experience for the clinician. Her philosophy becomes integrated, her knowledge and procedural skills are expanded, and her interpersonal relationships are cultivated and broadened. With no claim to sexism, we shall continue to refer to the nurse as "she" and the patient as "he" abiding by tradition.

The adaptation and integration of a particular personal philosophy predispose entry into the nursing profession. The theologian Fulton Sheen describes the nurse as having a sense of humor and an incision.[1]

A sense of humor, as he discusses it, is the ability to see beyond what is there; the ability to sense the invisible; the perception of a person beyond his wounds. How appropriate it is for the intensive care nurse to move beyond the disease and focus on the ultimate potential for high level wellness for her patient, spreading joy and gladness in life itself.

The incision, as Bishop Sheen describes it, becomes an appreciation and experiential understanding of pain. This may be developed by the nurse's experiencing pain herself, or acquired by her schooling herself in empathy and understanding of someone else's pain. Here lies the caring involvement with the patient we are often so afraid of.

In caring for the neurologic patient, the nurse must demonstrate advanced knowledge, refined competency of skills, and superior judgment. Observation and interpretation of overt and covert signs become essential in planning patient care. Intervention is based on a

---

[1] McFadden, Charles J., *Medical Ethics*, 3rd ed., Foreword by Fulton Sheen, Philadelphia: F. A. Davis, 1955.

knowledge of anatomy, physiology, and pathology; data obtained from assessment and physical exam skills; and technical competency. The professional nurse must interpret the data, problem-solve, plan, and evaluate the management of the neurologic patient.

Interpersonal relationships are cultivated and broadened when one is administering total patient care. These relationships contribute to the health of the patient and the personal growth of the nurse. The nurse becomes sensitive, perceptive, empathic, and caring. Often she is compelled to decide between recovery care and comfort care. In the resolution of this conflict comes the wake of growth.

The unique circumstances in the intensive care unit provide the means for a very close and protected relationship between the medical and nursing professions. In a team approach to patient care management, the two realms become complementary rather than competitive. It has been our experience with neurologists and neurosurgeons that these relationships can be satisfying, supportive, and productive.

We welcome the reader who is interested in dealing with the critically ill neurologic patient. We invite the nurse, with the many demands placed on her, to "grow," "be," and "become." May our book provide a sense of direction that will be personally and professionally rewarding.

JOAN DAVIS AND CEL MASON

CONTENTS

NEUROLOGIC CRITICAL CARE

1
PHILOSOPHY

INTRODUCTION

Theory

We all have a philosophy of life, a life-style, a set of religious beliefs; and our behavior is an expression of our basic, implicit philosophy. Each nurse also integrates a philosophy of nursing that governs his/her attitudes and nursing actions. We would support a humanistic, holistic philosophical theory in professionals preparing for intensive care nursing. Nurses do become intensely involved in therapeutic relationships with their patients and are impelled to consider the "whole" patient as a complex entity (his/her ecosystem or bio-psychosocial functioning). Regardless of the vocabulary in vogue, the ideal philosophy encompasses a significant nurse–patient relationship and a "corporate" view of the patient's entire "being."

Purpose

In 1961 the Kellogg Foundation Report defined the purpose of the intensive care unit as a provision of "high level nursing care for patients who require continuous, comprehensive observation and detailed, intensive care in an atmosphere of compassion and understanding."[1] Through a maze of tubing, machinery, and electronic modules, it is the capable, observing, and interpreting nurse who intervenes in the patient's behalf.

Intensive care of the critically ill is based on the fact that although there are thousands of pathological conditions, the mechanism of death is uniquely limited to a fairly small number of physiologic events. Basically, all medical care, including all nursing care, is designed to observe and preserve the vital functions of ventilation, circulation, assimilation, and elimination. In some instances these processes are amenable to control at least temporarily. Death can be prevented in many situations if time is gained to perform therapeutic measures and to allow the recuperative powers of the body to come into play. Recovery, which may have been impossible otherwise, may then be achieved. Intensive care units group critically ill patients under the care of specially trained staff members whose philosophy, education, and personality allow them to grant attention to minute physiologic variations. Units are developed

[1] W. B. Kellogg Foundation, *The Planning and Operation of an Intensive Care Unit*, Battle Creek, Michigan, September 1961.

for seriously ill patients who require extraordinary care and preferred treatment on a concentrated and continuous basis.

Policies and Procedures

The policies or guidelines of any critical care unit reflect its philosophy. Generally, there are multiple criteria for the admission of a patient into the area, usually based on a life-threatening illness with potential for recovery. There are a variety of units dealing with selected disease entities, e.g., renal disorders, heart problems, burns, and so on. There also exist units with multidisciplinary patients who benefit from close physician supervision, life support systems, monitoring, and intensive nursing care. Each institution provides the organizational structure appropriate for its size, number and type of patients, physician availability, and staffing. Limits of responsibility are designated, and efforts are directed toward evaluation of care, utilization review, and requisites for patient discharge from the unit. There are procedures established for admission and discharge of patients, as well as documented directions for specific technical procedures.

The wise nurse is aware of the philosophy, policies, and procedures of the unit in which she is employed and can seriously abide by them in accordance with her own beliefs.

PATIENT-RELATED OBJECTIVES

The Biopsychosocial Process

The following general goals have been established for the nurse in the intensive care unit:

1. Detection of and participation in the treatment of life-threatening crises;
2. Preservation of the patient's physiological defenses and prevention of further bodily complication;
3. Provision of comfort that does not conflict with the second objective and serves as a beginning implementation of the next objective;
4. Establishment and maintenance of meaningful communication with the patient, reflecting an attitude of respect for the person and his emotional reactions and concerns.[2]

There is also emphasis on utilization of the nursing process as a goal in planning patient care in the intensive care unit. The nurse must be capable of continuous rapid assessment, promptly integrating information from various

[2]Kintzel, Kay Corman, ed., *Advanced Concepts in Clinical Nursing*, 2nd ed., Philadelphia: J. B. Lippincott Co., 1977, pp. 232-233.

overt and covert clinical clues, establishing and maintaining priorities based on a threat to the patient's physiologic entity, initiating immediate action, performing specific procedures expertly utilizing very specialized machinery, and modifying care with respect to established outcome criteria.

The concept of nurturance, prevention, construction, coordination, and restoration may be interpreted as a general goal for intensive care personnel in relation to their patients' needs. Often only one or two phases receive attention in the critical care unit, though achievement of the entire process *depends* on continuity of care for the patient when he is transferred back to the wards.

Notice the high priority set on the preservation of life by meeting the patient's biological needs. If we consider that fear increases as the significance of the organ to the individual increases, we may then be able to comprehend the fear of loss of life itself. The alert, compassionate, available, and responsive nurse may offer something worthwhile to counter the emotional disharmony felt by the patient.

The spectrum of the "whole" person is complete when we direct our activities to include the patient's family. Although the patient has interacted with someone, in illness his social role has been impaired, with his communication and interaction quite limited. His perspective as a social being must be restored. There is an additional need displayed by a "hurting family." There is not always time for critical care nurses to deal with the problems posed by persons other than the patient. A sense of awareness and concern may be reflected, however, and possibly a pathway for resolution of problems discovered. This may appropriately be from resources available outside of the critical care unit.

Stress Adaptation

The impact of a serious illness on an individual depends on his health belief model. If he denies the existence of an imperfect biological entity that could threaten *his* well-being, the shock of a major health crisis in his life will be paramount. Disbelief may be replaced by a developing awareness of a physical problem, evolving into restitution and resolution. This adaptation process produces tension, requires energy, and demands a varying amount of time.

The patient's life may be in jeopardy, and the primary anxiety-producing stimulus may be the dissolution of the basic drive toward self-preservation. The nurse innately responds to the patient's physiologic stress, and all efforts are directed toward life support. There are also secondary anxiety-producing stimuli in the physical environment, which attract the patient's energy. The presence of machinery, the number of personnel involved in his care, the auditory sensory overload, the inevitable tubes and equipment, all are potential stresses superimposed on the patient by the atmosphere of the intensive care unit. If the nurse can reduce secondary anxiety by manipulating the environment therapeutically, the patient's energy may then be released to attend the process of adaptation and equilibrium.

NURSE-RELATED OBJECTIVES

The nurse in the critical care setting has additional responsibilities to the consumer of health care and to herself in her professional capacity: an improvement in the standard of patient care and the advancement of the nursing profession. The direction she chooses to take in achieving her objectives will influence her level of nursing practice as well as her professional goals. Nurse-related objectives may be organized in two models for our purposes here: the expanded role and the leadership role.

The Expanded Role

A transfer of responsibilities from the realm of medicine to the realm of nursing becomes increasingly evident in the intensive care unit, where the nurse fulfills expectations of increased education, increased technological training, and increased standard of care by becoming responsible and accountable for an unlimited series of actions traditionally reserved for the physician. Legally this comprises the entire scope of practice issue that has surfaced in recent years. Among the many factors entering into the determination of nursing liability are the expectations of: the nurse herself, the nursing profession, the institution, the medical staff, and the health consumer.

In the unit the nurse is considered a specialist and accountable in varying degrees for her actions. There are suggestions in nursing literature, by authors such as Martha E. Rogers and Rozella M. Schlotfeldt, that there be universal definition of roles for resolution of the legal authorization for practice. Perhaps this futuristic attitude is unrealistic, since nurses are presently practicing and adjusting to the dichotomy of medical versus nursing accountability. These nurses need our immediate support and attention in their individual and unique circumstances, support that perhaps would be more beneficial than an ambiguous role identification statement by law or profession that would inevitably become outdated in our rapidly changing society. Nuckolls states:

> Ultimately, the person who really determines what the nurse can do is the nurse herself. Her perception of her role and her expectations of herself will be the most important determinates of her behavior. Self expectations and role perceptions are determined by experience and interaction with others.[3]

[3]Nuckolls, Katherine B., "Who Decides What the Nurse Can Do?" *Nursing Outlook*, October 1974, pp. 626–631.

With her personal philosophy as a guide, the nurse may proceed toward the objective of improvement in the standard of patient care in an independent manner and begin to set precedents for the development of future concepts.

The Leadership Role

The achievement of the goal of advancement of the profession is in accord with the criteria established for a profession. The growth of a body of scientific knowledge depends upon the development of nurse leaders. We see these leaders as having certain qualities: technical skills, communication skills, and conceptual skills. To acquire these characteristics the nurse must be aware of and able to utilize data available from a variety of processes.

Technical Skills. The intensive care nurse must be familiar with all of the equipment in the department; often this responsibility includes troubleshooting for nonfunctioning machinery. She must be able to perform specialized procedures applying scientific principles and sound judgment. The faculty of interpreting data and determining nursing intervention requires practice and experience. A technical orientation is certainly an aspect of critical care nursing.

Communication Skills. The ability to communicate effectively is essential in a leader. The nurse must be aware of and interested in expanding her own knowledge base as well as promoting learning in her staff. She must utilize principles from other disciplines such as education in the teaching-learning process, as well as her human relations skills. Continuing education is also included in the professional criteria, and again we face the dilemma of legally defining continuing education as a factor in licensure.

In planning patient care the nurse utilizing the nursing process must be able to communicate the medical objectives to her patients and her peers. Interpersonal relationships correlate with the nurse's job satisfaction and job performance.

As a leader, the nurse attempts to move groups of people toward a goal, an effort in which the supervision/evaluation process becomes increasingly important. Again the utilization of human relations skills receives great emphasis. An understanding of change, values, motivation, and the like, tends to improve the leader's effectiveness.

Conceptual Skills. The ability to conceptualize is another asset for the nurse in a leadership role. In utilizing this ability the nurse becomes adept at applying principles from the decision-making process. The generation of problem-solving ideas, the selection of a possible alternative, and the implementation of the decision all require an unlimited amount of stamina. This is particularly true if the decision effects a major change in the *modus operandi.*

In the development of a construct the nurse may wish to take a scientific approach, and certainly the need for research in nursing cannot be denied. Not everyone is inclined toward experimenting or even collecting descriptive data; but think of the potential benefits to the patient if someone at the bedside were to investigate some critical problems in patient care within a research framework.

We have moved from the nurse with specialized skills to a nurse *educated* in her specialty with the purpose of advancing the nursing profession by becoming a leader.

DEATH AND DYING

A philosophy for working in the intensive care unit would be incomplete without some recognition of the myriad of problems imposed by the concept of "death and dying." Perhaps just probing the issue here will produce sufficient stimulation of thought and purpose for the nurse to investigate her own attitudes and declare a philosophical commitment.

Definition

The traditional maxim that "where there is breath, there is life" holds no substance in today's medical technology. Life can be maintained when the patient is no longer breathing spontaneously; life can be maintained when the heart is no longer pumping; life can be maintained when the brain is no longer discharging impulses. We have mechanically altered all of the human body's vital functions to a point where we face a dilemma—when has the patient died? Many definitions of death exist: natural death, biological death, clinical death, and legal death. Our role as nurses in determining when death has occurred may be indirect, but we certainly must explore what we believe constitutes *life*.

Criteria

Many disciplines have developed criteria for death; philosophy, theology, law, and medicine, to name only a few. The "Report of the Ad Hoc Committee of the Harvard Medical School to Examine the Definition of Brain Death" in 1968 is the most prominent proposal. The following criteria were described and presented in some detail:

1. Unreceptivity and unresponsitivity to externally applied stimuli and inner need
2. No spontaneous muscular movements or spontaneous respiration
3. No elicitable brain reflexes
4. Flat electroencephalogram[4]

[4]"A Definition of Irreversible Coma: Report of the Ad Hoc Committee of the Harvard Medical School to Examine the Definition of Brain Death," *Journal of the American Medical Association*, 205:337–340, 1968.

Some authorities appeal the conclusions of the report and encourage the clarification and revision of more appropriate criteria.

Elective Death

There is considerable discussion and some controversy regarding elective death. The nurse confronts the professional issue of recovery versus comfort care. Can she morally and professionally allow the patient to die with dignity? Can she accept the dictum of a living will declaring that no extraordinary means be used to sustain life? What becomes of the dedication to preserve life in these critical issues? Perhaps a reorganization of our thinking is necessary. Looking at death as a process rather than an event and declaring at some point along the biological continuum that life is gone may enhance our understanding of when to cease support measures and intervene with comfort measures.

Staff Psychodynamics

The nurse in the intensive care unit frequently deals with the death process. The way she copes with her personal feelings regarding death will reflect her congruent philosophy of life. A variety of emotional coping mechanisms utilized, such as depression, overactivity, detachment, frustration, anger, resentment, and even humor, may aid the person so susceptible to death saturation. The nurse must manage psychologically to endure a high stress level and to function competently and effectively in death situations. A unit that observes the morale of the nurses and the emotional atmosphere may subscribe to a variety of techniques for relief of tension and the maintenance of the nurses' mental health.

CONCLUSION

The philosophy adopted by the nurse in the intensive care unit is developed through critical thinking, exposure, and experience. Many factors influence its development, both internal and external. The purpose of our ministrations to the patient seems to evolve around an understanding of the biopsychosocial process and stress adaptation. In this concept we see nursing moving toward an improvement of patient care. Nurse-related objectives direct our pathway toward the pursuit of excellence in the nursing profession by exploring the expanded role of the nurse and the leadership role. The specialty of dealing with acutely ill patients deserves some philosophical background regarding death and dying. The nurse must determine her own conclusions and draw from them an eclectic philosophy. Perhaps in reading this chapter the nurse has discovered ways of relating to all people effectively enough to relieve suffering, increase security, promote health, and allow death in her care of patients.

BIBLIOGRAPHY

"A Definition of Irreversible Coma: Report of the Ad Hoc Committee of the Harvard Medical School to Examine the Definition of Brain Death," *Journal of the American Medical Association*, 205:337-340, 1968.

Baily, June L., and Karen E. Claus, *Decision Making in Nursing*, St. Louis: The C. V. Mosby Co., 1975.

Bernzweig, Eli P., *The Nurse's Liability for Malpractice*, New York: McGraw-Hill Inc., 1975, pp. 50 and 166-173.

Hudak, Carolyn, et al., *Critical Care Nursing*, Philadelphia: J. B. Lippincott Co., 1973, pp. 1-25 and 340-342.

W. B. Kellogg Foundation, *The Planning and Operation of an Intensive Care Unit*, Battle Creek, Michigan, September 1961.

Kintzel, Kay Corman, ed., *Advanced Concepts in Clinical Nursing*, 2nd ed., Philadelphia: J. B. Lippincott Co., 1977, pp. 231-249.

Meltzer, Lawrence E., et al, eds., *Concepts and Practices of Intensive Care for Nurse Specialists*, Philadelphia: The Charles Press Pub. Inc., 1969, Introduction, pp. XI-XXV.

Nuckolls, Katherine B., "Who Decides What the Nurse Can Do?" *Nursing Outlook*, October 1974, pp. 626-631.

Pattison, E. Mansell, *The Experience of Dying*, Englewood Cliffs, New Jersey: Prentice-Hall Inc., 1977, pp. 28-74, 245-251, and 316-325.

Silverman, D., R. Masland, M. Saunders, et al., "Irreversible Coma Associated with Electrocerebral Silence," *Neurology*, 20:525-533, 1970.

Wilcox, Sandra Galdieri, and Marilyn Sutton, *Understanding Death & Dying*, Port Washington, New York: Alfred Publishing Co., 1977, pp. 60-62, 44-59, and 352-367.

2
ANATOMY AND PHYSIOLOGY

INTRODUCTION

A human being is a unique entity with incredibly complex interrelationships and a blending of many elements. A major determinant of human behavior is the central nervous system, the most highly sophisticated system in the human body, which is responsible for all the complex processes that enable a person to adjust to both the internal and the external environment. This physiological apparatus moves us to do what we should and should not do by means of electricity, the source of power that keeps the system functioning.

The comprehension and interpretation of neurologic and neurosurgical symptomatology depends on an understanding of the anatomical structures, the physiological apparatus of the central nervous system, and of how a lesion might affect this complex machinery of the human body. We, therefore, approach this topic with a presentation of anatomy and physiology, with the intent of identifying and localizing lesions.

For the purpose of review and discussion, this chapter has been divided into: neurophysiology, with an emphasis on nerve impulse transmission; the central nervous system, with the head, brain, and vertebral column; and the peripheral nervous system, with the spinal nerves and autonomic nervous system. Generally, gross anatomy is the beginning point for instruction, but we selected this organization of material (neurophysiology first) because the entire nervous system is based on the operation of nerve cells.

NEUROPHYSIOLOGY

Cellular Anatomy

Brain tissue is basically composed of two main types of cells—neurons and neuroglia (glial cells). The neurons specialize in impulse conduction, while the neuroglia serve to support, nourish, and protect the neurons. Neuroglia will be presented first and then neurons.

Neuroglia. The glial cells, which outnumber the neurons ten to one, make up about one-half the mass of the brain. They serve to protect the neurons and act as a selective barrier to the brain. They may even be concerned with such functions as memory. Theoretically, the structure of the glial cells surrounding neurons changes markedly under different functional conditions, which

9

may enhance the synapses and, therefore, be the basis of memory. The three major types of glial cells are astrocytes, oligodendroglia, and microglia. Astrocytes are star-shaped cells with multiple processes that form a network around nerve cells; other processes attach and hold nerve cells close to their blood vessels. Oligodendroglia also intertwine between neurons and blood vessels. Microglia support nerve tissue and protect against infection. Usually small and stationary, in the presence of infection they enlarge and move around to carry on phagocytosis.

Neurons. The cerebral cortex is made up almost entirely of neurons; three-fourths of all neuronal cell bodies of the entire nervous system are located in the cerebral cortex. Although they may vary in detail, all neurons consist of a nucleus (cell body) and at least two processes—one axon and one or more dendrites. The cell body resembles other cells with a nucleus, cytoplasm, and various organelles.

The unique structures of the neuron are the dendrites, axons, neurofibrils, nissl bodies, myelin sheath, and neurilemma. The dendrites (the short processes), with their distal end in the receptors, conduct impulses initiated in the receptors, to the cell body of the neuron. The axon (a single, longer process) conducts impulses away from the cell body. Axons vary in length and diameter; those fibers with a large diameter conduct impulses more rapidly. Neurofibrils are fine fibers that bundle together and form a network in neuron cytoplasm. Nissl bodies with RNA granules specialize in protein synthesis and maintain and regenerate the neuronal processes. The segmented coating around a nerve fiber is called the myelin sheath, and the nodes of Ranvier fill the gaps in the segments of the sheath. The myelin sheath is developed from Schwann cells, which provide the covering for each section of the nerve fiber between the nodes of Ranvier. The peripheral nerve fibers have a continuous sheath, the neurilemma, which encompasses all of the fiber, including the myelin sheath with the nodes of Ranvier. The neurilemma is the essential part of peripheral nerve fiber regeneration. Brain and spinal cord fibers do not have this covering; therefore, if injury or disease occurs to these fibers, the destruction is permanent.

The entire neuron (including the processes) is enclosed in a cell membrane, which regulates the transport of substances in and out of the cell. All of these threadlike fibers connect with fibers from one or more other nerve cells, creating a communication network that reaches every part of the body. Impulses move through this network within the brain, from the brain to the body, and from the body to the brain. (See Fig. 2-1.)

Neurons are classified by the direction in which they conduct impulses and by the number of processes they have: sensory (afferent) neurons transmit nerve impulses to the spinal cord or the brain; motoneurons (efferent) conduct impulses away from the brain or spinal cord to muscle or tissue; interneurons conduct impulses from sensory to motor neurons. There are three types of

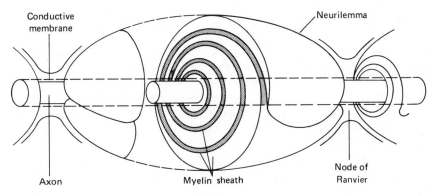

Fig. 2-1. Peripheral nerve.

neurons based on the number of proceses they have: multipolar, bipolar, and unipolar. Multipolar neurons have *one* axon and *many* dendrites; bipolar neurons have *one* axon and *one* dendrite; unipolar neurons have *one* process for a short distance from the cell body, from which *one* axon and *one* dendrite then become distinguishable.

Nerve Impulse Transmission

Membrane Potential. In a nonconducting neuron three significant differences exist: the concentration of sodium ions in extracellular fluid is much higher than in the neuron's intracellular fluid; the concentration of potassium ions in intracellular fluid is higher than in the neuron's extracellular fluid; and the outer surface of the neuron's membrane is 70–90 millivolts positive to its inner surface. The membrane is therefore polarized with a potential difference (difference in electrical charges), which is termed the *resting potential.* Diffusion generally occurs from an area of greater ion concentration to an area of lower ion concentration, equalizing the concentration gradient. Ions move from a more electropositive area to a less electropositive area down the electrical gradient. On this basis, diffusion across the cell membrane should equalize the ionic concentrations of extracellular and intracellular fluids, and the electrical charge on both sides of the membrane should equalize. These equalizations do not occur in a normal nonconducting cell. The sodium pump (still not completely understood) moves sodium out of the cell, maintaining a high sodium ion concentration in extracellular fluid; the movement of sodium ion by diffusion through the cell membrane back into the cell occurs only with difficulty. The potassium pump moves potassium into the cell, but the resting cell membrane is 50 to 100 times as permeable to potassium as it is to sodium; therefore, potassium moves by diffusion back out of the cell. The electrical potential difference is caused by diffusion of the potassium ions from intracellular to extracellular fluid, removing the positive charge from inside the cell while building up the positive charge outside the cell. Subsequently, the outer surface of the membrane is positive to the inner surface of the membrane. This concentration difference created by the movement of potassium determines the magnitude of the resting membrane potential.

A sequence of rapid changes occurs in the membrane potential when the permeability of the membrane to sodium and potassium ions is altered. These changes are called the *action potential*, and they occur in two stages: depolarization and repolarization.

In the first stage there is activation of the membrane, which causes a sudden increase in the membrane's permeability to sodium. Theoretically calcium binds the pores of the membrane, causing a resistance to the passage of sodium. When the calcium ions are dislodged, sodium rushes to the inside of the fiber, carrying positive charges within the fiber and depolarizing the membrane; with this increase in positive ions, a reversal potential is created. Normally membrane potential in a resting neuron is positive outside and negative inside; this condition is now reversed.

The second stage, repolarization, begins with the calcium ions binding the pores, prohibiting further passage of sodium into the fiber and returning the electrochemical balance back to the normal resting membrane potential.

Hypothetically, during the latter phase of the action potential, there is an increase in the conduction of potassium from within the fiber, with it moving through the membrane to the outside very rapidly. It is thought that the rapid diffusion of potassium is responsible for returning the membrane to its resting potential.

The sequence is as follows: resting membrane potential, action potential (altered calcium and the movement of sodium), depolarization, reversal potential, repolarization (primarily by the movement of potassium), and resting membrane potential.

The entire cycle occurs in a minute fraction of a second, and obviously any disturbance in the body's electrolyte balance of sodium and potassium will influence this series of events.

Propagation of Action Potential.   The action potential initiated at any one point of a membrane excites the point adjacent to it, causing a local circuit of current flow between the depolarized membrane and the resting membrane adjacent. As the cycle repeats itself with current flow from inward through the depolarized membrane and outward through the resting membrane, the process moves in both directions, progressing the full length of the nerve fiber. The action potential, or nerve impulse, is the transmission of the depolarization process or a self-propagating wave of negativity that travels along the surface of a neuronal membrane. Repolarization occurs at the point of stimulus first, and then, moving in the same direction as depolarization, spreads along the membrane in the same manner.

In reestablishing the ionic balance, the sodium and potassium pumps require energy. Active metabolism with the production of adenosine triphosphate for energy occurs within the neuron. As metabolism increases, the rate of production of heat by the nerve fiber increases. This is also influenced by the number of impulses per second that are transmitted. It is this increased energy that causes recharging of the nerve fiber and restores the action of the sodium and potassium pump to achieve their original balance.

An important aspect in the velocity of conduction of impulses is the structure of the neuron, with the segmented myelin sheath interrupted by the nodes of Ranvier. The myelin sheath is thick, and this insulation, which is nonconductive, prevents easy flow of ions into the nerve fiber, while the node of Ranvier presents an uninsulated area, where ions may flow with ease between extracellular fluid and the axon of the nerve fiber. On the myelinated nerve, impulses are conducted (or jump) from node to node rather than continuously along the entire nerve, as in unmyelinated nerves. This process, called saltatory conduction, influences the velocity of nerve transmission in myelinated nerves. (See Fig. 2-2.)

Velocity of transmission also varies directly with the diameter of the nerve fiber: the larger the diameter, the faster the conduction. Fibers with large diameter conduct at a rate of 100 meters per second, and fibers with a smaller diameter conduct about one-half meter per second.

The initiation of a second action potential cannot occur while the nerve fiber is still depolarized. This interval of inexcitability is called the absolute re-

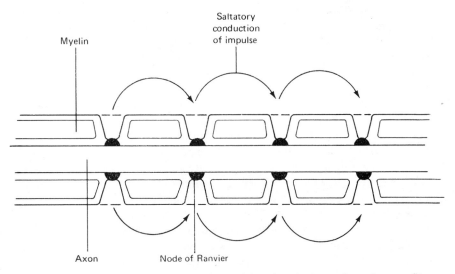

Fig. 2-2. Saltatory conduction, the process by which an impulse jumps down the nerve fiber.

fractory period. Even the introduction of a stimulus of maximum strength will not elicit a second action potential until the refractory period is over. This absolute refractory period lasts about 1/2500 second in a large myelinated nerve.

Synaptic Transmission. The junction between one neuron and the next is called a synapse. As we have said, the neuron is comprised of the cell body; the axon, which relays impulses away from the cell body; and dendrites, which relay impulses toward the cell body. Many axon filaments end in knobs or presynaptic terminals, which lie in contact with either a dendrite or the cell body of another neuron; the presynaptic terminal is separated from the other neuron body by a synaptic cleft. In the presynaptic terminal are hundreds of neurovesicles which secrete and release neurotransmitter substances.

In the transmission of the action potential over the presynaptic terminal, the neurovesicles release an excitatory transmitter into the synaptic cleft, which excites the membrane of the cell body, increasing its permeability to sodium, generating a new action potential in the next neuron. One known excitatory transmitter is acetylcholine in the autonomic nervous system. Within seconds cholinesterase, an enzyme, is released, which inactivates acetylcholine, prohibiting further synaptic conduction.

Certain presynaptic terminals release an inhibitory transmitter, which produces either a postsynaptic inhibition or a presynaptic inhibition at the synapse. It is believed the postsynaptic inhibition occurs by increasing the membrane's permeability to potassium rather than sodium, making the neuron less excitable and prohibiting initiation of the action potential. One substance thought to be a postsynaptic inhibitor is gamma-aminobutyric acid. In presynaptic inhibition, terminals lying on presynaptic nerve fibrils release the excitatory transmitter; the terminals become partly depolarized, preventing the release of normal quantities of excitory transmitters, therefore inhibiting synaptic transmission. This inhibition mechanism controls central nervous system input and output by selecting important signals and blocking others, minimizing the continual excitation of the brain from the peripheral neuromuscular junction.

The neuromuscular junction (or neuroeffector junction) is the place where the nerve fiber terminates in the motor end plate (Fig. 2-3). At the tip of the nerve fibers are sole feet; the synaptic cleft is the space between the sole foot and the muscle fiber membrane, and the synaptic gutter is formed by the numerous folds of the muscle membrane. The neurotransmitter acetylcholine is stored in the vesicles in the sole feet and released into the synaptic cleft. Within milliseconds, cholinesterase accumulated around the rim of the synaptic gutter destroys the acetylcholine. The muscle fiber is excited, but reexcitation does not occur, owing to the destruction of acetylcholine by cholinesterase. Normally each impulse at the neuromuscular junction creates a high end plate potential, and the muscle is stimulated, initiating the action potential.

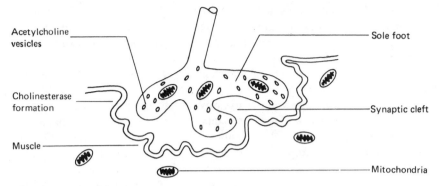

Fig. 2-3. Neuromuscular junction.

CENTRAL NERVOUS SYSTEM

The central nervous system will be discussed in relation to the head, the brain, and the vertebral column.

Head

Scalp. The covering of the head may be divided into five layers and abbreviated accordingly:

S —Skin
C—(Sub)cutaneous tissue
A—Adipose tissue
L—Ligament (galea aponeurosis)
P—Pericranium

It is recommended that the first three layers be considered as a single functional unit; they remain firmly connected when evulsed surgically or traumatically. The skin of the scalp is approximately 3 to 7 millimeters in thickness, which may be contrasted to other areas of the body, where skin averages 1 to 2 millimeters in thickness. The highly vascular subcutaneous layer is relatively dense, inhibiting inflammation and swelling.

The galea aponeurosis is the layer of greatest strength in the scalp. This flat tendon extends anterior-posterior from the glabella above the orbit to the occipital protuberance. The contracture of this ligament accounts for the gaping appearance of a transverse scalp wound; therefore, it must be included in the surgical closure of the wound for close approximation and healing.

The pericranium is the periosteum of the skull, differing somewhat from periosteum in that it has minimal bone-forming capacity. Because of its many small vessels which supply nutrients to the underlying bone, it is able to sustain a split thickness skin graft in the absence of more suitable closure material. A scalp wound can be expected to bleed profusely, since there is no vasoconstriction of the scalp blood vessels.

Cranium.   The word cranium is restricted here to mean the skull without the mandible and facial bones.

The cranium is a hollow but rigid bony structure, which serves to protect and support the sensitive central nervous system substance. The cranial bones are composed of external and internal tables of compact substance, separated from each other by the diploë, a middle spongy layer. The fact that this formation is hollow rather than solid gives the skull its structural integrity.

The cranium is made up of a series of bones united at immovable joints called sutures; these bones are the frontal, parietal (paired), occipital, temporal (paired), sphenoid (paired), and ethmoid (paired) bones.

The anterior aspect of the skull is formed by the frontal bone, which is the skeleton of the forehead. The region above the articulation of the frontal bone with the nasal bones and between the eyebrows is called the glabella. The elevation extending laterally on each side of the glabella is the superciliary arch.

The superior aspect of the cranium is formed by the frontal bone, right and left parietal, and occipital bones. The union between the frontal and two parietal bones is called the coronal suture; between the two parietal bones there is the sagittal suture; and between the two parietals and the occipital bone, the lambdoidal suture.

The posterior aspect of the cranium is formed by portions of the parietal bones and the occipital bone (lambdoidal suture). The occipital bone is composed of four parts arranged around the foramen magnum: a squamous part behind, a lateral part at each side articulating with the mastoid process of the temporal bone (occipitomastoid suture), and a basilar part in front.

The lateral aspect of the cranium is fashioned by portions of the parietal, temporal (parietomastoid or squamous suture), and sphenoid bones. The temporal bone is comprised of the squamous, tympanic, styloid, mastoid, and petrous parts. The sphenoid bones are comprised of a body and three pairs of processes or wings: greater wings, lesser wings, and pterygoid processes. Laterally the frontal, sphenoid, parietal, and squamous part of the temporal bones join closely in a small circular area called the pterion.

The inferior external surface of the cranium is complicated and irregular. It may be divided into anterior, middle, and posterior parts.

The anterior part is the bony palate formed by the palatine processes of the maxillae and the horizontal plates of the palatine bones separated by a cruciform suture.

In the median plane the posterior vomer separates the two posterior nasal apertures. Behind the vomer the body of the sphenoid is continuous with the basilar part of the occipital bone, extending downward to the foramen magnum.

Important openings in the greater wing of the sphenoid are the foramen ovale and foramen spinosum. The foramen ovale transmits the mandibular division of the trigeminal nerve; the foramen spinosum transmits the middle meningeal artery to the middle cranial fossa.

In the posterior plane of the inferior external surface of the cranium is the foramen magnum, which communicates between the posterior floor of the skull and the vertebral canal. The foramen magnum transmits the lower end of the medulla oblongata. The hypoglossal canal runs laterally and transmits the hypoglossal nerve. The jugular fossa transmits the glossopharyngeal, vagus, and spinal accessory nerves, and in its posterior part the internal jugular vein. Posteriorly the stylomastoid foramen transmits the facial nerve.

The cranial cavity lodges the brain, the meninges and their blood vessels, and portions of the cranial nerves. It is roofed by the superior aspect of the skull (frontal, parietal, and occipital bones). The floor is formed by the upper surface of the base of the skull (ethmoid, sphenoid, temporal, and occipital bones).

The inferior internal surface of the base of the skull is very irregular and may be divided into three levels by two prominent bony ledges on each side. The posterior border is called the "sphenoidal ridge" of the lesser wing of the sphenoid bone in front, and the superior border called the "petrous ridge" of the petrous temporal bone behind. Thus there is a natural division into the anterior, middle, and posterior cranial fossae.

The anterior fossa is formed by the frontal bone in front and each side. The floor is formed by the orbital parts of the frontal bone, the cribiform plate of the ethmoid bone, and the lesser wings and part of the body of the sphenoid bone.

The ethmoid bones are separated by a perforated strip known as the cribiform plate, which forms a large portion of the roof of the nasal cavity. The minute olfactory nerves pass through the perforations in the plate from the nasal mucosa to the olfactory bulb. Anteriorly a median elevation called the crista galli extends upward between the two cerebral hemispheres and attaches to a fold of the dura mater, the falx cerebri. The sphenoid bone completes the posterior region of the floor. The anterior fossa contains the frontal lobes of the cerebrum.

The middle fossa is bound in front by the lesser wings of the sphenoid; behind, by the petrous part of the temporal bones; laterally, by the squamous part of the temporal bones, the frontal angles of the parietal bones, and the greater wings of the sphenoid. Centrally the floor is formed by the body of the sphenoid bone. The optic canal runs between the lesser wing and the body of the sphenoid and contains the optic nerve, the ophthalmic artery, and meninges. The superior surface of the sphenoid, shaped like a saddle, is called the sella turcica; its surface is hollowed out and contains the hypophysis cerebri (the pituitary).

The superior orbital fissure transmits the ophthalmic veins and the oculomotor, trochlear, and abducens nerves. The foramen lacerum contains the internal carotid artery. The middle fossa contains the temporal, parietal, and occipital lobes of the cerebrum.

The posterior fossa, the deepest and largest of the three compartments, is formed by portions of the sphenoid, temporal, parietal, and occipital bones. The lowest part of the posterior fossa presents the foramen magnum, through which the medulla oblongata becomes the spinal cord. The internal acoustic meatus runs transversely, containing the vestibulocochlear nerves. The mastoid foramen transmits a meningeal branch of the occipital artery. The posterior fossa contains the cerebellum behind and the pons and medulla oblongata in front.

Meninges. The brain, as well as the spinal cord, is surrounded and covered by three fibrous membranes or meninges: the pachymeninges (large), or dura mater, and the leptomeninges (small), the arachnoid and the pia mater.

The dura mater is described as having two layers in the cranium: the external periosteal layer and the internal meningeal layer. The periosteal layer is lightly adhesive to the inner aspect of the cranial bones and is separated from the meningeal layer by the venous sinuses (see discussion of dural sinuses). This double-layered structure is absent in the spinal canal.

The meningeal layer of the dura mater folds and sends four processes internally: the falx cerebri, the tentorium cerebelli, the falx cerebelli, and the diaphragma sellae (Fig. 2-4):

1. *Falx cerebri.* This process lies in the longitudinal fissure between the two cerebral hemispheres. Anteriorly it is attached to the skull at the crista galli, and posteriorly it fuses with the tentorium cerebelli.

2. *Tentorium cerebelli.* This process supports the occipital lobes of the cerebral hemispheres horizontally, separating them from the cerebellum; it covers the cerebellum. This dural reflection, along with part of the sphenoid bone, forms the boundary of the tentorial notch, which is largely occupied by the upper brain stem. The free margin of the tentorium cerebelli surrounding the cerebral peduncles leaves an opening called the incisura tentori. The tentorium cerebelli, therefore, separates the posterior cranial fossa from the remainder of the cavity. Space-occupying intracranial lesions may cause herniation of the brain from one dural compartment to another through the tentorial notch and the incisura tentori. The tentorium serves as a line of demarcation when one is describing the sites of central nervous system lesions, dividing them simply as supratentorial and infratentorial.

3. *Falx cerebelli.* This process lies below the tentorium, and the anterior

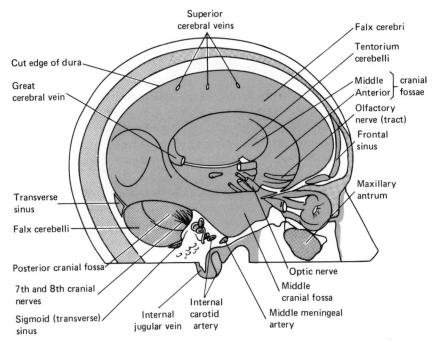

Fig. 2-4. Dural reflections. Note the placement of: the falx cerebri, tentorium cerebelli, falx cerebelli; anterior, middle, and posterior fossae.

border projects between the cerebellar hemispheres. The posterior border is attached to the occipital bone.

4. *Diaphragma sellae*. This circular and horizontal process forms a dural lining for the sella turcica covering the hypophysis cerebri.

The area between the meningeal layer of the dura and the arachnoid is the subdural space.

The arachnoid and pia mater (the leptomeninges) are described as two membranes, but they are united by weblike fibers. The arachnoid membrane surrounds the brain and is separated from the dura mater by the subdural space. The compartment formed by the arachnoid and pia mater is called the subarachnoid space. This space communicates with the fourth ventricle and provides a channel for cerebrospinal fluid circulation. The arachnoid membrane extends a large number of microscopic projections called arachnoid villi into the subarachnoid space. These projections form the structural mechanism for the absorption of cerebrospinal fluid.

The brain's larger blood vessels lie in the subarachnoid space, passing through the pia mater into the brain tissue and providing a large amount of the brain's blood supply.

There are areas where the arachnoid membrane does not follow the contour of the brain, thereby diverging from the pia mater and permitting the existence of larger subarachnoid spaces called cisterns. There are four large cisterns along the base of the brain. The most significant of these is the cisterna magna, which is between the cerebellum and the dorsum of the medulla. Since there is an increase of cerebrospinal fluid in the cistern, the cisterna magna is used as a puncture site for removal of cerebrospinal fluid for analysis.

The pia mater, the innermost layer of the meninges, covers and adheres intimately to the brain, dipping into the gyri. The pia mater forms the choroid plexuses of the ventricles—those structures responsible for the formation of cerebrospinal fluid.

The dural sinuses, created by the meningeal and periosteal layers of the dura, receive blood from the diploic veins of the skull, the emissary veins of the scalp, the meningeal veins of the dura, and the cerebral bridger veins of the brain. The thin-walled sinuses, devoid of valves, ultimately drain into the internal jugular vein. (See Fig. 2-5.)

The superior sagittal sinus lies in the convex border of the falx cerebri. It extends above the roof of the nose over the cranial vault, back to the occipital protuberance, ending in the confluence of sinuses.

The inferior sagittal sinus lies in the concave border of the falx cerebri and ends in the straight sinus.

The straight sinus lies at the junction of the falx cerebri and the tentorium cerebelli, ending in the confluence of the sinuses.

The occipital sinus lies in the attached margin of the falx cerebelli, beginning at the foramen magnum and ending at the confluence of sinuses.

The confluence of sinuses is the region at the internal occipital protuberance

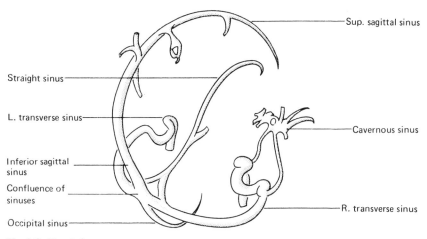

Fig. 2-5. Dural sinuses.

where the superior sagittal sinus, straight sinus, and occipital sinus end, and the right and left transverse sinus begins.

The transverse sinus begins in the confluence of sinuses, runs laterally and forward in the border of the tentorium cerebelli, and becomes the sigmoid sinus.

The cavernous sinus lies in the compartment bordered on each side by the sphenoid bone. In addition to this main venous channel, the compartment contains the internal carotid artery and the abducens, oculomotor, trochlear, and ophthalmic nerves. The cavernous sinus communicates with the transverse sinus and the internal jugular vein. The cavernous sinus is unique in that it is the only place in the body where an artery is bathed with venous blood. (This concept, historically developed, is now being questioned!)

Brain

The brain has been described as the most highly organized apparatus in the universe. It is a fabulous machine that receives, digests, and gives meaning to all experience and initiates and regulates all thoughts, emotions, and actions, whether conscious or unconscious. It is probably the most important organ in the body, since it is the means by which the human body becomes a dynamic, living being rather than a conglomeration of cells. It organizes, integrates, and controls the body, giving it purpose and meaning. It is the physical center of human behavior.

The brain weighs 1.96% of the total body weight. It receives aproximately one-sixth of the cardiac output and consumes approximately one-fifth of the oxygen utilized by the body at rest.

The following structures of the brain will be discussed: cerebrum, brain stem, and cerebellum, followed by discussion of the ventricular system and the cerebrospinal fluid.

Cerebrum. The cerebrum, contained in the anterior and middle cranial fossae, is the largest and perhaps the most important constituent of the central nervous system.

The surface of the cerebrum has irregular eminences called gyri or convolutions, which are separated from each other by larger furrows called sulci or fissures.

The longitudinal fissure, which partially separates the cerebrum into two large convoluted hemispheres, is a deep median cleft formed by the sagittal folds of the dura mater—the falx cerebri. The hemispheres are connected internally in the depths of the longitudinal fissure by a transverse band of white fibers called the corpus callosum. Each hemisphere contains a cavity known as the lateral ventricle.

The lateral sulcus—the fissure of Sylvius—begins on the inferior surface of each cerebral hemisphere, approximately one-third of the way from the anterior end of the cerebrum, and progresses diagonally upward, remaining parallel to the base of the cerebrum, ending about one-half of the distance into the posterior cerebrum. The central sulcus—the fissure of Rolando—begins at the superior border of each hemisphere, progressing curvingly downward and forward, ending about 2.5 centimeters above the lateral sulcus (Fig. 2-6).

The angular gyri, created by the sulci, are usually highly developed in only one cerebral hemisphere, the dominant one. The cerebral hemispheres, at birth, have the same capacity to develop. As the brain begins to function, the attention of the mind seems to be directed to one side at a time. One region begins to be utilized to a greater extent than the other and, therefore, becomes better developed, a situation that is perpetuated by the mind directing its attention further to the more fully developed region. This is one explanation of the dominant hemisphere in the adult.

Each cerebral hemisphere has an external layer of gray matter and an internal area of gray matter (gray due to lack of myelin deposit), the cerebral cortex and the nuclei of the basal ganglia, and a central core of white matter (due to myelin deposit) or medullary substance. Each sulcus or fissure of the cerebral surface corresponds to an infolding of the cortex, thereby tripling the square cortical surface area of the brain.

The cerebral cortex mediates the highest mental and behavioral activities of human beings. It receives and analyzes the impulses; receives and stores knowledge; controls voluntary movements, thought, association, discrimination, judgment, and memory.

The gray matter of the cerebrum includes not only the outer layer of cortical nerve cells, but also nuclei of the thalamus, the hypothalamus, and the

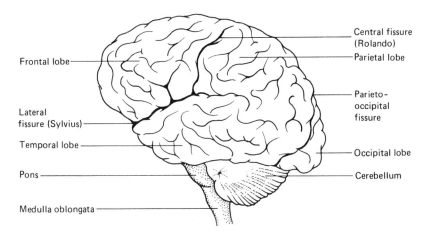

Fig. 2-6. Cerebral fissures.

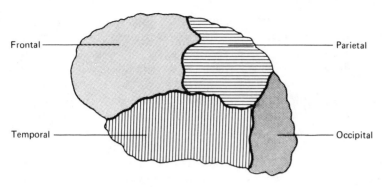

Fig. 2-7. Cerebral lobes.

basal ganglia. For each area of the cortex there is a connecting area of the thalamus. Activation of a minute portion of the thalamus activates the corresponding and much larger portion of the cerebral cortex; the thalamus, therefore, serves as a relay to critical cortical activities.

The central core of white matter consists of nerve fibers that lead from these cortical neurons to other parts of the nervous system. These association and projection pathways make up the rest of the brain.

The sulci of the cerebral surface divide the cortex of the cerebral hemispheres into frontal, parietal, temporal, and occipital lobes. These sulci establish limits for certain functional areas. The frontal lobe lies anterior to the central sulcus and anterior to the lateral sulcus; the parietal lobe lies posterior to the central sulcus and anterior to the lateral sulcus; the temporal lobe lies inferior to the lateral sulcus; the occipital lobe is posterior to the convergence of the lateral sulcus and at the base of the cerebrum (Fig. 2-7).

The cerebrum can be functionally divided into eight units: personality, behavior (social and moral), intellectual functions, the motor strip, the sensory strip, the auditory speech center, hearing and visual association.

The frontal lobe is the anterior part of the cerebral hemisphere, anterior to the central sulcus and anterior to the lateral sulcus.

The greater forward portion of the frontal lobe, the prefrontal area, is responsible for personality, behavior, higher intellectual functions, consciousness, learning, abstract and conceptual thought, problem solving, judgment, memory, volition, and social, moral, and ethical values. It has often been said (and indeed is true) that the frontal lobe makes man the poet and man the thinker.

The frontal lobe also contains higher-level centers for autonomic functions such as respiration, gastrointestinal activity, intravascular reactions, and emotional responses.

The area of the frontal lobe that lies anterior to the precentral gyrus is dividided into superior, middle, and inferior frontal gyri. The inferior frontal gyrus, bordered by the lateral sulcus, is known as the speech area of Broca and is almost always dominant on the left side of the brain. This region is associated with the motor element of speech, causing the formation of words.

The written speech center, located in the frontal lobe above the motor speech center, governs the ability to write words.

Right- or left-handedness is partially linked with cerebral dominance. The speech center is dominant in the left cerebral cortex in most individuals whether they are right- or left-handed.

The narrow uneven band of cortex lying anterior to the central sulcus is called the precentral gyrus, or primary motor area, or motor cortex. It is extremely important, since it initiates voluntary motor function. This area contains unusually large pyramidal-shaped cells—Betz cells, as described by Vladimir Betz in 1874. Fibers emanate from these cells and extend from the frontal lobe to the spinal cord and finally to muscle fibers in the body. This is the upper motor neuron. Groups of Betz cells control a particular muscle and initiate voluntary motion on the opposite side of the body. The left side of the brain controls the right side of the body, and the right side of the brain controls the left side of the body, since these fibers decussate (cross over) in the medulla.

The motor area on the cortex may be visualized by inverting an individual onto his head. The innermost portion of the motor area (toward the top of the cerebrum and on the medial aspect) stimulates the lower leg and foot; progressing downward in the motor area the muscles of the thigh are stimulated, the abdomen, thorax, shoulders, arms, hands, fingers, and finally the neck and head.

The upper motor neuron is described as a functional unit rather than an anatomical entity with its purpose being the initiation of all voluntary motion. The nerve fibers originate in the giant pyramidal cells of Betz in the motor cortex of the frontal lobe. These fibers gather together and descend through the internal capsule, a narrow band of white matter deep in the cerebrum, transverse the cerebral peduncles (large bundles on each side of the brain stem) and the pons, and enter the pyramids of the medulla oblongata. In the medulla a variable number of nerve fibers decussate the median plane of the spinal cord, and all descend the length of the spinal cord through the lateral white column, ending in the target cells of the gray matter of the spinal cord.

The upper motor neuron tract has a singular distinction in that most fibers descend without interruption (synapse) from the cerebral cortex to a termination point in the spinal cord white matter (Fig. 2-8).

The upper motor neuron has also been called the pyramidal tract, since the nerve fibers originate in the pyramidal Betz cells and pass through the pyramids of the medulla. In the past it was also frequently called corticospinal tract, since it traversed cortex to spine. Recently, and more correctly differen-

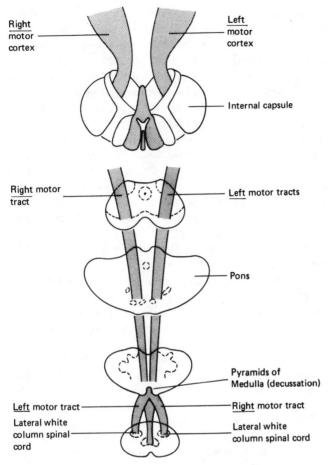

Fig. 2-8. Upper motor neuron. Note where the motor tracts decussate in the pyramids of the medulla.

tiating, the name upper motor neuron has been used to describe this tract; it is particularly popular in clinical parlance.

Injury anywhere in the upper motor neuron system causes a pattern of altered motor function that is unique.

The temporal lobe, which lies inferior to the lateral sulcus, is primarily reserved for the perception of sound and is called the auditory speech center. Each hemisphere receives impulses from both ears.

The function of interpretation of language by the temporal lobe is usually highly developed in only a single hemisphere—the dominant hemisphere.

The temporal lobe also interrelays inhibitive and primitive emotions (such as fear and sex) with other areas of the brain, such as the hypothalamus. The temporal lobe is often referred to as the "silent" area, since a lesion in this region may become quite extensive before making a clinical appearance.

The parietal lobe is bounded anteriorly by the central sulcus, inferiorly by a division of the lateral sulcus, and posteriorly by the parieto-occipital sulcus. The portion of the parietal lobe adjacent to the motor area but posterior to the central sulcus, is called the general sensory cortex, the sensory strip, or the somesthetic cortex. The senses that the parietal lobe receive and interpret are called somatic senses. These somatic senses exclude the "special senses" of hearing, taste, smell, and sight, which are mediated elsewhere in the brain.

The parietal lobe receives and interprets these sensory impulses from the skin, mucous membranes, muscles, joints, and tendons. Again one visualizes the inverted individual and associates the area of the hemisphere with the function of the brain.

Somatic senses dealt with by the parietal lobe include all of the following: recognition of size and shape (stereognosis), weight, texture, and consistency of objects; the ability to discriminate between two simultaneous skin contacts (two-point discrimination); and the interpretation of pain (some authors disagree on the accuracy of assigning pain interpretation to the general sensory cortex of the parietal lobe), touch, pressure, temperature, position, and vibration.

An important speech area of the dominant cerebral hemisphere, Wernicke's area, is located posteriorly in the parieto-temporal area of the cerebral cortex. It is a receptive language area, providing the ability to comprehend spoken and written language.

The occipital lobe lies posterior to the parieto-occipital sulcus. It contains the visual language center, which receives and interprets all of the sensations dealing with visual perception. It governs the ability to read with understanding. (See Fig. 2-9.)

The extrapyramidal tracts include all of the tracts (other than the pyramidal tract) that transmit motor signals from the cerebral cortex to the spinal cord.

The extrapyramidal system is a functional entity composed of subcortical nuclear masses of gray matter deep within each cerebral hemisphere, which have a neuronal connection with other parts of the nervous system, specifically the cortex, cerebellum, and descending pontine tracts. These paired structures, collectively called the basal ganglia, include: the claustrum, the caudate nuclei, the lentiform nuclei, divided into an internal globus pallidus and an external putamen (the caudate and lentiform nuclei are commonly grouped as the corpus striatum), and the amygdaloid nuclei. The substantia nigra and the red nuclei operate in close association with the caudate nuclei and the lentiform nuclei; they are considered to be the core of the basal ganglia system for motor control (Fig. 2-10).

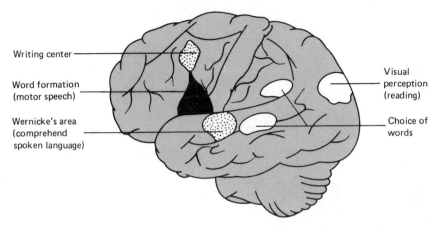

Writing center

Word formation
(motor speech)

Wernicke's area
(comprehend
spoken language)

Visual
perception
(reading)

Choice of
words

Fig. 2-9. Cortical areas. The cortical areas dealing with speech, writing, and reading.

The basal ganglia provide a circular route of neuronal pathways passing from the motor portions of the cerebral cortex through the extrapyramidal system and back to the cortex, serving as an integrator of motor function. There is also a circuit through which signals are passed from the cerebral cortex to the pons and cerebellum, and back to the cortex by way of the basal ganglia. The basal ganglia also have short neuronal connections among themselves. It is through these pathways that motor control signals are transmitted.

Functions of the extrapyramidal system include the integration or smoothing out of motion, the provision of automatic movements (swinging arms when walking, facial gestures when talking), and the maintenance of an upright posture.

In this feedback system the extrapyramidal tract exerts some control over the motor cortex by preventing it from "kicking" off too rapidly. Therefore, when it is interfered with, the result is that the motor area fires impulses rapidly and without being "checked," resulting in involuntary muscle contractions. A lesion in this area certainly produces characteristic symptoms.

There is an overall group of brain structures around the lateral ventricle surrounded by a ring of cerebral cortex called the limbic system. These structures are concerned with special types of behavior associated with emotions, subconscious motor and sensory drives, the intrinsic feelings of pain and pleasure, and memory. The affective qualities of sensory sensations are called reward and punishment or satisfaction and aversion.

The cerebral hemispheres play a role in the limbic system along with the subcortical gray structures: the thalamus, the hypothalamus, the hippocampus, the amygdaloid nucleus of the basal ganglia, the olfactory tract, and the mamillary bodies.

Brain Stem. The brain stem is a complex system of neuronal circuits con-

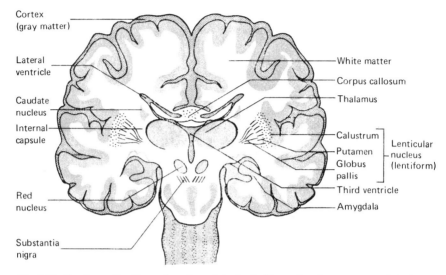

Cortex (gray matter)
Lateral ventricle
Caudate nucleus
Internal capsule
Red nucleus
Substantia nigra

White matter
Corpus callosum
Thalamus
Calustrum
Putamen
Globus pallis
Lenticular nucleus (lentiform)
Third ventricle
Amygdala

Fig. 2-10. Basal ganglia. Coronal section of the brain illustrating the structures of the basal ganglia.

necting the cerebrum above and the spinal cord below. The structures usually included for discussion are the thalamus and the structures below the thalamus: the hypothalamus, midbrain, pituitary, pons, medulla, and nuclei of the 12 pairs of cranial nerves. The deeper parts of the brain are not visible when one is viewing the intact specimen.

The thalami are two large ovoid masses of gray matter, clothed partially by white matter, situated on each side of the third ventricle. The main mass of the thalamus is divided into anterior, medial, and lateral parts, each containing a group of thalamic nuclei. Well-defined nerve bundles connect with the cerebral cortex, other thalamic nuclei, neighboring subcortical masses of gray matter, and pathways of the brain stem and spinal cord.

The thalamus is considered a relay and transmission center for sensations such as touch, pain, heat, cold, and muscle senses. The thalamus receives sensory data and magnifies or suppresses the impulses, while the specific and nonspecific thalamic nuclei filter sensations. The milder sensations are transmitted through to the parietal cortex, while the rougher ones are dealt with quickly by the thalamus without much time for consideration. Differentiation achieved on this basis allowed the cortex originally to be considered the cold center of reason and the thalamus the hot focus of emotion. This is certainly an oversimplification developed historically, as emotions do not arise from any one area of the brain, and many areas (including frontal and temporal cortex) play a closely related and complex role.

The thalamus, as a structure in the reticular activating system (discussed later), provides for generalized activation of the cerebral cortex and controls the ability to direct attention toward specific areas of the conscious mind.

The pineal body is located below the corpus callosum and is covered by the tela choroid of the third ventricle. Little is known of the function of this gland, but calcification often takes place; the organ may be visible radiographically.

The hypothalamus is the region below the thalamus functionally restricted to the anterior floor and lower lateral walls of the third ventricle. This region provides a major pathway for the limbic system, controlling impulses for the regulation of vegetative functions. These processes are necessary to sustain life; for example, arterial pressure, thirst, water conservation (synthesizes antidiuretic hormone), sexual functions, uterine contraction (synthesizes oxytoxin hormone), body temperature, hunger, feeding reflexes, and regulation of satiety.

In conjunction with the hypophysis cerebri, the hypothalamus offers brain control of the body's metabolic functions.

The hypophysis cerebri (pituitary) is a small endocrine gland that rests in the concavity of the sphenoid bone of the skull termed the sella turcica. It is connected to the hypothalamus by the hypophyseal (pituitary) stalk. The pituitary is not considered part of the brain, since it lies outside the blood-brain barrier. It is anatomically and physiologically divided into the anterior (adenohypophysis) and posterior (neurohypophysis) lobes.

Embryologically, the neurohypophysis is of neural origin, formed from the nervous tissue of the brain, and is considered an extension of the hypothalamus. Functionally, the neurohypophysis stores and releases two hormones: oxytoxin and antidiuretic hormone. Both of these hormones are synthesized by the hypothalamus.

Embryologically, the adenohypophysis, a glandular structure, is formed from the roof of the mouth. Functionally, the adenohypophysis controls the activity of the thyroid gland, the adrenal cortex, the gonads, and the mammary glands. It synthesizes and releases seven hormones of vital importance to the human body: somatotropin hormone (STH), adrenocorticotropic hormone (ACTH), thyroid-stimulating hormone (TSH), lactotropic hormone (LTH), follicle stimulating hormone (FSH), luteinizing hormone (LH), and melanocytic stimulating hormone (MSH).

Brain control of metabolic functions has been established since the discovery of the relationship between the hypothalamus and hypophysis cerebri. There exists a blood-borne portal system that carries substances from the hypothalamus to the hypophysis cerebri to stimulate or inhibit the release of various hormones.

The hypothalamus receives impulses from the internal and external environment and transmits messages via the hypophyseal stalk through nerve fibers, known as the hypothalamohypophyseal tract, to the hypophysis cerebri. In response to neuronal stimulus of the neurohypophysis and substances carried by the portal system to the adenohypophysis, both lobes release their hormones into the bloodstream, maintaining *Homo sapiens* in equilibrium.

The midbrain is located in the tentorial notch formed by a process of the dura mater, the tentorium cerebelli. It is composed of a ventral surface, the cerebral peduncles, and the tectum. The third cranial nerve, the oculomotor, and the fourth cranial nerve, the trochlear, emerge from the midbrain.

The midbrain relays impulses from the cerebral cortex above and the subcortical structures below. The origin of postural reflexes and the righting reflexes are located in the midbrain.

The pons (a word meaning bridge) connects the medulla, the midbrain, and the cerebellum. It is composed of gray matter (the pontine nuclei) and white matter (the descending corticospinal tract). The motor and sensory nuclei of the fifth cranial nerve (trigeminal), sixth cranial nerve (abducens), seventh cranial nerve (facial), and eighth cranial nerve (acoustic) are found in the pons. The pneumotaxic center is located in the pons and controls the rhythmic quality of respirations. The upper motor neurons descend to the spinal cord through the pons, as do the thalamic, cerebellar, and extrapyramidal tracts.

The medulla connects with the central canal of the spinal cord below through the foramen magnum. Above, it connects with the pons and widens to become the floor of the fourth ventricle. The ninth cranial nerve (glossopharyngeal), tenth cranial nerve (vagus), eleventh cranial nerve (spinal accessory), and twelfth cranial nerve (hypoglossal) all originate in the medulla (Fig. 2-11).

The vital centers for cardiac, respiratory, and vasomotor control are all located in the medulla, as well as the swallowing, gag, and cough reflexes.

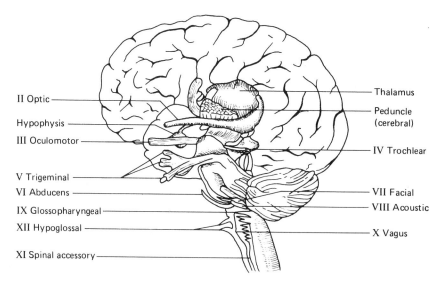

Fig. 2-11. Brain stem and origin of cranial nerves.

The medulla plays a role in the reticular activating system, which is essential for the initiation and maintenance of alert wakefulness.

The cortical motor tracts decussate in the median plane in the pyramids of the medulla. As previously mentioned, the right motor area of the frontal cortex initiates voluntary motion on the left side of the body; the left motor area of the frontal cortex initiates voluntary motion on the right side of the body, and so forth.

The reticular activating system extends from the medulla through the pons, midbrain, hypothalamus, and thalamus. The system is composed of cell bodies of neurons of various types, sizes, and shapes. These interlacing nerve fibers integrate afferent and efferent impulse pathways controlling the overall degree of central nervous system activity, including wakefulness and sleep. Reticular formation is primarily excitatory, causing an increase in muscle tone throughout the body; it is also inhibitory, causing decreased muscle tone throughout the body; thus our body is supported against gravity.

The thalamus plays a role in reticular formation, causing generalized activation of the cerebral cortex; it allows us to direct our attention to specific areas of our conscious mind (concentration).

Cranial Nerves.   The name, origin, and function of the cranial nerves may be found in Table 2-1.

Cerebellum.   Located in the posterior cranial fossa, the cerebellum lies behind the pons and medulla and is separated from the cerebrum by the tentorium cerebelli. It is divided into two cerebellar hemispheres connected by a thin, elongated, wormlike structure called the vermis. The cerebellar cortex of gray matter is tightly convoluted, its fissures lying in parallel lines. The three cerebellar peduncles connect the hemispheres to each other and to the various parts of brain stem. The inferior peduncles connect the cerebellum with the medulla; the middle peduncles connect it with the pons; the superior peduncles connect it with the midbrain.

The cerebellum has three functions, all related to coordination. These functions include monitoring and making corrective adjustments of body movement by a feedback system. The first function is to keep us oriented in space and to maintain equilibrium in the trunk; the second controls the antigravity muscles of the body; and the third is to damper volitional movements, i.e., to check or halt activity.

Ventricular System.   The ventricles or cavities within the brain (four in number) are described from above downward: the first and second ventricles, called the lateral ventricles with one in each cerebral hemisphere, the third ventricle, and the fourth ventricle (Fig. 2-12).

The lateral ventricles are irregular cavities situated in the interior of each cerebral hemisphere. Each ventricle consists of a body and three horns: the anterior horn, which extends into the frontal lobe; the posterior horn, which extends into the occipital lobe; and the inferior horn, which extends into the

Table 2-1. The Cranial Nerves

Number	Name	Origin	Function
1st C.N.	Olfactory	Olfactory bulb	Sensory—sense of smell
2nd C.N.	Optic	Lat. geniculate body	Sensory—vision and circuit for light reflexes
3rd C.N.	Oculomotor	Midbrain	Motor—pupillary constriction, elevation of upper eyelid, conjointly 3rd, 4th, and 6th C.N.—extraocular movement
4th C.N.	Trochlear	Midbrain	Motor—extraocular movement of the eyes downward and inward (oblique muscles)
5th C.N.	Trigeminal	Pons	Sensory: 1. ophthalmic—cornea of the eye and above 2. maxillary—cheek and upper lip 3. mandibular—lower lip and chin Motor—masseter and temporal muscles—biting down and chewing and lateral movement of the jaw
6th C.N.	Abducens	Pons	Motor—extraocular movement of the eyes laterally
7th C.N.	Facial	Pons	Motor—facial muscles around eyes and mouth, and forehead Sensory—taste receptors of the anterior two-thirds of the tongue
8th C.N.	Acoustic	Pons	Sensory: cochlear division—hearing; vestibular division—monitors and controls equilibrium
9th C.N.	Glossopharyngeal	Medulla	Motor—constrictors of the pharynx—used in swallowing Sensory—taste receptors of the posterior one-third of the tongue
10th C.N.	Vagus	Medulla	Sensory—pharynx and larynx Motor—pharynx and larynx, movement of soft palate and uvula; conjointly 9th C.N., 10th C.N. and 12th C.N.—the ability to speak clearly
11th C.N.	Spinal Accessory	Medulla	Motor—sternocleidomastoid, trapezius, and rhomboid muscles
12th C.N.	Hypoglossal	Medulla	Motor—tongue

temporal lobe. The lateral ventricles are separated by the septum pellucidum and communicate with each other and with the third ventricle through the interventricular foramen (foramen of Munro).

The third ventricle is a single narrow cleft situated between the two thalami. It communicates with the fourth ventricle through the cerebral aqueduct (the aqueduct of Sylvius).

The fourth ventricle is a diamond-shaped cavity located between the cerebellum posteriorly and the pons and medulla. From the fourth ventricle there are three openings into the subarachnoid space: the two lateral apertures (foramina of Luschka) and the medial aperture (foramen of Magendie). The fourth ventricle connects with the central core of the spinal cord at the cisterna magna (Fig. 2-13).

Cerebrospinal Fluid.   Cerebrospinal fluid fills the ventricles and the cranial and spinal subarachnoid spaces. The essential function of cerebrospinal fluid is the exchange of nutrients and waste materials between the blood and the cells of the central nervous system. It also protects the central nervous system from injury in its shock-absorbing action, reducing the force of impact. As a volume reservoir it assists in the regulation of blood volume within the cranium.

Vascular fringes of the pia mater project into all of the ventricles, forming an intricate network of fine blood vessels called the choroid plexus. It is generally accepted that cerebrospinal fluid is primarily manufactured by the choroid plexus through active transport and filtration through the capillary walls just like other tissue fluid. Under normal circumstances the rate of formation is relatively stable—approximately 0.4 milliliter per minute in the adult. On this basis a total volume replacement occurs about every six hours.

Cerebrospinal fluid flows from the lateral ventricles through the interventricular foramen (foramen of Munro) into the third ventricle. It leaves the

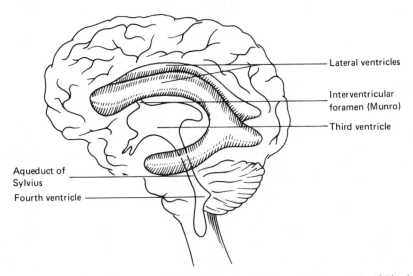

Fig. 2-12. Ventricular system. A sagittal view that depicts the ventricular system within the cerebral hemispheres and downward to the fourth ventricle between the brain stem and the cerebellum.

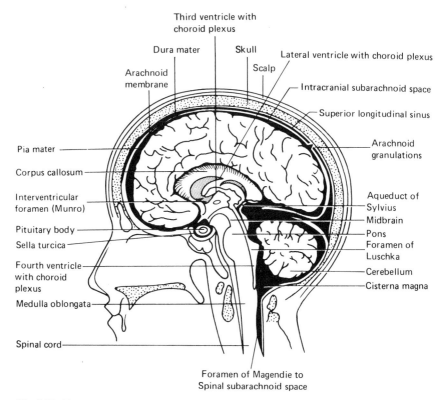

Fig. 2-13. Nervous system. A sagittal view illustrating the gross anatomy of the meninges, brain, and detail of the ventricular system.

third ventricle traveling through the cerebral aqueduct (aqueduct of Sylvius) into the fourth ventricle. Cerebrospinal fluid leaves the fourth ventricle through the lateral apertures (foramina of Luschka) and medial aperture (foramen of Magendie) into the subarachnoid cisterns. The inferior portion of the fourth ventricle is continuous with the central canal of the spinal cord.

There is approximately 120–140 milliliters of cerebrospinal fluid circulating in this closed system. Approximately one-half of the fluid is circulating in the ventricles and the intracranial subarachnoid space over the brain, and one-half in the spinal subarachnoid space to the level of the second sacral vertebra.

The majority of cerebrospinal fluid absorption into the blood takes place through the fingerlike granulations of the arachnoid villi in the dural sinuses (Fig. 2-14). The mechanism of absorption depends on the hydrostatic pressure and concentration of cerebrospinal fluid in the subarachnoid space being less than the hydrostatic pressure and concentration of the venous blood in the dural sinuses.

Cerebrospinal fluid is a clear, colorless, odorless liquid with a specific gravity of 1.007. Normally there are no red blood cells and few white blood cells. It does contain protein, which is affected by gravity; therefore the normal values vary according to the source of the specimen. The ventricular cerebrospinal fluid protein content is 5-15 milligrams %, which is lower than the lumbar cerebrospinal fluid protein content of 15-45 milligrams %. The cerebrospinal fluid glucose levels fluctuate with the serum glucose levels. The normal average is 60-80% that of the blood. The normal value of cerebrospinal fluid glucose is 40-80 milligrams/100 milliliters. The normal cerebrospinal fluid pressure in the lateral recumbent position is 80-180 millimeters of water, which is 6-13 millimeters of mercury.

Craniocerebral Circulation

There are several branches of the external carotid artery that supply the *cranium* (skull).

The occipital artery of the external carotid follows a course that eventually leads to the superficial fascia of the scalp, where it divides into numerous branches. The meningeal branch of the occipital artery enters the skull through the jugular foramen to supply the dura mater and bones of the posterior fossa.

The superficial temporal artery of the external carotid artery lies beneath the skin and fascia as it crosses the zygomatic process, and a pulse may be readily felt. It supplies the temporal region of the scalp and communicates with the orbital artery, creating an arterial anastomotic cross flow of blood. If this cross flow system is intact, circulation in the temporal region is preserved when one or the other of these vessels is injured.

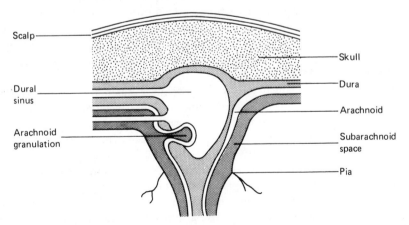

Fig. 2-14. Reabsorption of cerebrospinal fluid. Illustration of the fingerlike arachnoid granulation as it projects into the dural sinus.

The accessory meningeal branch may arise from the maxillary artery or from the middle meningeal artery and supplies the sphenoid bones (greater wings and pterygoid processes).

The internal carotid artery divides into the cerebral artery, which branches into a meningeal artery. It is a minute branch that supplies the lesser wings of the sphenoid, the dura mater, and the bone of the anterior cranial fossa.

Venous return of cranial blood is through the superficial temporal vein, the occipital vein, and the diploic veins.

The superficial temporal vein begins in a network that extends widely over the scalp. It unites with the maxillary to form the retromandibular vein and drains into the external jugular vein.

The occipital vein drains the posterior scalp. It joins with the posterior auricular vein and opens into the external jugular.

Diploic veins in the diploë of the cranial bones are large, thin-walled, and void of valves. They communicate with meningeal veins, the sinuses of the dura mater, and the veins of the pericranium. They are frontal diploë, anterior temporal, posterior temporal, and occipital; all drain through the internal jugular.

There are several branches of the external carotid artery that supply the *dura mater*: the occipital, which supplies the posterior fossa; the temporal, which supplies the temporal region; and the maxillary producing the middle meningeal artery, supplying middle, anterior, and posterior meninges. A branch of the internal carotid artery divides into the cerebral artery, which branches into another meningeal artery supplying the anterior dura and fossa.

The middle meningeal artery, a division of the maxillary branch of the external carotid artery, is of vital importance in its distribution to anterior, middle, and posterior dura and fossae, as well as its clinical significance in head injury. It enters the cranial cavity through the foramen spinosum in the sphenoid bone, running forward and laterally for some distance on the squamous portion of the temporal bone. In the middle cranial fossa it divides into the frontal branch, supplying the anterior dura, and the parietal branch, supplying the posterior dura.

The meningeal veins, which actually are sinuses, lie in and drain the dura. The lateral lacunae—a complicated venous network, situated on each side of the superior sagittal sinus—receives the venous blood of the meningeal veins and communicates with the superior sagittal sinus draining into the internal jugular vein.

The arterial blood supply to the *brain* originates from the two internal carotid arteries anteriorly and the two vertebral arteries posteriorly.

The cerebral branch of the internal carotid artery divides into the anterior cerebral and anterior communicating arteries and middle cerebral, posterior communicating, and anterior choroidal arteries, thereby supplying a major share of arterial blood to the interior of the cerebral cortex.

The vertebral arteries enter the posterior fossa through the foramen magnum and join together below the pons to form the basilar artery, which branches into superior cerebellar and posterior cerebral arteries, thereby, supplying the pons, cerebellum, and posterior cerebrum.

The arterial system of the brain provides an anastomosis between the two vertebral arteries and the two internal carotid arteries, forming an alternate means of arterial blood supply to the brain, assuring continuity of circulation in the event of occlusion of one of the vessels. This polygonal anastomosis, called the circulus arteriosus (circle of Willis), is formed by the posterior communicating arteries, posterior cerebral arteries, anterior cerebral arteries, and anterior communicating arteries. (See Figs. 2-15 and 2-16.)

The venous system draining the brain is divided into the cerebral veins receiving blood from the cerebrum and the cerebellar veins receiving blood from the cerebellum. All drain into the dural sinuses and ultimately into the internal jugular vein (Fig. 2-17).

The external cerebral veins receive blood from the superior cerebral vein (ends in superior sagittal sinus), middle cerebral vein (ends in cavernous sinus), and inferior cerebral vein (ends in superior sagittal sinus). The internal cerebral veins end in the straight sinus.

The cerebellar veins, superior and inferior, end in the transverse sinus.

Brain metabolism accounts for approximately 8% of the total oxygen consumption of the human body. The metabolism of carbohydrates and aerobic glycolysis (the oxidation of glucose) provide brain tissue with its vital source of energy. It has been proved that protein and fat metabolism have no role in energy production. The brain contains 7 milliliters of oxygen at any given mo-

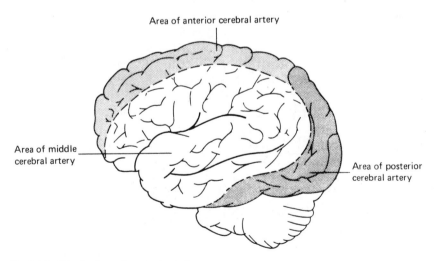

Area of anterior cerebral artery

Area of middle cerebral artery

Area of posterior cerebral artery

Fig. 2-15. Distribution of cerebral arteries.

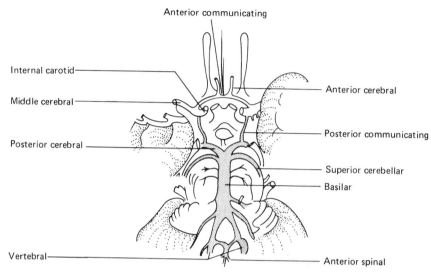

Fig. 2-16. Circle of Willis.

ment; with the usual rate of utilization this would be consumed in approximately 10 seconds. Normally there exists a metabolic autoregulatory mechanism that alters the diameter of the resistance vessels and changes the flow to meet the demands of the tissues. There is, however, a very short survival time for the brain in oxygen deprivation. Severe damage can occur if circulation is impaired for longer than three minutes.

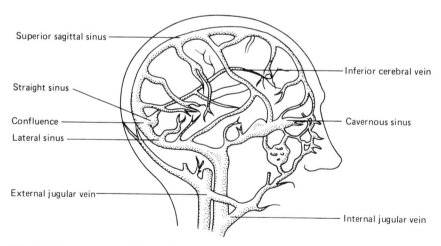

Fig. 2-17. Venous system of the brain.

Circulation in the brain is affected by certain factors: blood pressure head (the difference between arterial and venous pressure at the level of the brain) and cerebrovascular resistance.

The maintenance of a normal arterial blood pressure is under the influence of homeostatic mechanisms such as carotid sinus reflex and central control of peripheral vascular tone. Persistence of a mean arterial blood pressure at 70 millimeters of mercury is essential; below this level perfusion is seriously limited. The shock syndrome and orthostatic hypotension are clinical conditions that exhibit decreased arterial pressure with impaired perfusion.

Cerebrovascular resistance is affected by intracranial hypertension, viscosity of the blood, and vascular tone of the cerebral blood vessels.

As intracranial hypertension heightens, owing to increased cerebrospinal fluid pressure, cerebral blood flow decreases, a result probably due to obstruction of venous return by compression of the vessels in the dural sinuses. Pressure autoregulation automatically alters the diameter of resistance vessels, primarily venous, during changes in perfusion pressure. Autoregulation is impaired when intracranial presure is above 33 millimeters of mercury.

Changes in the viscosity of the blood affect circulation. Polycythemia reduces cerebral circulation by 50%, and severe anemia significantly increases cerebral circulation.

Vascular tone of cerebral vessels affects circulation. Very little vasoconstriction can be effected in cerebral arteries; cerebral vasospasm and vasodilation may, however, occur.

Blood-Brain Barrier.   The selective blood-brain barrier is a phenomenon that limits the free movement of substances from the blood to the brain tissue. The movement of substances from the blood into the brain occurs: (1) from the capillaries to the glial cells through the selective blood-brain barrier; (2) from the capillaries into the extracellular space of the brain; or (3) from the capillaries by way of the choroid plexus into the cerebrospinal fluid, from which a small amount may pass into the brain tissue. Passage of substances into the brain is relatively slow by comparison to passage into other organs.

The tissues that separate the blood and the neurons are: (1) the vascular wall; (2) the perivascular sheath, which is the internal and external layers of the leptomeninges (the fusion of the arachnoid and pia mater); and (3) the neuroglial cells of the brain substance. The perivascular sheath fuses at the level of the arterioles and venules and is replaced by an extra layer of glial cells, the neuroglial sheath. The capillary endothelial cells form a continuous layer of fusions or tight junctions, creating an externally applied basement membrane. The neuroglial sheath and the thickened basement membrane of the capillaries inhibit the process of diffusion between the blood and the brain.

This process provides a selective barrier, preventing the entry of toxic substances, plasma proteins, and other large molecules, and allowing entry of fluid, gases, and smaller molecular substances. The movement of inorganic substances, anions and cations (potassium and chloride), organic substances (glutamic acid), dyes, large molecules of insulin, and penicillin is all relatively slow; while the movement of water, gases, lipid-soluble compounds, glucose, and smaller molecular substances is all relatively fast. The transfer of these substances influences the level of metabolism and ionic composition of brain substance.

The blood-brain barrier is not fully developed in the infant, but becomes more competent with maturity. Consider the premature infant with a high bilirubin level. The infant brain is quite permeable to bilirubin, and kernicterus develops readily, whereas it does not exist with even greatly increased bilirubin levels in the adult.

The blood-brain barrier is significant in a number of situations:

1. Water reaches equilibrium within all regions of the brain and spinal fluid within 20 minutes. Urea as an impermeable substance reduces swelling when administered in a hypertonic solution, causing rapid movement of water from the ventricles to the blood, resulting in a temporarily decreased brain volume.

2. It is essential when administering medication to consider the rate of entrance to brain tissue as proportionate to the size of the molecules.

3. The brain scan as a diagnostic tool is effective based on the principles of the blood-brain barrier. Normally the blood-brain barrier inhibits the movement of a tracer into brain tissue. In the absence of a competent blood-brain barrier, the tracer permeates brain tissue. A tumor, for example, with the blood-brain barrier absent allows abnormal tracer permeability.

Vertebral Column

The vertebral column consisting of 24 movable presacral vertebrae supports the head and protects the spinal cord. There are 7 cervical vertebrae, 12 thoracic vertebrae, 5 lumbar vertebrae, 5 sacral vertebrae, and 3–4 coccygeal vertebrae. The consecutive central canals (spinal foramina) of the vertebrae form a long curved tube housing the spinal cord. The typical vertebra consist of: the body, which gives strength and supports weight; the arch, composed of the transverse process projecting laterally on either side, the lamina projecting dorsally and medially, and the spinous process projecting dorsally and caudally. Motion occurs between the adjacent body of the vertebra anteriorly and the articular process of the lamina posteriorly. A space exists between the vertebral bodies occupied by the intervertebral disc. This central core of cartilage has a soft, elastic, pulplike center called the nucleus pulposus. The intervertebral disc forms the conection between the vertebral bodies from the second cervical vertebra (C2) to the sacrum, joining bones and absorbing shock. This shock-absorbing mechanism equalizes stress and provides an axis for movement. Above and below each vertebral arch is an opening through which the spinal nerves exit, called the intervertebral foramen. (See Fig. 2-18.)

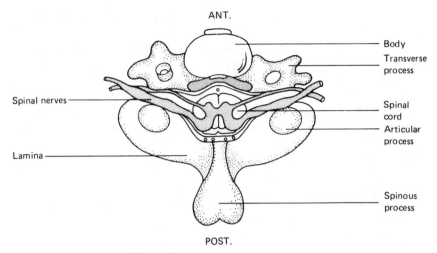

Fig. 2-18. Vertebrae. The nucleus pulposus lies between successive vertebral bodies.

Spinal Cord. The spinal cord, forming a continuous structure with the medulla oblongata, extends from the foramen magnum through the spinal foramina of the vertebral column to the upper portion of the lumbar region. The conus medullaris is the cone-shaped termination of the cord. The filum terminale, a fibrous-like band, descends from the apex of the conus, securing the cord to the coccyx. Extension varies from the 12th thoracic vertebra to the 2nd lumbar vertebra. The length of the cord remains fairly constant in adults: 45 centimeters in males and 43 centimeters in females.

The cord, weighing about one ounce and approximately 1½ inches wide, is elliptical in shape. It appears wider from right to left than anterior to posterior. The size and shape, however, do vary, depending on the vertebral region; for example, it presents cervical and lumbar enlargements, which are areas of nerve origin to the upper and lower limbs. There is a slight longitudinal groove on the posterior surface running the length of the cord, named the posterior median sulcus. The dorsal (posterior) root filaments enter this sulcus at regular intervals. There is a wider, shallower depression on the anterior surface running the length of the cord, named the anterior median fissure, occupied by the spinal artery and small veins. Anterolaterally, the ventral root filaments leave the cord at regular intervals.

A small oval-shaped central canal formed by white matter follows down the axis of the spinal cord and extends beyond the termination of the cord about 25 centimeters, ending at the 2nd sacral vertebra. The spinal cord is protected by three meninges, extending beyond the length of the central canal. Similarly, the spinal cord meninges have the same vascular spacings, with the subarachnoid space containing cerebrospinal fluid. The cord, terminating at the 2nd lumbar vertebra, but with meninges and subarachnoid space extending to the 2nd sacral vertebra, anatomically provides for an excellent region for the aspiration of cerebrospinal fluid for analysis.

The spinal cord, composed of gray (unmyelinated) and white (myelinated) matter, is supported by a framework of neuroglia. In cross section there is a round, oval-shaped structure formed by white matter with the middle gray matter roughly forming the pattern of an "H." The broader lower legs of the "H" correspond to the anterior (ventral) horns of the spinal cord. Efferent nerve cells of the *anterior* (ventral) *motor* root originate in the anterior horns. These nerve cells are essential for the voluntary and reflex motor activity in the muscles innervated by them. The thinner upper legs of the "H" correspond to the *posterior* (dorsal) horns of the spinal cord. Afferent *sensory* nerve fibers enter the posterior (dorsal) root, a segment of the spinal cord that is part of the cord to which a pair of dorsal roots and a pair of ventral roots are attached. The spinal cord has 31 segments. The crossbar of the "H" in the thoracic region extends from each side as the lateral horns give rise to autonomic nerve fibers. The motor and sensory nerve roots leave the vertebral column separately through the intervertebral foramina. Outside the column the motor nerve joins with the sensory nerve to form the spinal nerve. Autonomic nerve fibers join the spinal nerve, and together they constitute the peripheral nerve.

The white matter of the spinal cord contains groups of fibers or tracts called fasciculi. The three pathways or tracts are: (1) the posterior fasciculus, conducting sensation (touch, pressure, vibration) from one side of the body, crossing over in the medulla to the opposite side of the cerebral cortex (posterior fasciculus—ascending sensation pathway); (2) the anterolateral or spinothalamic fasciculus, conducting perception (pain and temperature) from one side of the body, crossing to the opposite side immediately upon entering the spinal cord, continuing to the thalamus and the cerebral cortex (anterolateral pathway or spinothalamic fasciculus—ascending perception); (3) the lateral fasciculus (pyramidal or corticospinal), conducting motor impulses from the cerebral cortex to the anterior horn cells on the opposite side of the body, crossing over in the medulla (lateral fasciculus—descending motor pathway).

An important function of the gray matter of the spinal cord is the part it plays in reflex activity. A sensory neuron leading from a receptor to its cell body in the dorsal (posterior) root ganglia outside the cord relays an impulse to a central neuron within the gray matter of the cord. Here the impulse synapses in a reflex arc with a motor cell body located in the (anterior) ventral horn and emerges from the ventral roots relaying a motor impulse leading to a gland or muscle. The incoming sensory impulse has now become an outgoing motor impulse in this reflex activity, in the absence of cerebral cortex mediation.

PERIPHERAL NERVOUS SYSTEM

Nerve fibers originating in the spinal cord receive and transmit impulses to and from the central nervous system from and to the periphery of the human body. The peripheral nervous system includes the spinal nerves and the autonomic nervous system.

Spinal Nerves

Each of the 31 segments of the spinal cord has a symmetrically arranged pair of spinal nerves, with one for each side of the body. Each spinal nerve is derived from the spinal cord by two roots: a sensory (dorsal) root and a motor (ventral) root.

Recall the cross section of the spinal cord with the middle gray matter roughly forming the pattern of an "H." The thinner upper legs of the "H" correspond to the posterior (dorsal) horns of the spinal cord. The sensory (dorsal) nerve root of the spinal nerve originates in this posterior (dorsal) horn of the spinal cord. A sensory (dorsal) root with afferent fibers relays sensory impulses from organs and muscles to the central nervous system. The broader lower legs of the "H" correspond to the anterior (ventral) horns of the spinal cord. The motor (ventral) nerve root of the spinal nerve originates in this anterior (ventral) horn of the spinal cord. A motor (ventral) root with efferent fibers relays motor impulses from the central nervous system to the skeletal muscles in the periphery. The motor and sensory roots leave the vertebral column separately through the intervertebral foramina, but immediately outside the column the fibers join together, forming a spinal nerve.

The spinal nerves are topographically divided into eight cervical pairs (C 1-8), twelve thoracic (T 1-12), five lumbar (L 1-5), five sacral (S 1-5), and one coccygeal (C). These nerves branch and interweave, forming three major plexuses or networks serving all parts of the body: the cervical plexus (C 1-4), brachial plexus (C 4-8 and T 1), and lumbosacral plexus (L 1-5 and S 1-3). The cervical plexus includes the cervical and thoracic nerves, which exit the spinal column in a horizontal course, sending motor impulses to neck muscles and diaphragm and receiving sensory impulses from the neck and back of the head. The brachial plexus nerves innervate the upper extremities. The lumbosacral plexus includes the lumbar and sacral spinal nerves, which group together resembling a horse's tail (the cauda equina), occupying the vertebral canal below the cord. They have an oblique course as they exit the spinal column and descend to innervate the lower extremities. This extension network of overlapping nerves in the peripheral distribution of spinal nerves allows the interruption of a single nerve without significant loss of sensory or motor function; an adjacent nerve in the network will serve the same area.

At the peripheral end of the sensory fibers of the spinal nerves are receptions for sensation of pain, touch, stretch, pressure, heat, and cold. The body surface has been divided into areas supplied by each nerve with each skin area corresponding to a spinal cord segment. These skin areas are called dermatomes and are significant in determining localization of spinal cord injury (Fig. 2-19).

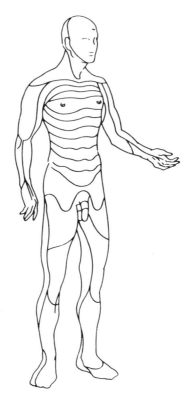

Fig. 2-19. Spinal dermatomes.

Autonomic Nervous System

The autonomic nervous system is a functional classification of a group of peripheral nerves governing involuntary activity on an unconscious reflex level. This system regulates the action of secretory activity of glands and the involuntary contraction of smooth muscle, as in the blood vessels, the ciliary bodies, the iris, the skin, the heart, the intestines, and the bronchial tubes. The autonomic nervous system also transmits pain sensations from vessels, viscera, and bones.

The higher centers of the autonomic nervous system are found distributed in the cerebral cortex, and the axons connect with the hypothalamus. The neuron link of ganglia and nerve fibers leaving the hypothalamus descends through the brain stem and spinal cord and forms a chain on each side of the bodies of the vertebral column. These autonomic fibers join the spinal nerve and constitute the peripheral nerve.

As the fibers descend from the hypothalamus through the brain stem and spinal cord, the axons end in association with three groups of cells: a group in the brain stem in relation to the 3rd, 7th, 9th, and 10th cranial nerve nuclei; a grouping in each segment of the thoracic and upper lumbar spinal cord; and a group in the sacral spinal cord.

The thoracolumbar unit or grouping forms the sympathetic division, and the craniosacral unit or grouping forms the parasympathetic division of the autonomic nervous sytem. There is dual automatic innervation, both sympathetic and parasympathetic fibers, of most visceral effectors (tissues and/or organs).

The autonomic nervous system tends to keep the body in balanced harmony by regulating the functioning of visceral effectors maintaining or restoring homeostasis. The sympathetic and parasympathetic divisions act in a reciprocal manner to bring about this effect by releasing pharmocologic transmitters. The sympathetic division liberates norepinephrine, which transmits impulses across the synapses and neuroeffector junctions and generally accelerates body function. The parasympathetic division liberates acetylcholine, a neurotransmitter, which tends to slow bodily processes and conserve bodily resources. These chemicals are continually released at the neuroeffector junctions of the doubly innervated visceral effectors. The response of these organs or tissues is determined by the algebraic sum of these opposing chemicals. If sympathetic impulses increase, there is an increase in the release of norepinephrine, and bodily functions are accelerated. This stimulating effect enables the body to respond energetically to a stressor in a "fight or flight" reaction. This explains the dominance of the sympathetic division under stressful situations. If parasympathetic impulses increase, there is an increase in the release of acetylcholine, which slows the heart rate and promotes digestion and elimination. This explains the dominance of the parasympathetic division of digestive tract glands and smooth muscle under normal conditions. In this manner the two divisions in antagonistic actions, depending on the algebraic sum of the opposing chemicals, maintain or restore the human body to a state of equilibrium.

The autonomic nervous system, despite its name, does not operate autonomously, but in conjunction with all parts of the nervous system. It is partly controlled by higher autonomic centers in the brain, notably the hypothalamus and limbic system. This higher autonomic center control plays a part in the expression of emotion.

Lower Motor Neuron

The idea of the lower motor neuron is identical to that of the upper motor neuron in that it is a physiologic concept; the anatomy of the lower motor neuron is more precise. Lower motor neuron refers to the aggregate of the neurons of the motor nuclei of the cranial nerves and the parent neurons of the anterior gray column of the spinal cord. These neurons along with the group of somatic muscle fibers innervated by them constitute a motor unit. Every neuron of this system is the final common pathway whereby all of the multiple influences of the nervous system on motor function are both integrated and transmitted to the effector muscle. In the spinal cord an aggregate of lower motor neurons at a given spinal cord segment constitutes the efferent limb of the spinal reflex arc. Thus this system includes the parent neurons of the anterior column along their axons coursing through the anterior spinal roots, spinal nerves, plexus, peripheral nerves, and the synaptic junction of the muscle (motor end plate). A lesion anywhere in this system produces characteristic symptoms of lower motor neuron paralysis.

CONCLUSION

A great deal of complex material has been covered in this chapter. Anatomy and physiology of the neurologic system have been presented in depth for the purpose of having the reader gain a strong, comprehensive background knowledge of the central nervous system and its components. Our bodies are truly "magnificent machines."

In focusing on normal structures and their relationships and healthy physiology, we should be able to identify pathophysiology and the resultant symptomatology when it exists.

It is from this basic knowledge that we, as nurses, can move toward understanding the problems of neurologic patients.

As other chapters are encountered by the reader, there should be frequent reference to this anatomy and physiology chapter for a clear understanding of the conditions being described.

BIBLIOGRAPHY

Blount, Mary, et al., "Obtaining and Analyzing Cerebrospinal Fluid," *The Nursing Clinics of North America*, December 1974.

Carini, Esta, and Guy Owens, *Neurological and Neurosurgical Nursing*, 6th ed., St. Louis: The C. V. Mosby Co., 1974.

Chusid, Joseph G., *Correlative Neuroanatomy and Functional Neurology*, 5th ed., Los Altos, California: Lange Med. Pub. Co., 1973.

Gardner, Ernest, Donald Gray, and Ronan O'Rahilly, *Anatomy*, 4th ed., Philadelphia: W. B. Saunders Co., 1974.

Greisheimer, Esther, and Mary Wiedeman, *Physiology and Anatomy*, 9th ed., Philadelphia: J. B. Lippincott Co., 1972.

Guyton, Arthur *Textbook of Medical Physiology*, 5th ed., Philadelphia: W. B. Saunders Co., 1976.

Lopez-Antunez, Luis, *Atlas of Human Anatomy*, Philadelphia: W. B. Saunders Co., 1971.

Luckman, Joan, and Karen Sorenson, *Medical Surgical Nursing*, Philadelphia: W. B. Saunders Co., 1974.

Mauss, Nancy K., and Pamela H. Mitchell, "Increased Intracranial Pressure: An Update," *Heart and Lung*, 5 (No. 6):19, November–December 1976.

Pansky, Ben, and Earl Lawrence House, *Review of Gross Anatomy*, 2nd ed., London: The Macmillan Co., 1969.

Warwick, Roger, and Peter L. Williams, *Gray's Anatomy*, Phildaelphia: W. B. Saunders Co., 1975.

Youman, Julian R., *Neurological Surgery*, Vols. 1, 2, and 3, Philadelphia: W. B. Saunders Co., 1973.

3
THE NEUROLOGIC ASSESSMENT

INTRODUCTION

This chapter is divided into three sections: the neurologic nursing history, the neurologic examination, and intracranial pressure monitoring. The first section deals with the relevant components of a nursing history and contains a suggested format for collecting data on the neurologic patient in the intensive care unit. The second section, on the neurologic examination, emphasizes the development of physical examination skills and includes a tool for rapid assessment. The last section deals with the physiology and related concepts of intracranial pressure monitoring.

SECTION I: THE NEUROLOGIC NURSING HISTORY

The purpose of the nursing history is to provide personalized and individualized care to the critically ill patient. This perhaps varies from the goal of the physician, where the history becomes a keystone for accurate diagnosis. The role of the critical care nurse is to assist the patient in reaching his optimal level of functioning. In this role she must understand his background, his strengths and weaknesses, his perception of his illness, his coping mechanisms, and so on. Basic nursing is no different in the critical care unit from elsewhere; it must not be intuitive, accidental, or haphazard, but must be rationally planned. In this manner may the nurse assist the patient and contribute to his health, recovery, or peaceful death.

Neurologic Nursing History Format

I. **Vital Statistics**
   Name
   Hospital Number
   Previous Admissions
   Age/Sex
   Marital Status
   Religious Preference
   Emergency Contact Person
      Telephone

II. **Admitting Vital Signs**
    Temperature   Heart Rate   Blood Pressure
    Respiratory Frequency   EKG Pattern   Pupils
    Level of Consciousness

III. **Medical Diagnosis**
    Surgery
    Surgical Diagnosis
    Medications

IV. **The Patient's Perception Of Illness**

V. **The Family's Perception Of The Patient And His Illness**

VI. **Initial Assessment**
    Status/Habitus
    Neurologic Assessment
      Speech Flow
      Cognitive Thought
      Level Of Consciousness
      Cranial Nerve Evaluation
      Reflexes
      Motion
      Coordination
      Sensation
      Autonomic
    Integumentary
    Head and Neck
    Respiratory
    Cardiovascular
    Genitourinary
    Gastrointestinal
    Musculoskeletal
    Mental Status; Psychological Status

VII. **Past medical history relating to patient's current diagnosis. Include medications the patient is taking.**

VIII. **Psychosocial history. Include educational level, occupation, status of family and friends.**

IX. **Critical Care Nursing Orders**
    Frequency And Type Of Neurologic Assessment
    Respiratory Orders
    Problem Areas
    Resuscitation Orders
    Special Monitoring Considerations

X. **Patient-Nurse Goals**

XI. **Factors That Might Influence Achievement of Goals**

XII. **Implementation Of Care Plan**

Conclusion

In gathering information for the nursing history, ask the questions in an objective and tactful way. Reassure the patient of the importance of the information and allay his anxiety regarding the answers to your questions. Be perceptive of his attending behavior and the process of interaction during the interview, and deal with it appropriately. It is essential that the nurse-patient relationship be established and preserved. Thus the nursing history becomes an important tool for establishing a basis of care for the patient.

SECTION II: THE NEUROLOGIC EXAMINATION

The neurologic examination identifies the integrity, capability, function and/or dysfunction of the nervous system at a given moment. The data collected become increasingly important when interpreted conjointly with the neurologic history.

Equipment

The clinician should have the necessary equipment for utilization at the bedside:

Aromatic agent	Ophthalmoscope
Percussion hammer	Otoscope
Sharp pin (on hammer)	Flashlight
Small brush (on hammer)	Cotton applicator
C-256 tuning fork	Stethoscope
Tongue blade	Tape measure

Mental Function

The neurologic examination begins when the nurse first greets the patient. At this time the examiner can observe the patient's speech, movements, and mannerisms, all of which may give clues to dysfunction. The nurse then proceeds to questions aimed at evaluating the patient's mental function. This process requires both tact and an objective demeanor. Begin by using frank inquiry into the patient's memory, such as: "Do you think that you have difficulty remembering things?" Further explore this area by having the patient answer questions regarding the date, recent news events, and so on. Test the patient's ability to think abstractly by quoting a familiar phrase to him and having him explain the meaning to you, such as: "A stitch in time saves nine." Continue by having the patient demonstrate his ability to calculate—for example, by asking him to subtract 7 from 100 in a series (100 minus 7, 93 minus 7, etc.). Language function may be tested by having the patient read a passage from a book, write a phrase, draw an object, and so forth.

Agnosia/Aphasia. Agnosia and aphasia are symptoms of disordered language function which are highly specific findings. They indicate a focal lesion involving the dominant cerebral hemisphere. Remember that language is an intellectual function which utilizes words as symbols and groups of words to convey meaning. It is a dual process: one must receive and recognize word symbols as well as express them.

Agnosia means the inability to recognize or understand the significance of stimuli, even though the perception of the stimuli is intact. Aphasia means the inability to understand or meaningfully communicate language in the absence of mental disability or motor dysfunction. Aphasia is usually accompanied by the inability to write (agraphia) or inability to read (alexia). Neither symptom is likely to occur alone from an isolated intracranial lesion.

Dysphasia is a mild degree of aphasia. It is manifested by occasional misuse of a word during a conversation. When speech is partially impaired, both primitive (such as exclamations) and automatic speech (such as salutations) are usually left intact. Symbolic speech conveying ideas rather than feelings is usually impaired to some degree in dysphasia.

Examples of such tests are: requiring the patient to name objects as they are shown to him; read aloud from a book; write a sentence to dictation; or carry out a complicated oral command. Extensive testing is necessary to help evaluate the patient suspected of having language difficulty.

Motor aphasia or expressive aphasia occurs when a patient is unable to say what he wishes. The patient may be alert, appear oriented, and understand what is said to him as well as what he reads; however, he cannot communicate the language normally. He is aware of and in fact frustrated by this difficulty. It represents a lesion anterior to the fissure of Rolando on the dominant frontal lobe.

Sensory aphasia, or receptive aphasia, is also called Wernicke's aphasia. Although it varies in details of presentation, it usually consists of the inability to understand spoken language (auditory verbal aphasia), the inability to understand written language (visual graphic aphasia), and the inability to write (agraphia). The patient can speak and is often loquacious. What he says becomes progressively disassociated from what was said to him. Since he cannot understand what he is saying, he talks in disjointed sentences. Occasionally this is accompanied by an amnesic aphasia in which he cannot name objects or describe their use, although he can recognize their names. Unlike the motor aphasic patient, the sensory aphasic patient does not recognize his disability. He becomes annoyed at those speaking to him rather than at himself. This speech and annoyed behavior may give one the impression that he is mentally disturbed. This aphasia occurs from a focal lesion that involves the posterior superior convex surface of the dominant temporal lobes or Wernicke's area.

Aphasias or dysphasias must be differentiated from other speech disorders controlled at a lower anatomical level: dysarthria, dysphonia, and mutism. Dysarthria, meaning deterioration of enunciation or articulation of speech, is due to motor dysfunction of the lips, tongue, or pharynx. Dysphonia is a loss of voice or hoarseness due to motor dysfunction of the laryngeal muscles. Mutism, which means the patient cannot speak, usually accompanies either hysterical reactions or the deaf-mute syndrome. The condition can be akinetic; that is, there is a loss of ability to talk that occurs with generalized severe motor impairment.

Levels of Consciousness

Any impairment of consciousness is a cardinal clinical finding, if one explains consciousness as being the highest function of the brain. Consciousness ranges in decreasing degrees from alert to comatose. The degree of consciousness, or level, is one of the most important items of assessment in intensive care units. The subtlest change may influence diagnosis, management, and prognosis of the patient. In order to ensure continuity of nursing care and evaluation, the ending and beginning shift nurses should jointly assess the patient's level of consciousness so that individual conjecture regarding a change in level does not affect judgment at a later time. When charting the level of consciousness, avoid using representative numbers or words, but rather describe the patient's behavior or wakefulness in clear, descriptive terms. The gradations of consciousness are alert, lethargic, stuporous, and comatose.

The Alert Patient. The normal and highest level of consciousness is alert wakefulness, which is characterized by appropriate responses to external and internal stimuli, including noxious or harmful stimuli. An alert patient will also be either oriented or disoriented. In evaluating him, the clinician should avoid using questions regarding time, place, and situation. When questions of this nature are used repeatedly, they tend to elicit programmed responses. Rather, ask pertinent questions about the patient's family, marriage, home, or occupation. This approach affords the clinician another means of establishing a positive rapport with the patient by becoming interested and involved in his world.

The Lethargic Patient. Lethargic means that the patient is somnolent and indifferent. His responses are quiescent, dull, delayed, or incomplete, and he may require an increased stimulus to evoke a response. He appears to drift back to sleep as soon as he is awakened, reflecting loss of consciousness rather than sleepiness. The lethargic patient will be oriented or confused. The word obtunded is sometimes used to refer to a dull indifference in which little more than wakefulness is maintained by the patient.

The Stuporous Patient. Stuporous describes a state in which a response is evoked only by vigorous and continuous noxious stimuli. The patient does not verbalize; however, his movements are still purposeful and intentional, showing a lesser degree of encephalization (cerebro-cortical influence) than the lethargic patient.

The Comatose Patient. Coma is described as a state in which psychological and motor responses are either reduced to reflex motor responses or completely lost: the term "moderately deep" coma is sometimes used when motor response to stimulation is reduced to reflex motor responses; when it is completely lost, the term "deep coma" applies.

Motor Responses in Coma. Abnormalities of motor function in patients in coma give evidence of the nature and localization of the lesion. These abnormalities can be classified as paratonic rigidity and mass response, which is decorticate and decerebrate. Motor responses in comatose patients may be elicited by providing some type of noxious stimuli. One easy and acceptable method of providing this noxious stimuli is for the examiner to rub his knuckles against the patient's sternum using increasing pressure as necessary or appropriate to evoke the response. We feel that this is advantageous over other methods which are apt to cause bruises or marks injurious to the patient or identifiable by the family.

Paratonic rigidity. Paratonic rigidity is an early, although nonspecific, indicator of cerebral subcortical motor dysfunction. It is characterized by an abnormal increase in resistance offered to passive motion, is intermittent, and is independent of the initial extremity position. It can range from slight failure to relax to intense rigidity of the entire body, and often mimics a patient voluntarily opposing every effort of the clinician to examine him.

Mass response: decorticate and decerebrate. Mass response is an inappropriate response showing stereotypes of movement and posture in response to noxious stimuli. The two types of mass response are decorticate and decerebrate.

Decorticate positioning consists of motor response to noxious stimuli by flexion of the arms, wrists, and fingers with adduction of the upper extremities, and extension, internal rotation, and plantar flexion in the lower extremities. This may be due to a lesion of the frontal lobes, internal capsule, or cerebral peduncles.

Decerebrate positioning consists of motor response to noxious stimuli by opisthotonus, adduction with extension and hyperpronation of the arms, and extension and plantar flexion of the lower extremities. It requires at least partial bilateral division of the midbrain and pons structures from influence from the cerebral hemispheres. Decerebracy is commonly found with lesions that destroy or depress the upper brain stem.

Cranial Nerve Evaluation

First Cranial Nerve: Olfactory. The olfactory nerves are sensory and innervate the sense of smell. Injury to these nerves is common, often following cribiform plate fractures and ethmoid bone fractures.

Test. To test the olfactory nerves, shield the patient's eyes and allow him to smell identifiable, nonirritating odors with first one nostril and then the other.

Normal/abnormal. If the nerve is injured, the patient will have anosmia —the inability to detect the odor presented.

Second Cranial Nerve: Optic. The optic nerves are the sensory tracts for vision and part of the circuit for the light reflexes. Injury to these nerves is common following trauma to the orbit, intracerebral clot, or lesion of the temporal, parietal, or occipital lobes.

Test: Vision. The visual fields are assessed by gross confrontation. It is a crude method of testing vision; however, it remains the most practical and accurate bedside test available. In this method the practitioner should observe the following steps: have the patient cover one eye and look at your eye directly opposite him or at a point straight ahead. Position yourself level with him and about two feet away. Close your other eye so that you may roughly superimpose your visual field on the patient's visual field. Wiggling your fingers, bring them from the periphery into his field of vision from several directions. Your wiggling finger should be equidistant between you and the patient except in the temporal field. In the temporal field start with your fingers a little behind the patient and in a location well within your own visual field. Have the patient identify your fingers as they appear, and compare his response with that of your own visual field. Repeat these actions on the other side, testing his other eye.

Normal/abnormal. The visual field of the normal eye is in the range of about 45° for vertical peripheral vision to about 80° for temporal peripheral vision. An abnormal finding would be a defect in the visual field as identified in gross confrontation. An example of an abnormal finding would be hemianopsia, which is loss of vision in one-half of the visual field.

Test: light reflexes. These tests are discussed in detail and illustrated under the evaluation of the third cranial nerve.

Test: auscultation. Although auscultation of the eyeball is not part of a cranial nerve evaluation, now is an opportune time for it. It is performed by placing the bell of a stethoscope directly on the eyelid over the eyeball.

Normal/abnormal. The abnormal finding would be the detection of a bruit, which may occur with cavernous sinus fistula.

Third Cranial Nerve: Oculomotor. The oculomotor nerves have both a sensory and a motor unit. The third, fourth, and sixth cranial nerves innervate the muscles for eye movement. The third also controls pupillary constriction and the muscles of the upper eyelid. Injury to this nerve is common, especially as the nerve is encroached on by other lesions, particularly when pressure is exerted on the third cranial nerve before it enters the cavernous sinus by a herniating uncus. Fracture involving the cavernous sinus may also produce the same effect.

Test: light reflexes. When you flash a light on the retina of the eye, it will cause reflex pupillary constriction of that eye, which is direct reaction to light. It will also cause pupillary constriction of the opposite eye, which is consensual reaction to light (Fig. 3-1). The sensory pathway is the retina, optic nerve, optic tract, diverging pathways in the midbrain through synapses to the third nerve, and the constrictors of the iris on either side. When testing light reflexes, use a bright light and a semidarkened room. Flash the light on each pupil in turn, and avoid flashing the light into the pupils simultaneously. Do not let the patient focus on the light because it will produce an accommodation reaction (explained on p. 56).

Normal/abnormal. If a right third nerve palsy is present, shining a light in the normal left eye will produce a direct pupillary reaction to light; i.e., the left pupil will constrict. The consensual reflex will be absent; i.e., the right pupil will not constrict when the light is flashed in the left eye. When the light is flashed into the affected right eye, the direct pupillary reflex will be absent; so the right pupil will not constrict. The consensual reflex is present; so the left pupil constricts.

Test: accommodation. Accommodation is the process in which a focused visual image is maintained as you move your gaze from a distant point to a near point. The sensory pathway for it is similar to that involved in vision and direct and consensual reaction to light. There are three components to this reaction: convergence of the eyes, pupillary constriction, and thickening of the lenses. The first two components are visible to the clinician. To test accommodation, have the patient look into the distance. Hold your finger 10 to 12 centi-

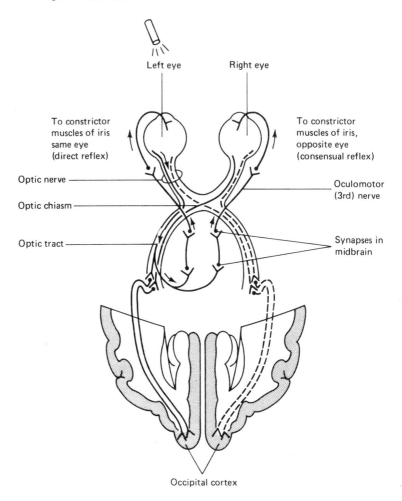

Fig. 3-1. Light reflexes.

meters from the bridge of his nose and then have him focus on your finger. Move your finger toward the bridge of his nose. This should cause the eyes to accommodate.

Normal/abnormal. Three things occur when the eyes accommodate normally: the eyes converge, the pupils constrict, and the lenses widen. The examiner observes the normal reaction of convergence at 5 to 8 centimeters from the nose, and he also observes pupillary constriction.

Test: autonomic function: ciliospinal reflex. The fibers that produce pupillary constriction and control the iris are parasympathetic nerve fibers. However, the iris is also supplied by sympathetic fibers, which travel through the sympathetic trunk and ganglia in the neck. Then they follow a nerve plexus around the carotid artery and its branches into the orbit. The reflex center is located in the brain stem. The integrity of this system may be tested by pinching the skin on the back of the neck. When these fibers are stimulated, dilatation of the pupils occurs.

Normal/abnormal.   Pinching the skin in the back of the neck should result in ipsilateral dilatation of the pupil. This reaction reveals that the brain stem sympathetic fibers are intact.

Third Cranial Nerve: Oculomotor.
Fourth Cranial Nerve: Trochlear.
Sixth Cranial Nerve: Abducens.

These three pairs of nerves, which are motor, have interrelated functions and are often examined together. All of them conjointly innervate the muscles for eye movement. The fourth nerve is not commonly injured, but may be damaged at its course around the basilar skull or following fracture of the orbit. The sixth nerve is frequently injured with cavernous sinus fracture or orbital fracture. Injury to the third nerve is described on p. 127.

Test: extraocular movements.   The movements of the eyes are controlled by the coordinated activity of six muscles. Each eye uses four recti muscles and two oblique muscles. The function of a muscle is tested by having the patient follow your finger with his eyes. You move your finger so that he will move his eyes in the six cardinal fields of gaze. If the patient is awake and cooperative, extraocular movements can be easily assessed.

In an unconscious patient, assessment is more difficult; therefore, instead of extraocular movements the assessment is based on the oculocephalic response or "doll's eyes" maneuver. The term doll's eyes originated with dolls with weighted eyes; when their heads are moved, their eyes move in contrast. The normal response will be described under "Normal/abnormal." To perform the test, hold the patient's eyes open and move his head to the right. The eyes move in opposition toward the left or center of his body. When the same is done moving the patient's head upward, the eyes move downward, and so forth. This is the coordinated action of the same muscles and nerves that control extraocular movements. In addition, the stimulus for the doll's eyes maneuver involves the labyrinthine vestibular system.

Normal/abnormal.   When one is observing extraocular movement, or the doll's eyes maneuver, there is a normal conjugate (parallel) movement of the eyes in a given direction. There appears to be confusion among nurses regarding the doll's eyes maneuver. The normal response is referred to as "doll's eyes present," meaning that the eyes move conjugately in all directions. The abnormal response is referred to as "doll's eyes absent," meaning that despite movement of the head, the eyes remain "fixed" in their position in the orbit. When one of the nerves is palsied, the eye cannot deviate fully into the corresponding field of gaze. Nystagmus, a fine rhythmic oscillation of the eyes horizontally, is also an abnormal response. A few beats of nystagmus on extreme lateral gaze is, however, normal. Sixth nerve palsy is accompanied by diplopia on lateral gaze.

Fifth Cranial Nerve: Trigeminal. The trigeminal nerves (Fig. 3-2) are motor and sensory. Injury to the fifth nerve is not commonly encountered neurosurgically. Occasionally direct injury to one of its terminal branches causes damage. This is particularly true of the second division, as it enters the roof of the maxillary sinus. The first sensory division, ophthalmic, supplies the cornea of the eye and above. The second sensory division, maxillary, supplies the cheek and upper lip. The third sensory division, mandibular, supplies the lower lip and chin. The motor division supplies the masseter and temporal muscles used in biting down and chewing, and in the lateral movement of the jaw.

Test. The sensory divisions are tested by having the patient close his eyes and then, with a pin, testing his forehead, cheeks, and jaw on each side for pain sensation.

If abnormality is found, confirm your findings by testing temperature discrimination. Using two test tubes filled with hot and cold water, touch the skin

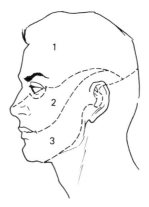

Fig. 3-2. Trigeminal innervation. Illustration of the ophthalmic, maxillary, and mandibular branches of the fifth cranial nerve.

and ask the patient to identify hot and cold. In addition to testing for temperature discrimination, you may follow by testing for light touch by using a brush as found on the percussion hammer, and asking the patient to respond whenever you touch his face.

The motor division of the fifth nerve is tested by palpating the temporal and masseter muscles in turn and asking the patient to clench his teeth. You will notice the strength of muscle contraction.

The corneal reflex is checked by approaching the patient's eye from the side and touching the cornea lightly with a fine piece of cotton.

Normal/abnormal.   If the sensory division of the fifth cranial nerve is intact, the patient will experience pain when tested with a pin and will be able to identify hot and cold sensations.

If the motor division of the fifth nerve is intact, the patient will be able to clench his teeth, and the clinician will be able to palpate the normal strength of the muscle contraction.

If the sensory portion of the fifth cranial nerve is intact, the patient will respond to touching of the cornea by tearing and blinking. Absence of any of the above findings may indicate lesion to that nerve.

Seventh Cranial Nerve: Facial.   The seventh cranial nerves are motor and sensory. The facial nerves innervate facial muscles (excluding the face's sensory receptors) and the taste receptors of the anterior portion of the tongue (excluding the muscles of the tongue). Injury to this nerve is common, resulting from fracture of the temporal bone, laceration or contusion of the parotid area, and intracerebral bleeds.

Test.   The motor portion of the seventh nerve is tested by observing the patient's face to note symmetry and movements. Have the patient do each of the following in turn: raise his eyebrows, frown, close his eyes tightly so that you cannot open them, show his teeth, smile, and puff out his cheeks.

The sensory division of the seventh cranial nerve supplies taste to the anterior two-thirds of the tongue, which it is impractical to test clinically.

Normal/abnormal.   Normally the patient can symmetrically move his face as described. Absence of any of these features, alone or in combination, as well as abnormal movements such as tics, indicates possible lesion. In Bell's phenomenon, there is paralysis of the facial muscles, causing the eye to remain open, the angle of the mouth to droop, and failure of the forehead to wrinkle.

Eighth Cranial Nerve: Stato-Acoustic.   The pair of stato-acoustic nerves is sensory. The eighth cranial nerve is commonly involved with seventh nerve lesions, especially following fracture of the petrous portion of the temporal bone. The eighth nerve has two parts (both sensory), cochlear and vestibular; the cochlear branch provides hearing, and the vestibular branch monitors and controls equilibrium.

Test. In children and uncooperative patients, these nerves can be tested by eliciting the startle reflex: suddenly slap your hands in front of and close to the patient's ear. This action normally startles the patient.

Hearing is tested by performing the Weber test (bone conduction). Place a vibrating C-256 tuning fork in the center of the forehead or on each mastoid protuberance. The sound should be heard equally well in both ears.

Normal/abnormal. If there is a defect, it can occasionally be lateralized by comparison of the Rinne test (air conduction) and the Weber test. If the defect is external (middle ear), the Weber test lateralizes to the affected (bad) side (meaning the bad side hears bone conduction best). Because the affected ear is not distracted by room noise, it detects bone conduction to a greater degree than normal. Bone conduction in this situation lasts longer than air conduction, since pathways of normal conduction through the middle ear are blocked. If the problem is inner ear (eighth cranial nerve), the Weber test and Rinne test lateralize to the good ear. Since the affected inner ear or eighth cranial nerve receives transmissions poorly arriving from any route, the sounds are heard best in the better ear. In an inner ear problem, air conduction lasts longer than bone conduction. The inner ear is less able to receive transmissions arriving from either route, so that the normal pattern prevails.

Test. The vestibular portion of the eighth cranial nerve is checked by observing for nystagmus (abnormal) and performing labyrinthine tests, such as caloric stimulation (the oculovestibular reflex). This test refers to reflex conjugate gaze or nystagmus induced by caloric stimulation of the labyrinth.

Elevate the head of the bed 30° so that the patient's lateral semicircular canal is vertical. In this position a maximum response can be evoked. Place a small volume (1 to 20 cc) of ice water slowly into the ear of the unresponsive patient. This test is usually performed by a neurologist or neurosurgeon.

Normal/abnormal. The normal response to ice water calorics is either horizontal nystagmus or tonic ocular deviation. Associated symptoms are nausea, vomiting, and vertigo. Interpretations of these responses is complex and should be reserved for the examiner.

Ninth Cranial Nerve: Glossopharyngeal.
Tenth Cranial Nerve: Vagus.

The pairs of glossopharyngeal and the vagus nerves are both sensory and motor. These nerves are responsible for such motor functions as swallowing, vocal cord movement, pharyngeal reflex, and upward movement of the soft palate and uvula. The ability to speak clearly, therefore, depends upon them. The ninth and tenth nerves are rarely affected in lesion of the brain. Extracranial lesions may cause destruction of these nerves, such as deep laceration of the neck or masses in the neck.

The motor portion of the ninth nerve supplies the constrictors of the pharynx and stylopharynx, which are used in swallowing. The sensory portion supplies the posterior third of the tongue and the soft palate. Autonomic functions include control of parotids and certain salivary glands.

The tenth nerve's motor branch supplies the pharynx and the larynx.

Normal/abnormal.   Dysfunction is manifested by nasal speech (from inability to elevate the soft palate), observed immobility of the soft palate, pharyngeal stimulation causing impaired gagging and increased mucus in the mouth from defective swallowing, hoarseness, and orthostatic hypotension. The latter is from lack of innervation by the ninth nerve to the carotid sinus, resulting in vasomotor inability to maintain blood pressure when upright.

Eleventh Cranial Nerve: Spinal Accessory.   The eleventh cranial nerves, spinal accessory, are motor. Injury rarely occurs, but may be associated with deep laceration of the neck. These nerves supply the sternocleidomastoid, trapezius, and rhomboid muscles.

Test.   These nerves are tested by three maneuvers: (1) Place your hand on the chin of the patient and have him push against your hand. Observe or palpate the contraction of the opposite sternocleidomastoid muscle. (2) Have the patient shrug his shoulders upward and against your hands. Observe the contraction and equality of the trapezius muscles. (3) Have the patient stretch out his hands and arms toward you.

Normal/abnormal.   (1) Lesion would be manifested by sternocleidomastoid weakness. (2) Lesion would be manifested by weakness of the trapezius. (3) If a lesion is present, the affected side seems longer, since the scapula is not "anchored."

Twelfth Cranial Nerve: Hypoglossal.   The twelfth cranial nerves supply motor innervation to the tongue. They are rarely damaged.

Test.   Have the patient protrude his tongue into each side of his cheek.

Normal/abnormal.   If damage has occurred, the tongue will move toward the middle of the mouth rather than the side of the cheek. If atrophy of the tongue occurs with lesion, increased wrinkling on the tongue surface will be noted. Also note any fasciculations (fine twitching movements) of the muscle bundles, which may also be a manifestation of lesion. Dysarthria and dysphagia may accompany bilateral lesions.

Ophthalmoscopic Examination

The ophthalmoscopic examination allows a unique opportunity to evaluate the fundus (retina and disc) of the eye. The optic disc (where the optic nerve joins the retina), the physiologic cup (inside the disc), the arteries and veins of the retina, the fovea centralis (tiny pit inside the macula), and the macula lutea (a depression marking the central point of vision) are all visualized and examined. The practitioner is expected to be skilled in the funduscopic examination and capable of identifying abnormal findings. This competency will become more refined and information will become more meaningful only through practice.

Mydriatic drugs are used to dilate the patient's pupils, thereby aiding the examination; however, this is not recommended for the neurological patient. Mydriatics could mask important changes in the pupils and retinal field. There is some risk involved in a patient with glaucoma, one with recent intracranial hemorrhage, and especially a patient with trauma. Observation of serial changes in the fundus is critical in planning intervention.

Adjust the lens wheel of the ophthalmoscope at +8 or +10 diopters. (A diopter is a unit that measures the power of a lens to converge or diverge light rays.) Darken the room. Use your right hand and right eye to examine the patient's right eye and your left hand and left eye for the patient's left eye. Grasp the ophthalmoscope with your right index finger on the lens disc for adjusting. Place your opposite thumb on the patient's eyebrow, gently pulling up the upper eyelid; ask the patient to look straight ahead or a little toward the side you are examining. Place the ophthalmoscope firmly against your face or glasses and look directly through the slight hole. Continue to rest your index finger on the lens disc so that you may adjust the diopters when necessary.

Position yourself about 15 inches away from the patient and about 15° lateral to his line of vision. Shine the light on the patient's pupil, using +8 or +10 diopters as previously set. Note the orange glow, which is the red reflex caused by light refracting off the retina. Note any opacities that serve to interrupt the orange glow. The light illuminates the retina so that any opacity or obstruction to the emerging light will be seen as a dark spot or shadow against the orange background.

Funduscopic examination. Relax your eyes and keep both of them open, gazing into the distance. Gradually move in toward the patient's eye on the 15-degree line, stopping about 8 centimeters from his eye. Continue to hold his eye open with the thumb of your free hand. Adjust the lens disc toward 0 diopters. The retina should now be in view in the vicinity of the optic disc, which is a round or oval structure located centrally and on the nasal side of the retina. Refocus the instrument until you can clearly see the details of the optic disc (the optic nerve head). Observe the size, shape, color, clarity of margins, and physiologic depression of the optic nerve.

If you encounter an elevated disc (papilledema), use the following procedure for estimating the degree of elevation: Focus the ophthalmoscope on the highest part of the disc (adjust the diopters) and note the number of the lens wheel. Move approximately two disc diameters nasally, and refocus the instrument on the retina (adjust the diopters); note the number on the lens wheel. Note the difference between the diopter number when focusing on the disc and the diopter number when focusing on the uninvolved retina. This number indicates the amount of elevation of the disc.

The physiologic cup, or depression, is a yellowish-white area on the inner temporal side of the disc. It is devoid of nerve fibers and therefore forms a depression. Identify the physiologic cup, noting size and shape, which may vary even in normal eyes.

Examine the retina, which is normally transparent. The amount of pigment varies with the patient's complexion and race. The retina is thinner in the nasal region, causing it to be paler. Occasionally there is a highlight of color, which follows the pattern of nerve fibers.

The fundus is the only area of the body in which blood vessels can be directly observed. The retina is supplied by four pairs of blood vessels, which emerge from and enter the disc. They should be examined in the following order: superior nasal vessels, inferior nasal vessels, inferior temporal vessels, and superior temporal vessels. Follow these vessels out as far as possible without having the patient move his eyes. Then have the patient look up, up and in, directly toward his nose, down and in, directly down, down and out, directly outward, then finally up and out. By these movements, you cover eight overlapping zones of the peripheral fundus. The course of the vessels may vary on the disc. The retinal vessels appear to be slightly sinuous and divide at approximately right angles, crossing each other without any obvious indentations. The arterioles are lighter in color than the veins, are about one-fourth as wide, and do not pulsate. The veins lack a stripe and normally pulsate on the retina.

When you are ready to complete the examination, have the patient look directly at the light so that you can visualize the central retina and macular area. The macula lutea is on a horizontal plane with the disc and can be found two to three disc diameters toward the temporal side. It is a small, darker red area lying in the retina, and is apart from the vessels. It shows a slight depression, called the fovea centralis, which marks the point of central vision and appears as a small, bright dot. This part of the ophthalmoscopic examination is usually done rapidly because using direct light is uncomfortable for the patient.

Normal/abnormal.   The optic disc, with convergent vessels, lies centrally and toward the nasal area in the retina. It is yellowish and round or vertically oval. The perimeter of the disc is reddish-orange, owing partly to nerve fibers. The disc margins are clearly defined, but may vary from gradual emergency into surrounding retina to a sharp demarcation with a small scleral ring. Pigmentation may be noted along the disc border; this is a normal pattern of myelin on the nerve fibers. Proliferation around the disc is a normal finding; it is viewed as semiopaque white patches emerging from the borders of the disc and spreading into the retina. The retinal borders may appear frayed, and thus may obscure the vessels underneath. If the disc is small, the nasal border may be blurred.

Three major pathological conditions will be presented: optic atrophy, papilledema (Fig. 3-3), and papillitis.

Optic atrophy.   In primary optic atrophy the disc appears white with sharply defined borders. Disc vessels are absent. The physiologic cup is visible, and vessels are within normal limits. Primary optic atrophy occurs in tabes dorsalis, taboparesis, and other conditions causing compression of the optic nerve in the absence of increased intracranial pressure. Occasionally it occurs in patients with pernicious anemia.

In secondary optic atrophy the disc appears white but has a very indistinct margin. The physiologic cup is not visible. There may be gray (pigmented) patches in the retina, which represent hemorrhages or exudates. It occurs with increased intracranial pressure, such as with an intracranial tumor.

Papilledema.   Papilledema, also called a choked disc, is a swelling of the tissues of the optic nerve. It is caused by increased pressure in the cranial vault,

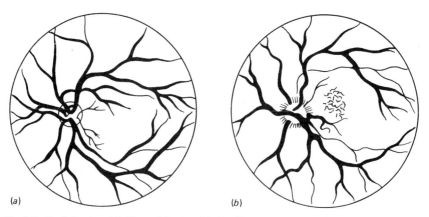

(a)

(b)

Fig. 3-3. Optic fundus. (a) Normal fundus. (b) Papilledema.

causing the cerebrospinal fluid in the subarachnoid nerve sheath to compress the central vein of the retina, which prevents venous return of blood. As you may recall, the subarachnoid space around the optic nerve is continuous with the intracranial subarachnoid space. A rise in pressure here allows fluid to transudate from the capillaries of the disc to the surrounding tissue. Many other mechanisms have been used to explain papilledema, although this one is apparently the most widely accepted. Since the optic nerve is rarely functionally disturbed, vision remains unimpaired. *The earliest ophthalmoscopic sign of papilledema is spontaneous loss of venous pulsation in the central retinal vein.* In early papilledema, the upper and lower disc margins are blurred. As the edema persists, the temporal margins blur. The *temporal blurring of the disc margins is a cardinal finding,* since some degree of nasal disc blurring is normal. The temporal blurring extends to diverging vessels; veins become engorged and bend sharply as they pass over the margin of the disc. Late edema may cause loss of vision. The physiologic cup is obscured. One to seven diopters is the expected disc elevation in papilledema. There may be a cystic elevation of the macula, and a "star figure" is seen in the macular area. This is a result of edema of the retina causing the formation of traction folds, which appear as white lines radiating from the macula. Hemorrhage may appear first on the disc and later on the retina; concentric folds surround the disc from the fluid of edema leaking from the disc.

Papillitis. Papillitis is visibly similar to papilledema, but it differs clinically. Both cause edema of the disc. Papillitis causes visual loss from optic neuritis. The optic disc is hyperemic with blurred margins. It is elevated above the retina +1 or +2 lens corrections. The physiologic cup is viewed as smaller than normal. Common causes of optic neuritis include: local inflammation such as uveitis and retinitis; systemic diseases such as multiple sclerosis, meningitis, sinusitis, pneumonia; metabolic conditions; and acute ethanol poisoning. A summary of optic pathology is found in Table 3-1.

Motor System

Motor testing can be difficult in the intensive care unit, considering how frequently one deals with the unconscious patient. However, it is certainly an integral portion of the neurologic examination. The motor system functions according to the anatomic and physiologic state of muscles as well as the condition of the motor nerves.

General principles. Observe the patient first for positioning of the extremities, flaccidity, loss of tone, spasticity, contractures, and movements such as decerebrate or decorticate rigidity. When the patient is responsive, he may be asked to move all four extremities and squeeze the examiner's hands. When

Table 3-1. Summary of Optic Pathology

Pathological Condition	Disc Color	Disc Elevation	Physiologic Cup	Retinal Vessels	Hemorrhage	Vision
Primary optic atrophy	Bone or white	None	Loss of outline	Normal	None	Intact
Papilledema	Pink or hyperemic	1–7 diopters	Not visible	Engorged, pulseless	Flame: disc and retina	Intact
Papillitis	Hyperemic	1–2 diopters	Smaller than normal	Normal, full	Frank: disc and retina	Lost

the patient is unresponsive, apply noxious stimuli, such as rubbing the sternal area, to determine motor function. The patient should withdraw the extremities when stimulation is applied. Paralysis of the arms can be ascertained by lifting them simultaneously and then releasing them. The paralyzed arm will fall more quickly and in a flail-like manner. Paralysis may also be determined by placing the elbows on the bed and at right angles to the forearm. The paralyzed arm will fall faster and often strike the face. This same test may be carried out on the legs by flexing them with the heels on the bed. When released, the paralyzed leg falls to an extended position with the hip in outward rotation; the unaffected leg maintains posture for a few moments and then gradually returns to its original position.

The pronator test may also demonstrate paresis or paralysis. With his eyes closed, have the patient extend his arms directly out in front of him with his hands supinated. When an arm is paresed or paralyzed, it will spontaneously pronate. This is an extremely valuable aid to motor testing, as it will illustrate even a slight paresis that could be missed if one were only evaluating grips.

Muscle atrophy. In assessing atrophy always examine corresponding concentric muscle masses, comparing their circumference with a tape measure at the same level. Bilateral atrophy may be present and is often difficult to assess. The examiner must rely on his knowledge of normal anatomy and its many variations.

Muscle tone. Muscle tone is observed by moving a limb so that resistance to passive motion can be felt. Experience teaches the examiner the feel of normal muscle tone; this must be learned and practiced in order to readily observe and evaluate abnormalities as described below.

Abnormalities. Cogwheel rigidity occurs from extrapyramidal tract disease and results in increased tone of the limb, which is released in degrees, causing a jerky (cogwheel) motor response to passive motion.

Leadpipe rigidity, or plastic rigidity, is also caused by extrapyramidal tract disease. As in cogwheel rigidity, there is an increase in tone in skeletal musculature; the result is constant resistance to passive motion, making the limb appear "stiff," resembling a lead pipe.

Jackknife spasticity, or the clasp-knife phenomenon, is an important pathologic motor response in upper motor neuron paralysis. There is an increased tone of stretched muscles. When the affected limb is moved against these spastic muscles, the resistance suddenly ceases, giving the jackknife effect.

Upper motor neuron lesion always is the cause of spasticity; extrapyramidal lesion causes rigidity, or hypertonus; and *lower motor neuron lesion may result in hypotonus.*

Muscle strength. Have the patient grasp your fingers; then, if possible, have him contract his muscle while you pull against it. Abnormality may range in a continuum from flaccid paralysis to paresis, to slight weakness. The difference may be graded, although grading is somewhat arbitrary. The examiner is encouraged to describe motor strength in simple, succinct terms and demonstrate the findings to the oncoming nursing team members.

Abnormal muscle movements:

Tremors. Tremors are involuntary contractions involving muscle groups, which produce oscillating motion. They may be classified as fine or coarse, rapid or slow, rhythmic or arrhythmic. Regardless of type, they disappear during sleep.

Fine rapid tremors can be associated with thyrotoxicosis, hypoglycemia, and chronic alcoholism.

Resting tremors are coarse, slow, alternating tremors that are most severe at rest and may be either totally or partially relieved by voluntary movements. Frequently seen with resting tremors is the "pill-rolling" tremor, which is alternating tremors of the fingers. Resting tremors are commonly seen with Parkinson's disease (paralysis agitans).

Familial tremors occur at rest but are augmented by volitional movement. Intention, end-point, or action tremors are initiated by voluntary motion and sustain a slow, wide-amplitude oscillation. They may be seen in multiple sclerosis or cerebellar diseases.

Choreiform movements. Choreiform movements are random, purposeless, jerky, rapid movements involving many parts of the body and preventing the normal progression of body movements. They may be spontaneous, but are increased during voluntary motion. They occur in extrapyramidal disease, such as Huntington's chorea and Sydenham's chorea, from destruction of the caudate nuclei and putamen.

Athetoid movements. Athetoid movements are slower and more writhing than choreiform movements and occur in peripheral parts of the body. They are a manifestation of extrapyramidal disease due to destruction of the globus pallidus.

Myoclonus. Myoclonus is a sudden jerking in either slow or rapid succession; it occurs with grand mal seizures, encephalitis, and other diseases exhibiting cerebral damage, such as hypercarbic or hypoxic encephalopathy, and nearly all metabolic encephalopathies.

Clonus. Clonus is to be differentiated from myoclonus and is discussed under "Reflexes," p. 70.

Tetany. Tetany occurs when the threshold of muscle excitability is lowered, causing involuntary spasms. If the tetany occurs in the hands and feet, it is labeled carpopedal spasm. In carpal spasm the wrist is flexed, metacarpophalangeal joints are flexed, the interphalangeal joints are extended, the hyperextended fingers are adducted to form a "cone," and the thumb is flexed on the palm. Chvostek's sign is elicited by tapping the facial nerve against the bone just anterior to the ears. When present (pathological), it produces ipsilateral contraction, or tetany, of the facial muscles. It is an important observation to be made in the intensive care unit. It can signify parathyroid disease, hyperventilation, or hypomagnesemia. It is a cardinal finding in hypocalcemia. (Tetany from hypocalcemia can lead to laryngeal stridor, tonic and clonic contractions, seizures, and eventually death.)

Fasciculations. Fasciculations are commonly found in lower motor neuron disease and consist of fine twitching in a resting muscle.

Reflexes

Stretch reflex and the reflex arc. A deep tendon reflex is elicited by briskly tapping a partially stretched tendon. This stimulates a special sensory ending and sends an impulse through an afferent nerve fiber. This afferent or sensory nerve fiber, travels with other sensory and motor nerve fibers on its journey toward the spinal cord as a peripheral nerve. Peripheral nerves are organized on a segmented basis, containing 31 pairs of spinal nerves: 8 cervical, 12 thoracic, 5 lumbar, 5 sacral, and 1 coccygeal. In the vertebral canal these spinal nerves separate into a dorsal and ventral root, the dorsal root containing the sensory fibers. This sensory fiber carries the sensory nerve impulse for the deep tendon reflex into the spinal cord where it synapses with the anterior motor neuron. After the impulse crosses the synapse, it is transmitted to the ventral (anterior) motor root, then the spinal nerve, and finally the peripheral nerve. It then crosses the neuromuscular junction and stimulates the muscle to contract briskly, completing the reflex arc. Deep tendon reflexes then are not tendon reflexes, but rather stretch reflexes. They are dependent on intact sensory nerves, functioning synapse in the spinal cord, an intact motor nerve, an intact neuromuscular junction, and a competent muscle. Although not dependent on higher reflex centers in the brain, deep tendon reflexes can be influenced by them.

General principles. Strike a sudden blow with the rubber hammer, preferably over the tendon insertion of the muscle. The muscle should be slightly stretched (by the position of the limb) and should be relaxed. The reflexes may be graded, but the nurse is urged to concentrate on the equality of the responses as well as the comparison of her findings with those of other staff members. Grading can be done as follows:

0	absent
1+	diminished, but present
2++	normal
3+++	normal
4++++	hyperactive

Superficial reflexes. These reflexes have reflex arcs whose receptor organs are in the skin rather than the muscle. They are elicited by stroking or touching. They are lost with upper motor neuron lesion.

Midabdominal skin reflex. Stroke the flank toward the midline at the level of the umbilicus. There should be an ipsilateral contraction of the muscles in the abdominal wall.

Cremasteric reflex. Stroke the inner thigh toward the scrotum. This should cause contraction of the cremaster muscle with prompt elevation of the ipsilateral testis.

Reflexes in upper motor neuron lesion. In upper motor neuron lesion, deep tendon reflexes will be normal or increased caudal to the level of the lesion. Superficial reflexes will be suppressed caudal to the level of the lesion.

Clonus. Clonus is caused by hyperactive reflex and is an abnormal response to the stretch reflex. It consists of a rhythmic contraction and relaxation of muscles, elicited by stretching. Clonus may be unsustained or lasting momentarily despite continued stretching; or it may be sustained, lasting as long as you apply stretch. Clonus is most commonly encountered in the ankle. To elicit it, flex the knee and grasp the foot and dorsiflex it. If clonus is present (pathological), rhythmic contractions of the gastrocnemius and soleus result, causing dorsiflexion and plantar flexion. This test can also be performed on the patella and wrist.

Babinski's sign. Babinski's sign when present is abnormal. Grasping the ankle with the left hand, stroke the sole of the foot near its lateral border with a blunt object with moderate force from the heel upward toward the toes. The stimulus should not be painful. The triad response (if complete) must consist of: (1) dorsiflexion of the great toe with fanning of the other toes; (2) dorsiflexion of the ankle; (3) flexion of the knee and hip. Any of these responses in itself, but especially dorsiflexion of the great toe, is pathognomonic of upper motor neuron lesion. Make sure that you accurately record the details of the response.

Oppenheim's sign and Chaddock's sign. These signs are two eponymic or alternate methods of eliciting Babinski's sign: Oppenheim's sign is elicited by stroking the skin on the pretibial area with thumb and index finger or knuckles; Chaddock's sign is elicited by scratching a path (with a dull point) along the lateral malleolus and then along the lateral aspect of the dorsal foot. Responses are as for Babinski's sign.

Grasp reflex. Stroke the patient's palm; if the patient will grasp your index finger between his thumb and index finger, the grasp reflex is present (pathological).

Hoffman's sign. Hoffman's sign is elicited by holding the patient's pronated hand with fingers extended. Supporting his extended middle finger with your right index finger, use your thumb to press his fingernail and flex the terminal digit while stretching the flexor. The pathological response is flexion with adduction of the thumb and flexion of the other fingers.

Signs of meningeal irritation. Posterior fossa tumors, subarachnoid hemorrhage, meningitis, or increased intracranial pressure cause abnormal muscle spasms as described below.

In nuchal rigidity the patient is unable to place his chin on his chest, and passive flexion of the neck is limited by involuntary muscle spasm.

Kernig's sign occurs when you passively flex the hip to 90° while keeping the knee flexed at about 90°. This is done with the patient supine. For the pathological situation, keeping the hip flexed and then attempting to extend the knee causes pain in the hamstrings as well as resistance to further maneuvering. Although it is a reliable sign of meningeal irritation, it also occurs with herniated nucleus pulposus and other disorders of the spinal cord and spinal nerves.

Brudzinski's sign is elicited with the patient supine and the limbs extended. If meningeal irritation is present, passive flexion of the neck produces flexion of the hips.

Coordination

The total integration of agonist and antagonist muscle groups as well as other muscle function is called coordination. It is primarily mediated through the cerebellum. Eupraxia describes the perfect performance of skilled motor acts; apraxis is loss of previous ability of performance. The loss of coordination in maintaining posture is called ataxia.

Coordination may be partially tested by the finger-to-nose test and heel-to-knee test. In the finger-to-nose test the patient is asked to extend his elbow and then quickly bring his index finger in a wide arc toward his nose. This should be done with eyes open and then with eyes closed. Tremor may accompany this maneuver; or with the eyes open, inaccuracy may accompany it, which indicates loss of sense of position. In the heel-to-knee test, have the patient lie supine, extend his legs, and lift one heel to place it on the opposite knee. He should then be instructed to glide the heel up and down the skin of the tibia. When cerebellar disease is present, the path of the heel to the knee can be shaky or jerky, or the patient can overshoot the target.

Gait. Although observation of gait is an important portion of the neurologic examination, it is difficult and, at times, impossible to execute in a critical care setting. For the purpose of completeness it will be discussed briefly.

Perhaps the most common form of ataxia encountered neurologically is cerebellar ataxia, a staggering, wavering, lurching walk. Movements can be in all directions (midcerebellar lesion) or staggering and pulling toward the affected side (cerebellar lobar lesion). This ataxia can be steadied to some degree by either standing or walking with the legs apart.

To elicit Romberg's phenomenon, the patient stands erect with legs together and eyes closed. Stand with your arms around, although not touching him. The patient with cerebellar disease may fall to either side, forward, or backward.

Sensory System

The routine physical examination does not usually include assessment of sensory functions. If a patient offers a history of localized pain, numbness, tingling, or motor deficits (including spinal cord injury), then a detailed sensory examination should be performed. Before you begin sensory testing, make sure that you are closely familiar with the diagrams showing cutaneous nerve and dermatome distributions (Fig. 2-19). Needless to say, the patient must be alert and oriented to complete such an examination successfully.

Examination of the cranial nerves includes sensory testing on the face; for the rest of the body, cutaneous pain, touch, pressure, position, and vibration should be tested. If deficit of any of these senses is encountered, then evaluate his sensibility for temperature.

Sense of pain. With the patient's eyes closed, have him indicate whenever he feels a prick, specifying dull or sharp. You may use both ends of a straight pin, both ends of a safety pin, or both ends of the pin attachment on the percussion hammer. Using equal degrees of pressure, compare symmetric zones of innervation. The patient's sensibility to pain may be normal, reduced (hypalgesia), absent (analgesia), or increased (hyperalgesia). Deep pain is elicited by producing pressure on the tendons, on the supraorbital region, or as described previously by rubbing the knuckles on the sternum (p. 53).

Sense of position. Testing the sense of position is done by grasping the medial and lateral side of the patient's toe and flexing or extending it. This is done with the patient's eyes closed; he should be able to indicate the position of his toe. Pressure applied dorsally or on the plantar surface should be avoided, as it gives him clues as to what is happening.

Vibratory sense.   Set the handle of a C-256 tuning fork in vibration on a long bony surface of the patient and ask him to tell you with eyes closed when it stops vibrating. Compare the vibrating sense on two symmetric surfaces.

Temperature sense.   Place cold water in one test tube, warm water in another. Make sure by testing on yourself that neither temperature is extreme enough to cause pain. Have the patient close his eyes and distinguish one test tube from the other when they are placed against his skin.

Tactile sense.   Have the patient close his eyes; then stroke his skin with a brush on symmetric areas of skin innervation. Have him indicate when you touch him. The result may be graded as normal, anesthetic, hypesthetic (decreased), or hyperesthetic (increased).

Pressure sense.   Have the patient distinguish between pressure over joints and pressure over subcutaneous aspects of bones, using the head of a pin and your fingers.

Stereognosis.   Stereognosis is a higher integrative function that represents the patient's ability to distinguish forms; place objects in his hands for identification with his eyes closed. Have him identify coins, pens, pencils, wood, cloth, glass, and other familiar objects.

Graphesthesia.   Graphesthesia is tested by drawing larger than 4-centimeter numerals on various parts of the patient's skin and having him identify them with his eyes closed.

Autonomic Testing

Temperature.   Disturbances of temperature include hyperthermia (usually high cervical cord or hypothalmic lesion) and hypothermia (insulin shock, myxedema).

Vasomotor disorders.   Dermatographia is an autonomic reflex that can be elicited by lightly stroking the skin, which normally produces a limited white line. In the pathological response there may appear a bright red or cyanotic line, or a red mottled flare around the red line, or even a 1- to 2-millimeter wheel. The finding is of little diagnostic significance.

Perspiration.   Localized areas of perspiration on the body occur with certain diseases, e.g., syringomyelia. Anhidrosis means lack of sweat. It occurs, for example, caudal to the lesion following transverse cervical cord transection.

Pilomotor response.   Normally if you scratch the midaxillary skin, it produces pilomotor erection (goose flesh). In transverse spinal cord lesion this response is lost below the level of the lesion.

Vital Parameters

Respiration.   Respiratory abnormalities are common with neurologic disorders. Many lesions of the cerebrum and basilar skull induce changes in respiratory frequency and rhythm. Diseases of the lower basilar skull and spinal cord interfere with respiration and ventilation and often produce respiratory failure, which is often the most serious aspect of such diseases.

Posthyperventilation apnea.   Breathing is affected by lesion or depression of the brain at nearly every level. The function of normal ventilation in the alert patient depends on nonchemical neuronal stimuli. Hence, when the neurologically intact patient is asked to hyperventilate briefly, he should continue to breath rhythmically after such hyperventilation even though oxygen and carbon dioxide are in a state of suspended activity. This function is automatic. In patients with bilateral cerebral dysfunction, posthyperventilation apnea can be demonstrated after the patient takes five or six deep breaths. The apnea usually lasts 10 to 25 seconds. This phenomenon can be used to differentiate a disoriented patient with cerebral dysfunction from a neurologically intact patient experiencing behavioral problems.

Cheyne-Stokes respirations.   As damage progresses, the nonchemical regulation of respirations can be negatively influenced to a greater degree, and, in fact, the patient's responsiveness to chemical stimuli may be altered. Such alteration occurs with Cheyne-Stokes respirations. The patient shows an increased respiratory responsiveness to chemical stimuli and, as a result, has a cyclic pattern of gradual increase in respirations to hyperpnea and a gradual decrease to apnea. The timing of such oscillations is dependent on stimuli reaching the respiratory system and, therefore, exhibits a cycle length equal to twice the lung-to-brain circulation time. If the hyperpneic phase is brief, and the apneic phase is prolonged, this type of breathing is usually a manifestation of severe lower brain stem injury at the level of the pons.

Central hyperventilation.   If the posterior hypothalamic or midbrain area is affected, the result can be pulmonary edema and a pattern of hyperpnea, causing a low arterial carbon dioxide tension combined with hypoxia. True central hyperventilation is a less common manifestation of midbrain or upper pons lesion. The pattern is usually seen only in patients who are unconscious. It is important that central hyperpnea be distinguished from other conditions which cause hyperpnea with loss of consciousness, such as hypoglycemia, hypoxia, and hepatic coma.

Irregularly irregular respiratory patterns.   If damage (including pressure) is incurred at or below the pons, irregularly irregular patterns of respiration occur. This irregularly irregular pattern may be present in many forms, none of which are conducive to viable arterial oxygen and carbon dioxide tensions.

Damage to the upper pons may result in apneustic breathing, also called pneumotaxic breathing or apneusis. It is a condition in which the patient maintains inspiratory activity that is unrelieved by expiration, and the inspiratory effort becomes prolonged and cramplike.

Cluster breathing is a type of respiration in which the patient's breaths are taken in groups interspersed with periods of apnea. It is distinguished from Cheyne-Stokes respirations in two ways: there is no gradual incline or decline in the pattern, and breathing is not cyclic.

Biot's pattern is characterized by irregular periods of apnea that alternate with periods of respiration when the patient takes four or five breaths of identical depth.

Ataxic respirations are abnormal. The respirations are extremely irregular, and the timing and depth of a respiration cannot be predicted from the previous pattern.

Other abnormalities of respiration and ventilation.   Gasping may also occur with other forms of irregularly irregular breathing. When medullary function is interfered with, hypoventilation and/or apnea may occur.

Pulmonary edema may result from injury or lesion of the brain by what is commonly referred to as the Cushing reflex. It occurs when injury to the brain results in systemic arterial hypertension, accompanied by displacement of blood from the systemic vasculature into the pulmonary circuit. Marked pulmonary venous and arterial hypertension with pulmonary edema is the net effect.

Heart rate, blood pressure, and the Cushing triad.   There has been inappropriate emphasis placed on the importance of prompt nursing recognition of the Cushing triad, which is bradycardia, bradypnea, and hypertension. These signs have been erroneously explained as a result of increased intracranial pressure when, in fact, they are a sign of early strangulation of medullary centers. Although these "classic signs" may call for immediate intervention to relieve pressure, it should be pointed out that most experts consider them as late symptoms and quite unreliable.

Hypertension. Hypertension in itself is an important finding in patients suffering from neurologic disorders. It is nearly always associated with increased intracranial pressure, commonly from cerebral edema, subarachnoid hemorrhage, or intracranial hemorrhage. Arterial hypertension may be the actual cause of cerebral edema (hypertensive encephalopathy).

Temperature derangement. Following any damage or injury to the brain, particularly the hypothalamus, derangements in body temperature may occur; hence, temperature must be a close and integral part of the neurologic assessment.

Hyperthermia is commonly precipitated by subarachnoid hemorrhage and other pathologies such as bacterioendocarditis, pneumonitis with resultant hypoxia, heat stroke, and exhaustion.

Hypothermia is frequently a result of metabolic or toxic diseases causing unconsciousness. This is particularly true when one encounters brain stem lesions, insulin coma, myxedematous crisis, barbiturate or phenothiazide overdose, and overdose of other central nervous system depressants. Prolonged exposure must be ruled out as a cause of hypothermia as well, especially in the unconscious victim.

Electrocardiogram. Monitoring of the electrocardiogram has rightly become an important tool for nursing assessment in the intensive care unit. This section will not be devoted to the interpretation of arrhythmias, but rather to a discussion of arrhythmias and of 12 lead changes that you may anticipate.

Arrhythmias that are thought to occur as a result of central nervous system damage include sinus tachycardia, paroxysmal atrial tachycardia, atrioventricular junctional tachycardia, and bradyrhythms from supraventricular and ventricular foci.

Lesions that affect the basilar skull and hypothalamus, subarachnoid hemorrhages, and strokes cause electrocardiographic features superficially similar to those changes that occur with an anterior myocardial infarction. Following intracerebral and subarachnoid bleeds, the following changes have been reported:

T waves: flat or inverted in limb leads
QT interval: prolonged
U wave: same prominent U wave as occurs with hypokalemia

Although these changes may present some confusion to the clinician, enzyme studies and history would be useful aides for the physician in differentiating a diagnosis.

Interpretation of vital parameters.   Vital parameters should be monitored frequently in the intensive care unit. Judgment should be made on the patient's total neurologic status considering the broad spectrum of assessment rather than a singular aspect of his condition. Significant changes should be identified and interpreted in relation to the patient's general state of wellness and promptly reported to the physician as deemed necessary.

Rapid Neurologic Assessment

Priorities dictate the time to be spent with any particular patient in critical care. Often the necessity of frequent assessment rules out the practice of lengthy assessment procedures. If a patient requires neurologic evaluation every 30 minutes, certainly a lengthy assessment is not in order.

Before presenting a guide for rapid neurologic assessment, it should be stressed that details of such an examination must always be discussed with the attending physician. It is the physician who will illustrate which areas of the patient's neurologic system are most likely to become altered or deranged when a particular patient develops a complication. This practice will greatly aid the management of valuable time spent in assessing versus caring (physically and emotionally) for the patient and his family.

Areas of greatest concern are:

Level of consciousness
Pupillary reaction, extraocular movements
Motor function
Pathological reflexes

This rapid assessment may be done on a flow sheet, which saves time recording and reporting. A format is shown in Table 3-2 and a prototype in Table 3-3.

SECTION III: INTRACRANIAL PRESSURE MONITORING

Purpose and Indications

Continuous or intermittent intracranial pressure monitoring has become a popular and informative means of aiding in the diagnosis, treatment, and prognosis of neurologic patients. The intracranial screw (developed by Vires in the early 1970s) allows for absolute intracranial subarachnoid pressure measurement as opposed to relative pressure measurement via a lumbar puncture. The procedure is useful in determining variations in intracranial pressure in patients with acute head injuries, space-occupying lesions, intracranial hypertension, Reye's syndrome, and hydrocephalus. In general, invasive monitoring may be utilized on any patient suspected of developing increased intracranial pressure. The intracranial pressure screw provides a vehicle for

Table 3-2. Rapid Neuro Assessment   FORMAT

TIME	LEVEL OF CONSCIOUSNESS ALERT STUPOROUS LETHARGIC COMATOSE	PUPILS SIZE AND D & C* R | L	EOM'S R | L	MOTOR RESPONSE	REFLEXES	OTHER COMMENTS
		D C				
		D C				
		D C				
		D C				

D

C

D

C

*(+) reactive, (−) nonreactive; state pupil size: 2, 4, 6, 8 mm.

Table 3-3. Rapid Neuro Assessment Prototype

TIME	LEVEL OF CONSCIOUSNESS ALERT LETHARGIC STUPOROUS COMATOSE	PUPILS SIZE AND D&C* R	L	EOM'S R	L	MOTOR RESPONSE	REFLEXES	OTHER COMMENTS
0100	Alert, oriented.	D: +/4 C: +/4	D: +/4 C: +/4	+	+	Moves all extremities; is purposeful	DTR's present & symmetrical. No pathological reflexes	VS stable (VSS) See flow sheet. HR 70 R 20 B/P 116/70
0200	Lethargic, difficult to arouse. Oriented.	D: +/4 C: +/4	D: +/4 C: +/4	+	+	Status quo.	Status quo.	B/P 114/70 HR 72 R 24. Called Dr. Doe @ 0202
0215	Status quo.	D: +/4 C: +/4	D: +/4 C: +/4	+	+	Status quo.	Status quo.	VSS. Head shaved, permit signed. TXm. 4 units, family here.
0230	Stuporous; arouses to painful stimuli only.	D: +/4 C: +/4	D: −/8 C: +/4	+	+	Still moves all extremities; is purposeful.	DTR's symmet. Bilat. Babinski's.	VSS. B/P 118/70 HR 72 R 18. Neurosurgeon here (Dr. Doe).

0235		OR check list completed; to surgery.						
	D							
	C							
	D							
	C							

*(+) reactive, (−) nonreactive; state pupil size: 2, 4, 6, 8 mm.

draining cerebrospinal fluid, for testing intracranial volume compensatory mechanisms, and for instillation of a contrast medium.

Physiology

Intracranial compensation is a term used to describe the adaptive mechanism for pressure changes in the cranial vault and spinal canal vault. The volume of cerebrospinal fluid, the brain, and the blood varies slightly, but the total intracranial volume and intracranial pressure remain relatively constant. An increase in one volume is compensated for by a slight decrease in the other, since the skull (which is nondistensible) is not a closed system, owing to the foramina of the basilar skull, which provide outlets for the cranial nerves, spinal cord, blood, and cerebrospinal fluid. The intracranial cerebrospinal fluid volume is decreased by shunting the cerebrospinal fluid to the spinal subarachnoid space. This reduction of cerebrospinal fluid volume is a normal response to physiologic changes in the body. A commonly quoted example of this occurs during normal sleep when carbon dioxide retention takes place producing cerebral vasodilatation, thus increasing the blood volume and intracranial pressure. The body compensates for this increase by displacing intracranial cerebrospinal fluid into the spinal subarachnoid space, thereby reducing intracranial volume and returning the intracranial pressure to normal. Intracranial pressure monitoring (ICPM) is used to evaluate this compensatory mechanism, as well as volume-pressure relationships, compliance, pulse pressure, pressure waves, cerebral blood flow, and cerebral perfusion pressure.

Volume-pressure relationship: As the intracranial volume rises in early stages, the intracranial pressure remains normal, primarily owing to the simultaneous reduction in cerebrospinal fluid and blood volumes. However, this small margin of compensation is soon exhausted, at which point intracranial pressure begins to rise. If the intracranial pressure is already elevated, a relatively minor increase in intracranial volume produces a major rise in intracranial pressure. When this occurs, cerebral decompensation and death follow. However, although the volume-pressure relationship is dramatically true for a rapidly expanding lesion, it is not necessarily true of slow-growing lesions, such as tumors, and in fact in such cases compensation may be prolonged compliance.

Compliance in this text refers to the degree of compensation that exists within the system. This adaptive mechanism is tested by instilling, or withdrawing, a small amount of known fluid volume (approximately 2 milliliters) from the ventricle and measuring the change in volume per unit pressure change. When the ventricles are large, this test is unreliable, since the ventricular volume becomes an influencing factor.

Pulse pressure: Pulse pressure also indicates the degree of compensation. Pulse pressure refers to the amplitude of the oscillations that are reflected from cardiac pulsations. These cardiac pulsations are damped by patent intracranial outflow channels, which allow cerebrospinal fluid to escape and therefore maintain a normal intracranial pressure. Because the measurement is influenced by the sensitivity of the transducer, an isolated pulse pressure measurement has little significance. Measuring pulse pressure as the intracranial volume changes does have significance, however. As the brain exhausts its compensation, intracranial pressure rises, and pulse pressure widens, primarily owing to cerebrospinal fluid and blood outflow reduction. As the intracranial volume continues to increase, this reduction occurs to a greater degree, increasing the pulse pressure and intracranial pressure. In the terminal patient, blood flow is markedly reduced, thus decreasing pulsations from the choroid plexuses. The pulse pressure then drops, and death is usually imminent.

The *pressure waves* created by the intracranial contents are abnormal spontaneous variations in intracranial pressure and have been categorized in three patterns: A, B, and C. Only the A waves were found to have any clinical significance.

A waves are divided into two types: 15- to 30-minute-interval rhythmic fluctuations in pressure and plateau waves that last for longer periods of time. Plateau waves are increases in the intracranial pressure between 50 to 100 millimeters of mercury lasting 5 to 20 minutes. Their etiology is not understood, but they may be caused by transient blood volume alterations and intermittent cerebrospinal fluid obstruction. Plateau waves may be caused by respiratory changes, or indeed these changes may be the effect of these same plateau waves.

B waves, on the other hand, are sharp rhythmic oscillations that have a characteristic sawtooth pattern and occur every ½ to 2 minutes, increasing intracranial pressure as much as 50 millimeters of mercury.

C waves are associated with respiratory influences in blood pressure and have questionable significance. The C waves are also called Traube-Hering-Mayer waves.

Cerebral blood flow can be regionally or diffusely impaired by increased intracranial pressure. It is now possible to measure cerebrospinal fluid simultaneously from many regions of the brain by using isotope clearance techniques. The cerebrovascular system maintains autoregulation of adequate cerebrospinal fluid by constriction and dilatation of cerebral vessels. In fact, cerebral vasodilation will maintain cerebral blood flow until mean arterial (systemic) pressure falls to 60 millimeters of mercury. Hypercapnia, hypoxia, decreased cerebral venous pressure, hyperthermia, and elevated intracranial pressure all evoke cerebral vasodilation when autoregulation is intact. When compensatory mechanisms are exhausted, or if intracranial pressure is high, however, cerebral vasodilation tends to increase intracranial pressure to critical or irreversible levels. This is but one important reason to avoid hypercapnia, hypoxia, and so forth, by meticulous nursing care in critical care.

Cerebral perfusion pressure (CPP) is determined by the difference between inflow pressure or mean arterial pressure and the outflow pressure or cerebral venous pressure. With increased intracranial pressure, cerebral venous pressure approximates intracranial pressure. The normal cerebral perfusion pressure is 80 to 90 millimeters of mercury, and cerebral blood flow begins to fail when the cerebral perfusion pressure reaches 40 millimeters of mercury. Irreversible hypoxia occurs when the cerebral perfusion pressure is below 30 millimeters of mercury. Cerebral blood flow ceases when intracranial pressure equals the mean arterial pressure, (the cerebral perfusion pressure is zero and perfusion pressure has been abolished). A poor prognosis is indicated by a combination of factors: cerebral perfusion pressure of less than 30 millimeters of mercury, rising intracranial pressure despite treatment, and loss of compliance.

Technique

Intracranial pressure monitoring is accomplished by use of a sensor, transducer, and recording instrument. The scalp is incised and a twist-drill hole made in the skull. The subarachnoid screw with a sensor tip is threaded into the hole and through a nick made in the dura mater. The proximal end of the screw communicates directly with the subarachnoid space. The scalp is then sutured closed with the screw in place. A transducer is attached to the screw and converts cerebrospinal fluid pressure transmitted by the sensor to electrical impulses. These electrical impulses are received and visualized on the oscilloscope or transferred to a chart as they are recorded.

The technique of intracranial pressure monitoring may vary with the equipment available. A catheter may be used with high pressure tubing, a three-way stopcock, flushing solution, and a manometer. Regardless of the variations in the assembly, there is obvious benefit to the neurologic patient in direct measurement of intracranial pressure.

Normal intracranial pressure ranges from 50 to 200 millimeters of water (4 to 15 millimeters of mercury). Pressures are affected by cardiac pulsations (transmitted to intracranial pressure by the choroid plexus), intra-abdominal pressure changes, and intra-thoracic pressure changes caused by breathing, coughing, or straining.

Special Considerations

It is suggested that the patient and family be introduced to the intracranial screw and equipment whenever possible. Fear of the instrument's puncturing brain tissue is prevalent. There is no physical alteration of the body when the screw is removed. The psychological implications of the procedure need to be dealt with appropriately.

Patient Response

Primarily the patient's increased susceptibility to infection must be considered. The intracranial pressure screw permits a direct route to the intracranial contents for the invasion of bacteria. Sterile dressing technique is used around the incision site, and cultures may be obtained prophylactically.

The duration of the monitoring system is determined by the patient's condition and response to therapy. The removal of the screw is expedient, and the insertion site heals with routine care.

CONCLUSION

In the intensive care unit the clinician is expected to complete the neurologic history and examination competently. This procedure illustrates the accepted, expanded role of the nurse in neurologic and neurosurgical nursing.

The patient is usually seriously ill and often unconscious. The biopsychosocial needs are met as completely as possible. Often life-death priorities prevail. However, consideration must be given to the safety and security needs of the patient as well.

It is important to focus on the distinction between technician and clinician. Either may perform the neurologic history and examination, but it is the clinician's communication skills and primarily her judgment in evaluating and interpreting the data obtained that allow her to make the decisions necessary to plan comprehensive patient care.

BIBLIOGRAPHY

Bates, Barbara, *A Guide to Physical Examination*, Philadelphia: J. B. Lippincott Co., 1974.

Beeson, Paul B., and Walsh McDermott, *Textbook of Medicine*, Vols. I and II, Philadelphia: W. B. Saunders Co., 1975.

Cropp, J. G., and G. W. Manning, "EKG Changes Simulating Myocardial Ischemia and Infarction Associated with Spontaneous Subarachnoid Hemorrhage," *Journal of Circulation*, 22:25, 1960.

DeGowin, E. L. and DeGowin, A. L., *Diagnostic Examination*, London: MacMillan, 1976.

Delp, Mahlon H., and Robert T. Manning, *Major's Physical Diagnosis*, Philadelphia: W. B. Saunders Co., 1975.

Elliot, Frank A., *Clinical Neurology*, Philadelphia: W. B. Saunders Co., 1971.

Fisher, C. M., "The Neurologic Examination of the Comatose Patient," *ACTA Neurological Scandanavia*, 45, Suppl. 36, 1969.

Gillian, L. A., *Clinical Aspects of the Autonomic Nervous System*, Boston: Little, Brown and Co., 1954.

Gillies, Deeann, and Irene B. Alyn, *Patient Assessment and Management by the Nurse Practitioner*, Philadelphia: W. B. Saunders Co., 1976.

Johnson, Marion, and Judith Quinn, "The Subarachnoid Screw," *American Journal of Nursing*, March 1977, pp. 448–450.

Judge, Richard D., George D. Zuidema, et al., *Methods of Clinical Examination: A Physiologic Approach*, Boston: Little, Brown and Co., 1974.

Plum, F., and J. B. Posner, *Diagnosis of Supor and Coma*, Philadelphia: F. A. David Co., 1966.

Tilburg, Mary S., "The intracranial Pressure Screw," *Nursing Clinics of North America*, 9 (No. 4):641–644, December 1974.

Youmans, Julian R., *Neurological Surgery*, Vols. I, II, and III, Philadelphia: W. B. Saunders Co., 1973.

4
DIAGNOSTIC MEASURES

INTRODUCTION

The patient awaiting neurodiagnostic studies is under considerable stress. These procedures are ominous, and the outcome is threatening. The nurse is in a unique position to provide information and offer psychological support to the patient. If the circumstances allow, the time before the procedure can best be utilized in patient teaching.

Explanations should be given simply and questions answered with professional judgment. Procedure permits usually need to be signed, depending on hospital policy. Attention should be focused on pre-procedure, intra-procedure, and post-procedure phases, which may present problems for the patient.

We have separated the studies into those dealing with spinal fluid, those dealing with X-ray exposure including use of radioactive isotopes and dyes or air, and other special techniques. The intent is to familiarize the nurse with the purpose, the indications for the test, the techniques themselves, special considerations, and the patient's possible responses to the studies.

CEREBROSPINAL FLUID EXAMINATION

Lumbar Puncture

Purpose. A lumbar puncture, when performed skillfully, is a valuable neurologic procedure. It consists of making a percutaneous puncture of the spine below the termination of the spinal cord (L-2) and entering the subarachnoid space surrounding the cord. The purpose of this technique is the procurement of cerebrospinal fluid for analysis and the measurement of cerebrospinal fluid pressures. This common diagnostic test may be employed safely (although not without hazard) and with a minimum of discomfort to the patient.

Occasionally a lumbar puncture is performed for the purpose of reducing intracranial pressure which may follow as a result of a spontaneous subarachnoid hemorrhage. Formerly this mode of reducing intracranial pressure was common with postoperative craniotomy patients; however, since it may precipitate cerebellar tonsillar herniation, it is considered hazardous by most physicians. Other methods of controlling cerebral edema such as the use of steroids have gained popularity.

This procedure also provides an aseptic channel into the subarachnoid space for the introduction of contrast media for both pneumoencephalography and myelography. These diagnostic procedures will be explained later in this chapter.

Therapeutically, the lumbar puncture is used for the intrathecal injection of anesthetics, antibiotics, chemotherapeutic agents, and radiotherapeutic drugs.

Indications.   Indications for a lumbar puncture include differential diagnosis of: diffuse or disseminated infections of the nervous system or the meninges, a subarachnoid hemorrhage, and demyelinating diseases; and for detecting the degree of subarachnoid block, e.g., the presence of a neoplasm.

Contraindications.   A lumbar puncture is contraindicated when clinical evidence of increased intracranial pressure is thought to be due to an expanding lesion, e.g., a subdural hematoma following craniocerebral injury. If an expanding lesion is present, the removal of spinal fluid decreases intracranial pressure and allows the lesion further to consume space, rapidly expanding the hematoma. Fatal cerebellar tonsillar herniation and medullary compression may occur. Careful consideration should be given to the potential risk of doing a lumbar puncture on a patient with a suspected spinal cord tumor or a brain tumor for the same reason.

Any cutaneous or osseous infectious process in the lumbar area absolutely contraindicates the use of a lumbar puncture.

Technique.   A lumbar puncture is performed with rigorous sterile technique while the patient remains in the lateral recumbent position for accurate pressure determinations. The vertebral spines should be parallel to the examining table; a rolled towel may be used under the flank to prevent dorsolumbar sag. The patient is assisted in arching his back and bringing his knees up to his chin. This position provides maximum lumbar flexion, widening the interspinous processes. After preparation of the skin and injection of a local anesthetic, the lumbar puncture needle is introduced into the 3rd, 4th, or 5th lumbar interspace. Upon entry into the subarachnoid space, some cerebrospinal fluid is allowed to escape, and then the needle is attached to an Ayer manometer by a three-way stopcock. While the patient relaxes, initial pressure determinations are made. Samples of cerebrospinal fluid are obtained for analysis and must be promptly taken to the laboratory to prevent morphological changes in the fluid. If a Queckenstedt test (to be explained) is not done, a closing pressure determination is recorded, and the needle withdrawn. A sterile dressing is applied to the puncture wound.

A summary of abnormal findings may be found in Table 4-1.

Table 4-1. Cerebrospinal Fluid

PATHOLOGY	PRESSURE	APPEARANCE	CELLS	PROTEIN	GLUCOSE
Within normal limits	Lateral recumbent 60–180 mm water	Clear	0–5 Lymphocytes	15–45 mg/100 ml	60–80% of true blood sugar 40–80 mg/100 ml
Intracranial tumor	Elevated	Clear	Increased	Increased	Within normal limits
Intracranial abscess	Elevated	Within normal limits unless abscess ruptures	Within normal limits to increased	Within normal limits to increased	Within normal limits to decreased
Cerebral infarct	Elevated	Within normal limits	Slightly increased	Slightly increased	Within normal limits
Subarachnoid hemorrhage	Within normal limits to extreme increase	Pink to grossly bloody	Red blood cells increased White blood cells increased	Increased	Within normal limits to marked decrease
Acute bacterial meningitis	Moderate to extreme increase	Clear to grossly purulent	White blood cells increased 10,000–50,000	Increased	Decreased

Special Considerations

Queckenstedt test. The Queckenstedt test is performed when a spinal-subarachnoid block exists or is suspected, due to tumor, vertebral fracture, or dislocation. With the lumbar puncture needle in place in the subarachnoid space, compression of the jugular veins is carried out by an assistant. Compression is maintained for 10 seconds and suddenly released. The resulting pressure changes are noted on the manometer and recorded at 10-second intervals. If no cerebrospinal fluid has escaped, one can expect a prompt rise in pressure to a figure of 100–300 millimeters of water greater than the opening fluid pressure. Although bimanual compression of the jugular veins can be done, usually a sphygmomanometer is used, inflating the cuff initially to 20 millimeters of mercury for 10 seconds. If a lesion is present, obstructing the spinal cord, cerebrospinal fluid pressure rises slowly. If the block is complete, no secondary elevation occurs. This test may be hazardous, especially when intracranial pressure is elevated, and is therefore used with caution.

Complications. The most serious complication of lumbar puncture is cerebellar tonsillar herniation and medullary compression. Other complications include: fever; meningitis; puncture site pain, edema, or hematoma; nerve root irritation; epidural abscess; subdural abscess; and/or chronic subdural hematoma. Perhaps the incidence of post-puncture headache is the most common aftermath of a lumbar puncture.

Patient response. The normal anxiety with a procedure may be minimized for the patient by a thorough explanation by the nurse of why the procedure is being done and what the procedure involves, including any adverse reactions. These explanations may be made when the patient is signing the procedure permit.

Special consideration should be given to positioning the patient for his comfort and for the facilitation of entry into the canal. The nurse should assist the patient in maintaining this position throughout the procedure. Discussing the effects of the local anesthesia with the patient may be helpful in achieving a level of relaxation. An effort should be made to assess the patient's breathing pattern and have it as close to normal as possible. Physical contact and reassurance throughout and following the procedure are essential. Following the lumbar puncture, frequent neurologic assessment is required; and if there is clinical evidence of herniation, the intensive care unit staff must be prepared for cardiorespiratory failure and/or immediate surgical intervention. Generally, the patient is kept in a horizontal position for a period of time to diminish the possibility of a post-puncture headache, and the puncture site is observed for edema, hematoma, and cerebrospinal fluid leakage.

Cisternal Puncture

Purpose and indications. The introduction of a needle into the cisterna magna (the subarachnoid space between the cerebellum and the medulla) is done: to reduce intracranial pressure, to procure cerebrospinal fluid for analysis in the presence of a subarachnoid block, to provide information when a lumbar puncture is contraindicated, and to introduce contrast material for diagnostic tests.

Technique. A cisternal puncture is performed under sterile technique by introducing a short beveled needle to an approximate depth of 5 centimeters into the cisterna magna below the occipital bone and between the first cervical lamina and the ridge of the foramen magnum. The patient is positioned at the edge of the bed on his side, with a sandbag slipped under his head to keep the cervical spine and head in line with the thoracic spine. His head is flexed and held in place by the nurse, the skin is prepared by cleansing and shaving in the midline up to the external occipital protuberance, and a local anesthetic is then administered. The needle is introduced, fluid is removed for examination, and the opening and closing pressures are recorded.

Special Considerations

Complications. The complications of cisternal puncture are few, in fact, even post-puncture headache rarely occurs. Medullary collapse from herniation may occur and the patient must be assessed frequently for this reason.

Patient response. A procedure permit must be signed, and, as with the lumbar puncture, a thorough explanation by the nurse to the patient is essential. Anxiety may be at a peak, for some patients are extremely fearful owing to the proximity of the puncture to the brain. Patient cooperation in positioning and remaining still during the procedure is important. A post-procedure headache is uncommon, and the patient may have no ill effects from the procedure, thus being able to resume normal activities soon after completion of the study.

NEURORADIOLOGY

Patients admitted to the intensive care unit require specialized care and are often seriously ill. If this is kept in mind, it makes sense to recommend that an R.N. accompany the patient to the X-ray department. Use your judgment on behalf of the patient. If the patient is in respiratory distress, is intubated, has a suspected cord injury, has an altered state of consciousness, is suffering possible cerebellar tonsillar herniation, or has any serious difficulty that may require intervention by a qualified nurse, then by all means have a competent person in attendance and ICU emergency equipment available.

Skull Films

Indications. Skull films are indicated with head and neck trauma, coma of unknown etiology, suspicion of a cranial defect, or as part of a routine neurologic workup. When there are questionable findings from plain skull films, other radiological techniques will be utilized.

Technique. When routine skull films are ordered, four projections are usually obtained: lateral, half-axial (Towne's), axial, and posterolateral. Each of these projections shows particular structures to best advantage; e.g., a calcified pineal gland should be at midline in the posteroanterior view and may be more readily identified in the half-axial view.

Tomography and zonography have become increasingly popular as radiologic techniques. Tomograms are X-rays in which selected horizontal and vertical layered exposures are taken at differing measured depths. This technique is essential in evaluating various components of the optic and auditory canals. Zonography provides a sharp view of a thicker anatomic section. These two techniques, when sequentially reviewed, are valuable in providing information about dimensional shapes of lesions, e.g., an abscess or a tumor.

Patient response. As the radiologic techniques become more refined and the nomenclature more scientific, the patient becomes increasingly disadvantaged in his capacity to understand what is happening to him. Again, a thorough explanation is essential even for the skull films. Fear of the procedure may be the overt effect, with fear of the diagnosis the covert effect. Communication skills and rapport with the patient may relieve his apprehension.

Brain Scanning: Radionuclide Imaging Studies

Purpose and indications. The development of radiopharmaceuticals and radiation-detecting instrumentation has provided a simple, safe, and accurate modality for the diagnosis of neurologic disease. In the detection of intracranial disease, brain imaging has been very successful in detecting meningiomas, some astrocytomas, and oligodendrogliomas; metastatic lesions, medulloblastomas, and certain other astrocytomas; cerebral infarction; A-V malformation; intracranial bleeds; and abscesses. Brain scanning is frequently done as a follow-through procedure on post-craniotomy and post-radiotherapy patients.

Technique. Radioisotope brain scanning is done by the intravenous injection of a radioactive element, a radionuclide. Rays (alpha, beta, and gamma) emitted by the isotope (tracer) are then measured electronically, and the radioactive uptake is transmitted to films or an imaging screen. Originally, detection and localization of radioactivity were by means of a Geiger-Müller counter; however, scintillation cameras developed in the 1950s replaced that instrument. The scintillation cameras have a greater sensitivity for gamma rays and view the entire field at one time, shortening the length of the procedure.

All tracers are albumin substances tagged with a radioactive isotope. The most widely used radionuclide for isotope brain scanning is chelated Technitium or sodium pertechnetate. It has a physical and biological half-life of approximately six hours, making radiation hazard negligible.

Tracers tend to concentrate more readily in pathological areas than in normal brain tissue. The most widely accepted explanation for this phenomenon utilizes the concept of the blood-brain barrier. Normally a radioactive isotope is not permitted entry into brain tissue; therefore, concentration in abnormal tissue is a result of alteration or probable absence of the blood-brain barrier.

Patient response.   Probably the most frequent patient response to radioisotope brain scanning is fear of radioactivity. The procedure is safe, and there is no radiation hazard. This information may be given the patient verbally, along with written instructions about the procedure. Though instrumentation has minimized the time needed for filming, there may be return trips to X-ray for late views over a period of time, even into the next day. There is no specific post-procedure care necessary.

Brain Scanning: Computerized Transaxial Tomography (CAT)

Purpose and indications.   Computerized transaxial tomography is a recent radiographic technique permitting visualization of cranial contents and structure without the use of a radionuclide element. As you may recall from the explanation of tomography, views of the skull are taken horizontally and vertically at measured depths. The scanner employs a narrow X-ray beam to film a series of horizontal slices. The scanner is rotated through 180° until the entire skull has been exposed. These layered views permit visualization of X-ray dense cranial structures and the cranial contents.

Technique.   The procedure may be carried out by a piece of equipment called an EMI scanner and may be referred to as an EMI, a CAT (computerized axial tomography), or a CTT (computerized transaxial tomography). It is necessary for the patient to remain in position for about 20 minutes as the X-ray beam is moved through a path on one side of the head and a detector crystal moved along the other side.

Special considerations.   A radiopaque contrast medium may be injected IV, which, when absorbed, allows visualization of an area for some minutes. A scan is done before and after injection of the contrast medium for differentiation.

Patient response. The patient needs to know that computerized transaxial tomography does not involve the use of a radioactive isotope, but that he may receive a radiopaque substance IV for contrast utilization. If possible, describe the equipment and the procedure to the patient beforehand, and accompany him to X-ray if necessary.

Cerebral Angiography

Purpose and indications. Cerebral angiography is a radiologic study of cerebral vasculature done by introducing radiopaque dye into the arterial bloodstream. It is used to detect abnormalities in the cerebral circulation such as: subdural hematoma, epidural hematoma, mass intracerebral lesions, cerebral edema, carotid-cavernous sinus fistula, and aneurysms.

Technique. The patient should be fasting six hours prior to the procedure. The neck is shaved and surgically prepared for bilateral percutaneous puncture of the carotid arteries. The patient may receive a sedative such as Nembutal one-half hour before the procedure. Atropine may be given to protect the patient against the carotid sinus effects of the barbiturate and to avoid reaction to local anesthesia if it is used. Patients with a head injury should receive a minimum of premedication to avoid depressing their level of consciousness and masking other signs and symptoms. Since the radiopaque contrast media contains iodine, sensitivity testing is recommended. However, bear in mind that the absence of a reaction to the test dose does not preclude an anaphylactic reaction to a full dose intraarterially. If this occurs, vigorous therapy is instituted and the procedure terminated. The dye may be injected manually or by a pressure injector. The patient needs to be aware that it is usual to experience a burning sensation behind the eyes and in the teeth or jaw, or the tongue and lips. Reassure him that this is a usual response and that it will subside momentarily. During injection of the dye, rapid serial films are taken from different angles. The arterial through venous phase occurs in about 6 seconds. A bolus of dye is injected again, and subsequent exposures are taken.

Special Considerations

Complications. A cerebral angiography is not without complications. Reaction to the iodine preparation has already been discussed. Most complications occur from vasospasm or local hemorrhage. Symptoms are manifested by a change in level of consciousness, aphasia, hemiplegia or hemiparesis, general prostration, seizure activity, or intensification of focal symptoms. Post procedure, the patient is observed closely for hematoma formation at the injection site, which may cause tracheal compression with resultant airway obstruction. Ice may be used to reduce edema and provide comfort to the patient. A tracheostomy tray must be readily available. A neurologic assessment is performed frequently, with an appraisal of the patient's respiratory status and the injection site and observation for any latent dye reaction. A delayed reaction may present with vomiting, numbness, weakness in the extremities, diaphoresis, or any altered state of consciousness.

Head trauma patients whose symptoms have progressed indicating a bleeding process require emergency angiography. It is important to consider that they are likely to go directly from the radiology department to the operating room for surgical decompression. Anticipate this possibility and have the proper permits signed, a type and cross match done, and a patent IV in the patient; and advise the family as soon as possible.

Patient response. The conscious patient needs to be taken through the procedure verbally and as simply as possible. Risks do need to be explained, but to what detail is left to your discretion in consultation with the physician. It is wise to discuss beforehand the sensory input during the procedure. If the patient knows it is usual to experience burning and has identified the noise of the machinery, he may be less apprehensive. An explanation of the presence of the tracheostomy tray may or may not reduce his fear. Breathing patterns are often altered, and the fact that the procedure occurs very near the throat is extremely frightening. A nurse who reflects feelings with empathetic responses and who answers questions with judgment is most helpful to the patient and to the family.

Encephalography

Generally, encephalography may be used to describe neurodiagnostic techniques used in the visualization of cerebrospinal fluid circulation. We will discuss pneumoencephalography, ventriculography, and myelography.

Pneumoencephalography

Purpose and indications. This procedure has largely been replaced by angiography, but remains the diagnostic test of choice for certain types of mass lesions.

Technique. A sedative may be ordered prior to the procedure. A lumbar or cisternal puncture is performed with the patient in a sitting position or in a special hydraulic chair. Small amounts of air are introduced into the subarachnoid space; and the air rises to outline the ventricular system. The patient is positioned for visualization of the ventricular system and meningeal spaces on X-ray. In noting the closely observed vital signs, one may expect to see an increase in blood pressure, heart rate, and respiratory frequency.

Special Considerations

Complications. The introduction of air into the subarachnoid space with or without the removal of cerebrospinal fluid is the first phase of a series of events that may lead to a shift in the position of the brain; and if a mass lesion exists, it further jeopardizes the patient's condition. When a mass lesion is identified, immediate surgery may be necessary.

Other complications of pneumoencephalography are: air embolization, extracerebral hematoma (especially subdural hematoma), mild to moderate aseptic meningitis, and, though rarely, chemical or bacterial meningitis.

Patient response. Severe headache seems to be the universal symptom following encephalography. The air injected into the subarachnoid space rises and tends to pocket in the ventricles. The ventricles provide no means for reabsorption of the air; therefore, it is necessary to assist the patient in moving from side to side every two hours while he is flat. In this way the air is returned to cerebrospinal fluid circulation pathways and is reabsorbed there in 24–36 hours. Failure to implement this nursing measure will delay the patient's recovery. If the patient is not nauseated, forcing fluids, including beverages high in sodium, may be helpful in promoting the reabsorption of air and the replacement of cerebrospinal fluid. A close observation of the patient's neurologic status is necessary for about two days. He is kept flat, and any of the following symptoms are reported: evidence of increased intracranial pressure, seizure activity, shock, prolonged or intractable headache, nausea and vomiting, chills or fever.

Both patient and family should be aware of the risks involved in a pneumoencephalogram. Pre-procedure teaching of post-procedure nursing interventions will help.

Ventriculography

Purpose and indications. The introduction of air or dye into the ventricle itself may be done for the following reasons: to establish ventricular drainage, to relieve pressure when lumbar or cisternal punctures are contraindicated, to demonstrate patency of the ventricular system, to localize tumors (especially posterior fossa tumors), or to detect cerebral anomalies.

Technique. Ventriculography is usually done in the operating room under local anesthesia with the patient sitting in a chair. After the head is shaved, an incision is made through the scalp, and a small trephine opening (either a burr hole or twist drill hole) is made on each side of the head. A short beveled ventricular needle is introduced through this opening directly into the lateral ventricle. Cerebrospinal fluid is removed and replaced by air or dye. X-rays are taken in various positions to verify free communication between the lateral ventricles and all portions of the ventricular system.

Special considerations. A craniotomy frequently follows ventriculography; therefore, appropriate preoperative preparation of the patient and family is important.

Complications. Complications of ventriculography include: epidural hematoma, intracerebral hemorrhage, porencephalic diverticula along the suture line, shock, and respiratory collapse.

Patient response. The patient must be observed frequently for increased intracranial pressure. A lumbar puncture set must be kept in the room for emergency puncture and release of cerebrospinal fluid pressure. The head of the bed is elevated, and food and liquids are given as tolerated. Usually nursing actions are implemented for relief of a headache.

Myelography

Purpose and indications. Myelography is the introduction of a contrast medium of a radiopaque substance or gas into the subarachnoid space of the spinal column. The purpose is for the identification of a space-occupying lesion of the cord. It is also useful in diagnosing a herniated nucleus pulposus.

Technique. Though this test is not commonly employed for intensive care patients, it does have neurologic significance. The procedure is similar to a lumbar or cisternal puncture. Introduction of dye through the lumbar route is used almost exclusively. The fluoroscopic flow of dye within the spinal subarachnoid space is observed, and radiographic exposures taken.

Special considerations. Information regarding the specific procedure is necessary to determine the post-procedure nursing intervention. Basically, the variables that must be considered are: the point of entry into the spinal canal (lumbar or cisternal), the type of contrast medium used (positive contrast medium—dye; or negative contrast medium—air or gas), and the approximate amount of medium remaining in the spinal subarachnoid space.

Patient response. The principles for post-procedure care remain the same as for pneumoencephalography with one exception, the position of the head of the bed. The patient may be flat, lateral, or elevated, depending on the information obtained regarding the specifics of the procedure. If a positive contrast medium has been used and completely removed, the patient will remain flat; if it has not been completely removed, then the head of the bed will be elevated to prevent passage of the dye into the intracranial spaces causing meningeal irritation. If a negative contrast medium is used, the patient's head is kept lower than his trunk for a period of time, to prevent the light air from rising and being trapped in the intracranial spaces. The patient is assessed frequently for neurologic changes.

OTHER NEURODIAGNOSTIC TESTS

Electroencephalograhy

Purpose and indications. An electroencephalogram is a measurement of the electrical activity of the brain. The variations in electrical potential discharged by the brain are measured and recorded on a graph, which is used for providing information on the localization of brain lesions in the diagnosis of epilepsy.

At present there is controversy regarding the Harvard Medical School report, *The Criteria for Death*, which stated that an isoelectric encephalogram, repeated with no change in 24 hours, confirms, in conjunction with other criteria, clinical death. Further exploration of the philosophical and ethical question of determining and defining death may be found in Chapter 1.

Technique. An electroencephalogram is made in a quiet environment where the patient is free from distraction. Electrodes are placed on the unshaven scalp and connected to a recording machine. The patient needs assurance that the machine is recording the electrical activity in the brain and is not discharging electricity into the body. The patient may be asked to hyperventilate during the procedure or to perform some mental function. Generally a resting, relaxed state is desirable for an artifact-free recording.

Special considerations. Brain waves are characterized by many factors including frequency. The frequency bands of electrical activity include delta—low frequency during sleep; alpha—less than moderate frequency during relaxed wakefulness; and beta—high frequency during mental activity and alertness. Although electroencephalography interpretation does not fall into the realm of nursing practice, this simplified explanation may be useful to intensive care nurses.

Patient response. The patient may not receive any anticonvulsive medication for 48 hours prior to the test; therefore, diligent observation for seizure activity is necessary. If a sleep recording is requested, the patient will receive sedation. The patient usually remains on his normal eating pattern with no stimulants (e.g., coffee) or depressants, unless specifically ordered. It is recommended that the patient's hair be clean and free of spray for effective electrode application. The test is harmless and painless, and no specific postprocedure nursing measures are indicated.

Echoencephalography

Purpose and indications. Echoencephalography is the use of an ultrasound beam projected through the head with the returning echoes converted to electrical impulses recorded on an oscilloscope screen. The procedure is used to determine the cerebral midline position of structures and for estimating the size of the ventricles. It is particularly useful in managing patients with rapidly expanding intracranial lesions in the absence of localizing neurologic deficits when either time or facility is lacking for contrast studies. Midline distortion is predicted without risk or discomfort to the patient.

Technique. An ultrasonic beam is passed through the intact skull, in the temporoparietal region, transversing the third ventricle. The echoes produced and recorded (called M-echoes) originate from the pineal gland, the septum pellucidum, the interhemispheric fissure, and particularly the posterior third ventricle. If the midline echo is displaced more than 3 millimeters, it is considered pathological in adults.

Patient response. Echoencephalography is a safe and reliable aid in differential diagnosis and creates no specific problems for the patient. Bear in mind, however, that fear of an unknown diagnosis may be a concern of the patient and should be perceived and dealt with honestly.

Electromyography

Purpose and indications. Electromyography (EMG) is a study of the electrical activity produced by the muscles. It reflects the muscle action potential (or nerve impulse) induced by muscle stimulation.

The test is done for diagnosis and localization of lower motor neuron disease. It is also used to detect the earliest evidence of peripheral nerve reinnervation.

Technique. The procedure is done by inserting a needle electrode into a skeletal muscle, with the electrical activity recorded on an oscilloscope for audio and visual analysis.

Observations are made upon entry of the needle into the muscle, specifically the electrical activity of the resting muscle and the electrical activity of the muscle during voluntary contraction.

Patient response. The electromyogram is usually well tolerated by the patient with only slight tenderness in the area of the muscles examined.

CONCLUSION

In some instances we have only covered the surface of neurodiagnostic studies. We hope that the reader has gained some information that will stimulate further study where necessary. It is our belief that the nurse is best prepared to instruct patients having these examinations by attending and observing the procedures personally.

Psychological support for the patient is viewed as necessary for his well-being and the success of the procedures. A patient does not enter the hospital alone; his fears and problems are usually shared by others. The nurse has to take time for explanations and reassurance for the family. Her kindness, empathy, and compassion need to be extended to the patient's entire ecosystem.

BIBLIOGRAPHY

Donohue, Katherine M., Mary Blount, and Anna Belle Kinney, "Cerebral Circulation and Cerebral Angiography," *Nursing Clinics of North America*, 9 (No. 4):623–630 December 1974.

Kinney, Anna Belle, Mary Blount, and Katherine Donohue, "Cerebrospinal Fluid Circulation and Encephalography," *Nursing Clinics of North America*, 9 (No. 4):611–621, December 1974.

Luckman, Joan, and Karen Sorenson, *Medical-Surgical Nursing A Psychophysiologic Approach*, Philadelphia: W. B. Saunders Co., 1974.

Mandrillo, Margaret P., "Brain Scanning," *Nursing Clinics of North America*, 9 (No. 4):633–639, December 1974.

Mayo Clinic and Mayo Foundation, *Clinical Examinations in Neurology*, 4th ed., Philadelphia: W. B. Saunders Co., 1976.

Nursing in Neurological Disorders, Contemporary Nursing Series, New York: American Journal of Nursing Co., 1976.

Wilcox, Sandra G., and Marilyn Sutton, *Understanding Death and Dying*, Port Washington, New York: Alfred Publishing Co., 1977, p. 49.

5
TRAUMA

INTRODUCTION

The frequency and the seriousness of trauma incurred from motor vehicle accidents have for a long time forced persons involved in health care delivery to study the problem and the appropriate care of trauma patients.

Accidents are the number one cause of death in young people in nearly all the countries of the world. In fact, in some countries, Canada for example, accidents account for more deaths between infancy and middle age than does any other condition.

Sixty percent of all vehicular accidents involve injury to the head. Perhaps more impressive (or frightening) is the fact that 70% of fatal accidents involve head injury, and in 66% of these cases, head injury is the *actual cause of death*.[1]

In addition to automobile accidents, patients sustain head injuries at sports, work, and home, collectively producing a frightening number of injuries.

The survivors of these accidents sustain catastrophic physiologic and mental handicaps, with consequent serious loss for the social and economic community.

Obviously, this is a major health problem, requiring more than the attention of the intensive care nurse alone. Within a conceptual framework of nurturance, prevention, coordination, restoration, and construction, all nurses must become more adaptable and flexible in establishing goals and objectives for these patients.

In administering care to head injury patients, the critical care nurse will need to rediscover the nursing process. She will need to increase her knowledge, refine her technical skills, develop more accurate assessment techniques, identify new problems, plan more appropriate intervention, and evaluate with a newer, less familiar sense of modification.

DEFINITION OF TERMS

As knowledge of a subject develops, concepts are communicated by new terms which become incorporated into the medical vocabulary by connotation. As the subject area is further explored, these rapidly changing terms may convey a different, poorly understood concept. Therefore, we will define

---

[1]Luckmann, Joan, and Karen Sorensen, *Medical-Surgical Nursing*, Philadelphia: W. B. Saunders Co., 1974, p. 515.

terms in order to avoid confusion and to clarify the context of this chapter. The terms are placed alphabetically for quick reference.

Acceleration: A *change* in the rate of velocity (speed) of a moving body. Acceleration is used in this text to express an *increase* in the velocity of an object.

Compressive Strength: The ability of an object to resist *squeezing* forces or inward pressure.

Concussion, Brain: A clinical syndrome characterized by *immediate* and transient impairment of neural function, such as *alteration of consciousness*, disturbance of vision, equilibrium, etc., due to mechanical forces.[2]

Consciousness: A state of general wakefulness and responsiveness to the environment. Impairment of consciousness may be of any degree of severity. Terms such as lethargy, drowsiness, stupor, semicoma, and coma are commonly used with varying connotations to describe levels of consciousness. There is no unanimity of opinion on the precise meaning of these terms.[3] See Chapter 3 for further clarification of consciousness.

Contrecoup Injury of the Brain: An injury occurring to the brain beneath the skull opposite to the area of impact.[4]

Contusion (Bruise), Brain: A structural alteration of the brain usually involving the surface, characterized by extravasation of blood and death of tissue, with or without edema. Clinical manifestations of the contusion depend on the area and extent of the injured tissue.[5]

Deceleration: A decrease in the velocity of an object.

Elasticity: An object's ability to return to its previous size and shape after removal of stretching or compressing forces.

Injury, Head, *Closed*: A head injury in which continuity of scalp and mucous membranes (paranasal sinuses, middle ear) is maintained.[6]

Injury, Head, *Open*: A head injury in which there is loss of continuity of the scalp or mucous membranes (paranasal sinuses, middle ear). The term is sometimes used to indicate a communication between the intracranial cavity and the exterior.

Lesion: A broad term used to describe any damage to brain tissue caused by injury or pathology.

Lesion, Focal: A single intracranial area diseased within definite limits causing discrete, recognizable, neurologic deficits.

Lesion, Generalized: Diffuse intracranial irritation or disease causing multiple indiscrete neurologic deficits.

[2]"Glossary on Head Injury," prepared by a committee of the Congress of Neurological Surgeons.
[3]Ibid.
[4]Ibid.
[5]Ibid.
[6]Ibid.

Momentum: The kinetic force of a moving body; the product of mass and velocity.

Shearing, Shear Stress: Forces occurring across a plane with objects slipping relative to each other.

Tensile Strength: The inherent ability of an object to *resist stretching forces.*

Wound, Penetrating: An open wound in which the dura mater is pierced.

PHYSIOLOGIC, DYNAMIC, AND BIOCHEMICAL FACTORS INFLUENCING TRAUMA

The response of various intracranial contents to trauma is primarily dependent on the following considerations:

1. *General strength* characteristics of tissue: tensile strength, elasticity, and compressive strength.
2. *Dynamic factors* influencing trauma: the magnitude of forces and location of impact.
3. *Specific biomechanical* response of tissue.

Although all of these considerations are closely interrelated, they will be presented separately for the sake of clarity and to provide a deep understanding of the factors influencing trauma.

General Strength Characteristics of Tissue

The response of the skull and its contents to trauma is closely related to the mechanical characteristics of the tissue. All tissue has different strength or loading capabilities. These general strength characteristics are tensile strength, elasticity, and compressive strength.

Tensile strength. Tensile strength refers specifically to the amount of tension a tissue can withstand. It refers to the ability of tissue to *resist stretching* forces. When a structure reaches its maximum tensile strength, failure occurs, resulting in fracture or tear.

Elasticity. Elasticity is the inherent ability or memory of a bodily substance *to resume its previous shape and size* after being stretched.

Compressive strength. Compressive strength is the ability of tissue to *resist squeezing* forces or inward pressure. When a structure reaches maximum stress or loading, compressive failure occurs, resulting in fracture or tear.

Dynamic Factors Influencing Trauma

A head injury is a function of pure physics, not only from the moment of impact, but immediately following impact. The injury is produced by mechanical and physical changes of the cranial vault and its contents in relation to the environment.

Forces. A classification of forces that may injure the head includes deformation (e.g., a hammer blow), acceleration (e.g., an uppercut blow such as delivered by a boxer), and deceleration (e.g., a moving head striking the dashboard in a car) (Fig. 5-1). These forces apply stresses to the head and brain that result in structural damage.

Stresses. The stresses that produce tissue damage are compressive-decompressive, tensile, shearing, and high-velocity impact. They will be considered independently, but reality dictates the rarity of a single intracranial stress. Indeed, it is the *combination* of these stresses that produces devastating injury to the human head.

Compressive-decompressive stresses. Forces of large magnitude applied in a small local area, such as a hammer blow, result in compression of the skull or bony deformation. The impacted area of the skull inbends, imposing compressive stresses, and adjacent areas outbend, imposing tensile stresses. The skull's tensile strength is considerably less than its compressive strength, and *bony failure occurs at the outbending site of tension,* initiating a fracture line. The magnitude of compression is determined by the momentum of the impacting agent and its size.

Compression of the skull also produces shock waves that travel throughout the contents of the cranium. Deceleration of the moving head produces positive pressure at the impacted location of brain–skull interface. Accordingly, negative pressure develops at the brain–skull interface at the *opposite pole.* This occurs in the brief time (a few milliseconds) following impact when the *brain velocity remains constant* despite deceleration of the skull. When the negative pressure is low enough, the brain interstices release gas bubbles (cavitation). It is thought that this phenomenon of cavitation partially explains contrecoup (opposite side) injury of the brain, which is so common in head injury patients.

Tensile stress. Compression may cause swirling of the cerebral hemispheres, subsequently tearing the bridging veins between the pia arachnoid and the longitudinal sinus. This tearing, representing tensile failure of vessels, is sometimes called traction injury. Since the bridger veins enter the sagittal sinus in the subdural space, subdural hematoma is the outcome of such an

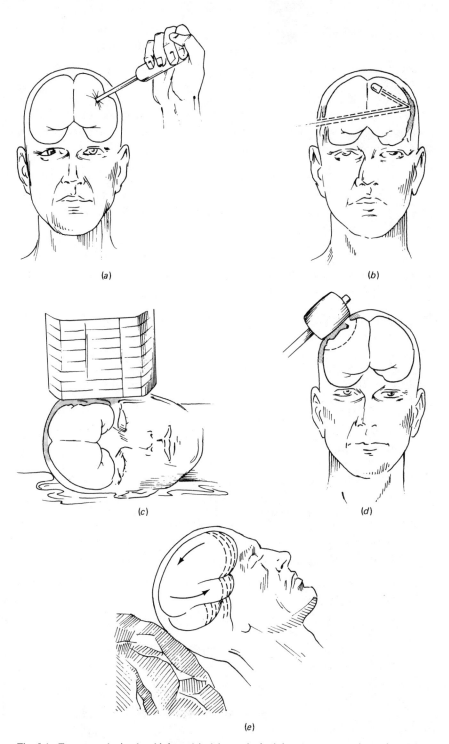

Fig. 5-1. Forces producing head injury. (a) A low-velocity injury by a penetrating object. (b) A high-velocity injury by a high-velocity object (missile). (c) A crushing blow producing gross deformation. (d) A more localized deformation injury produced by a hammer or mallet. (e) Acceleration–deceleration produced by a moving head striking an object.

injury. Cranial nerves are also susceptible to tensile failure, particularly when it occurs abruptly. Practically any object that is stretched abruptly is more apt to fail structurally than if it is stretched slowly. If the brain is rotated violently within its vault, tensile failure may occur to the brain stem. This tensile failure is due in part to stress seeking the place of least resistance (the foramen magnum), causing stretching of the brain stem.

Shearing stress. Shearing stress is caused by movement of contacting objects sliding or moving relative to each other. The head is connected to the body by structures that are functionally mobile: the cervical vertebrae with their axis and atlas. These structures when set in motion tend to produce rotational movement of the head. Shearing stress is usually encountered following rotational acceleration or deceleration. It results in tough fibrous material actively opposing brain substance. Areas of relative anatomic entrapment, such as the temporal lobes, are commonly contused or lacerated by the tough sphenoid ridge below.

Although severe central nervous system damage from shear stress is usually encountered with motor vehicle accidents, it may also occur in other ways. The blow of a boxer's *uppercut* is an example of a blow delivered with tremendous momentum causing a sudden change in movement and a complex rotation of the skull and brain. The result may produce far greater damage than if the blow had been dealt in a more *direct* fashion.

High-velocity impact. Stresses are of a different nature when induced by a high-velocity foreign body such as a rifle bullet. The impacting bullet imparts a shock wave to both the skull and the brain. It may cause extensive destruction of tissue at the entry site and even at some point distant from the actual trajectory of the missile. The reason for this is that the shock wave extends in a conical form from the point of entry, expanding outward. When this shock wave reaches sufficient proportion, implosion of intracranial contents occurs. This type of trauma causes massive brain destruction, and patients rarely survive.

Specific Biomechanical Response of Tissue

The preceding information will now be specifically related to all of the structures of the cranial vault and its contents.

Scalp. The scalp, which is 3-7 millimeters in thickness, offers some resistance to compression and in fact allows for partial if not total absorption of a mild blow, probably because of its ability to distribute the forces over a large area. In this manner it adds to the total structural integrity of the head.

Its elasticity prevents the majority of blunt objects from being disruptive. A violent-enough blow or a highly concentrated blow will certainly penetrate the scalp.

Skull. The skull represents an entirely different mechanism for protecting its contents. First of all, the skull is architecturally well designed with its three layers: the inner and outer tables with the diploë layer in between. This low-density middle layer, the diploë, adds considerable stability and acts as a shock absorber.

The skull has a high compressive strength, nearly twice its tensile strength. Although it is a rigid member, it is also somewhat elastic. As previously explained, following impact during which the skull is compressed, outbending (stretching) occurs in adjacent areas. Tensile failure occurs in these outbended areas, with a fracture produced when the areas are subjected to stress. It will usually extend from the tensile failure point toward the location of impact further and in a line of less resistance downward toward the base of the skull.

Meninges. The meninges offer a tough barrier to cerebral hemispheric and brain stem movement. They are also thought to maintain pronounced elasticity, as they easily extend a few millimeters.

The pia arachnoid membrane is believed to possess tremendous tensile strength, and when tested (even severely) probably prevents the brain from rupturing.

The dural reflections offer some protection to the brain. The falx cerebri, that portion of dura passing vertically between the cerebral hemispheres, is quite durable. The tentorium cerebelli covering the cerebellum is sufficiently strong to withstand nearly any stress applied to the skull. However, these reflections may also offer resistance to the moving brain and can alone cause contusion.

Cerebrospinal Fluid. The cerebrospinal fluid serves to cushion impacts and absorb shock, providing protection to the brain.

Cranial Nerves. The cranial nerves are particularly vulnerable to tensile failure and injury, especially the first, second, third, and eighth cranial nerves. Remember that nerve rupture upon stretching is primarily dependent on the *rate* of extension. Slow stretching (over a period of years) produces remarkable extending capabilities, while rapid stretching results in functional alteration or rupture.

Brain. When impact causes rotational motion of the head, the brain is often damaged.

The skull is ovoid in shape with a flat base. The internal surface is not uniform, but has definite prominences, which protrude and present obstacles for a smooth rotation of the brain. The two prominent ridges that divide the cranial cavity into anterior, middle, and posterior cranial fossae are the sphenoid ridge and the temporal ridge.

The sphenoid ridge, separating anterior and middle cranial fossae, presents a very sharp edge that protrudes into the middle cranial fossa near the tip of the temporal lobe. A rotational acceleration of the head causes this tough fibrous sphenoid bone to present opposition to brain substance. This tremendous shearing stress commonly results in contusion and/or laceration to the brain itself. In recent years the sphenoidal injury (injury to the temporal poles of the brain by the sphenoid bone) has been nicknamed "dashboard injury."

The temporal ridge, separating the middle and posterior cranial fossae, is larger and stronger than the sphenoid ridge, but does not have a sharp edge and does not contuse or lacerate the brain. It does, however, play an important role in the direction of skull fracture, since it is a large buttress and offers much resistance to fracture lines.

The rough frontal bone and orbital margins offer coarse resistance to the frontal lobes, resulting in contusion and/or laceration of the frontal poles. In fact, injured frontal and sphenoidal cerebral areas produce the majority of complications following acceleration-deceleration head injury.

The rotary motion of the skull may result in tensile stress. This tensile stress may cause rupture of small blood vessels; however, more commonly it results in spasm of the vessels, which can result in severe ischemia. The small vessels of the brain stem are particularly susceptible (because of their size) to such stress, and this phenomenon accounts for the severe brain stem sequelae seen following head injury.

FRACTURES

Factors Influencing Fractures

The following factors predict the type and severity of fractures: velocity of injuring agent, momentum of injuring agent, direction of injuring agent, and location of impact.

Velocity of Injuring Agent. The greater the velocity (speed) of the injuring agent, the more likely it is that compressive and tensile failure of the bone will occur. An injuring agent with a slower velocity will usually cause a linear fracture because of the ability of the skull to withstand the lesser compression.

Momentum of Injuring Agent. The momentum (kinetic force of a moving body) of the injuring agent is more important in determining the degree of injury than velocity. Physiologically, momentum must be considered as the ability of an injuring agent to *impart* its energy.

Direction of Injuring Agent. The more directly an object impacts the skull, the more the object is able to impart its energy to the skull and brain.

A glancing projectile carries the majority of its velocity on with it after impact, obviously imparting far less energy than if it impacted the skull at a right angle or directly.

Location of Impact. Areas of greater thickness in the skull, such as buttresses, offer greater resistance on impact than thinner areas.

A summary of head trauma is given in Table 5-1.

Table 5-1. Summary of Head Trauma

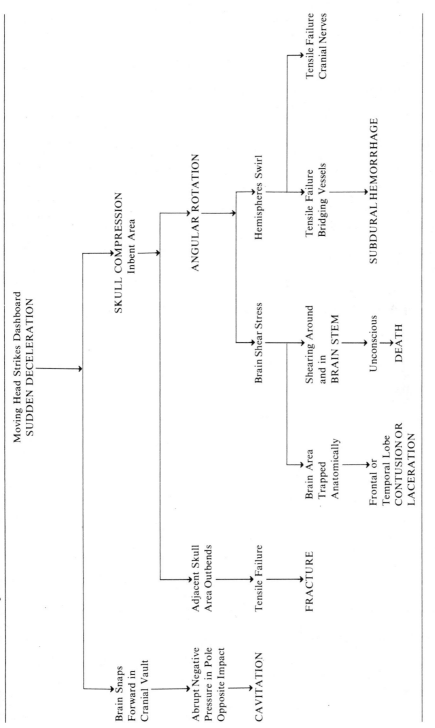

Classification of Fractures

Fractures of the skull may be linear, comminuted, or depressed. A fracture may be closed or open, depending on the presence of a laceration of the scalp or an extension of the fracture into the middle ear or paranasal sinuses.

Linear Fracture. The vast majority of skull fractures are linear or in a line. Such a fracture occurs as a result of compressive and tensile failure, and appears as a simple crease or a break in the bone. It follows thick to thin bone without crossing buttresses and moves toward the base of the skull. In order of common occurrence, such fractures appear in middle skull, frontal, and occipital regions.

Low-velocity injuries usually produce linear fractures owing to tensile failure in the surrounding areas. As velocity increases, the impacting agent may strike with sufficient force to cause local bone to fail and fragment. Therefore, as the injuring agent's velocity increases, there is an increase in energy imparted and an increase in the severity of the fracture. *The extent of a linear fracture may be a relatively good index of the severity of the blow, as well as a rough measure of the severity of damage incurred.*

Basilar skull fractures usually result from an extension of a fracture line from the vault above. The fracture proceeds to the point of least resistance below. However, it may also result from impact from below; a fall on the buttocks may produce such an impact by driving the vertebral column against the occipital condyles, distributing stress and consequently failure to the basilar skull.

Comminuted Fracture. A comminuted fracture is one in which there is a fragmented interruption of the bone, usually from multiple linear fractures. The bone may be splintered or crushed.

Depressed Fracture. A depressed fracture occurs when there is a sufficient concentration of energy to cause local failure of the bone with resultant fragmentation and inward displacement.

Types of depressed fractures are: perforating depressed fracture, penetrating depressed fracture, depressed fracture with linear fracture, and depressed fracture associated with avulsion.

Perforating depressed fracture. A perforating depressed fracture is caused when a small object moving at a high velocity (e.g., a rifle bullet) perforates the skull. High-velocity impact usually perforates the skull without additional bony deformity, but severe parenchymal damage results from shock waves produced by the object moving rapidly through the brain.

Penetrating depressed fracture. A penetrating depressed fracture is caused by an object moving at a moderate velocity with high momentum, penetrating the skull and causing further bony deformation. Such an object may drive bony fragments into the brain. A tire lever might cause such an injury.

Depressed fracture with linear fracture.   A depressed fracture with linear fracture is caused by an object moving at moderate velocity and low momentum (e.g., a baseball). Most of the momentum imparted is absorbed by the skull. The depressed area presents as a linear fracture with other associative fracture lines.

Depressed fracture associated with avulsion.   A depressed fracture associated with avulsion occurs when bone and intracranial contents become avulsed as the impacting agent continues to move.

Specific Manifestations of Fractures

Fracture of the skull is not as important as injury to the brain. However, the diagnosis of fracture is significant, since fractures indicate that injury has been sustained. The extent and nature of a fracture often influence ensuing developments and treatment. An example would be a fracture across the dural sinus, which would expose the patient to the risk of the extradural hemorrhage. Also, fractures that communicate with any of the paranasal sinuses provide an entry for infection. The location, symptoms, and/or sequelae of commonly encountered fractures are discussed below.

Frontal fractures are particularly hazardous to the patient because they may expose the brain to the entrance of foreign bodies and bacteria through the frontal sinus. These fractures can be associated with air in the forehead tissues (communicated from the frontal sinus), cerebrospinal fluid or cortex rhinorrhea (drainage from the nose), or pneumocranium (air filling ventricular and subarachnoid spaces from frontal sinus).

Orbital fractures are manifested by periorbital ecchymosis (racoon eyes). If one excludes the possibility of direct glabellar or orbital trauma, this symptom only develops with orbital fracture.

Temporal fractures are manifested by a boggy temporal muscle, which occurs when bleeding from the fracture extravasates into the temporal muscle (area of least resistance). The development of a Battle's sign (gravitation ecchymosis) is also a sign of temporal fracture. A Battle's sign occurs when bleeding from the fracture gravitates downward to the large air cells of the mastoid process (area of least resistance). It appears as a benign oval-shaped bruise behind the ear in the mastoid region. Cerebrospinal fluid or cortex otorrhea (drainage from ears) may also accompany temporal fracture.

Parietal fractures may be manifested by deafness, cerebrospinal fluid or brain otorrhea, blood or cerebrospinal fluid bulging the tympanic membrane, facial paralysis, loss of taste, and a Battle's sign.

Posterior fossa fractures are often compounded by occipital bruising resulting in cortical blindness, visual field defects, and rarely ataxia and other cerebellar signs.

Basilar skull fracture should be suspected when cerebrospinal fluid or brain otorrhea is found; blood or cerebrospinal fluid bulges the tympanic membrane; a Battle's sign, tinnitus, or hearing difficulty is present; fracture lines are apparent on the external auditory canal; or facial paralysis, nystagmus, conjugate deviation of gaze, or vertigo is encountered.

MAXILLOFACIAL INJURY

Introduction

As Americans (indeed people worldwide) have taken to the highway as an accessible means of transportation, the number of neurosurgical trauma patients has increased significantly. These patients rarely escape maxillofacial injuries. The intensive care nurse must therefore be prepared technically, academically, and emotionally to provide quality care for both craniocerebral and maxillofacial injury patients.

Maxillofacial injuries occur most frequently with motor vehicle accidents, but also with injuries from fast-moving machine parts (industrial) and hostile-action missile injuries, athletic and recreational accidents, fist fights, motorcycle accidents, and falls.

In automobile accidents facial impact may occur against the windshield or the dashboard. In this manner the face is in opposition to a very rigid surface which may cause both craniocerebral and maxillofacial injury.

Approximately two-thirds of maxillofacial injuries involve the mandible alone, one-fourth the maxillae and associated bones, and one-tenth both mandible and maxillae. The mandible is involved in three-fourths of all facial fractures. The middle third of the face (nasal bones and zygoma) is involved in one-third of facial fractures.[7]

These injuries alter or destroy the functions of chewing, eating, talking, breathing, and seeing. They are likely to affect appearance, identity, emotional expression, and even basic physiognomy.

Assessment and Priority Intervention *Maxillofacial Injury*

Rapid systematic assessment and intervention are required for the vital safety of the patient with maxillofacial injury. While absolute rules do not apply in all circumstances, experience dictates the relative importance of assessing the

---

[7]Ballinger, W., Robert B. Rutherford, and George Zuidema, eds., *The Management of Trauma*, Philadelphia: W. B. Saunders Co., 1973, p. 256.

following clinical priorities: ventilation, facial fractures, major coincidental injuries, shock syndrome, and the neurologic assessment.

Ventilation.   Upper airway obstruction is the major cause of death in patients with maxillofacial injuries. Damage caused by cerebral hypoxia may be more threatening to the patient than the initial injury. The existence of a patent airway with adequate ventilation becomes the primary objective in assessment and priority intervention.

To determine the presence of respiratory obstruction, the nurse should consider the following:

1. Ask the patient if he is having any difficulty breathing. Observe for dyspnea. Record respiratory rate, depth, and rhythm.

2. Note the existence of stridorous or stertorous breathing. All noisy breathing represents obstruction.

3. Observe the patient for restlessness, struggling efforts, or attempts to move his head off the examining table.

4. Check the patient's color.

5. Check for laryngeal or tracheal compression from a neck injury. This can produce a severe mechanical obstruction, which requires immediate intubation or tracheostomy.

6. Check for patency of the nasal passages. Each side of the nasal cavity should be checked for adequacy by alternately blocking each nares. Observe the position of the nasal septum and mobility of the nasal bridge.

7. Quickly examine the chest for size, shape, symmetry, excursion, expansion, retraction, and paradoxical movements.

8. Determine the presence or absence of a pneumothorax.

Intervention based on abnormal findings in the initial respiratory assessment will include the following to relieve respiratory obstruction:

1. Handle the patient's head and neck gently because of the possibility of cervical vertebra fracture. A dislocated fracture may convert a patient with a minimal spinal cord injury to a permanent quadriplegic.

2. Facilitate opening of the jaw with a bite block, if necessary.

3. Remove all clots and foreign bodies. Keep the throat and mouth clear of blood and vomitus. The patient should be cautiously positioned on his side with his face downward. Suction frequently and insert a nasogastric tube as soon as possible to prevent aspiration of gastric contents. (See p. 141.)

4. The airway may be improved by pulling upward and forward on the posterior angles of the jaw, bringing the base of the tongue forward.

5. If the mandibular arch is fractured, the base of the tongue may obstruct the laryngeal opening. If this occurs, a towel clip is passed through the anterior tongue, and traction is applied to bring the tongue and mandibular arch

forward (Fig. 5-2). An immediate onrush of air should result if mandibular arch fracture is the problem.

6. The examiner should inspect the position of the maxilla and soft palate. In severe injuries they may be impacted downward and backward. If this is the case, the examiner's fingers are passed up behind the free edge of the displaced soft palate, and forceful forward elevation of the fractured obstructing bone and soft tissue is attempted.

7. If the above measures do not immediately relieve airway obstruction, the vocal cords should be inspected with a laryngoscope for damage and an endotracheal tube inserted.

8. Finally, in some situations in which expediency does not allow detailed evaluation of the patient, an immediate tracheostomy and coniotomy must be performed (Fig. 5-3).

Facial Fractures. When ventilation is effectively restored, examine the patient for facial fractures. Maxillae or mandibular fractures are commonly manifested by malocclusion of the teeth. If the patient is conscious, he will usually offer the information that his "teeth don't fit right." If he is unconscious, the jaws may be brought together to check the meshing together of the upper and lower teeth. If the patient is edentulous, his dentures may be reinserted to check for malocclusion.

Fractures of the facial bones usually exhibit localized tenderness to palpation. The examiner should also look for increased mobility and asymmetry or crepitus to detect displacements in the bony skeleton of the face.

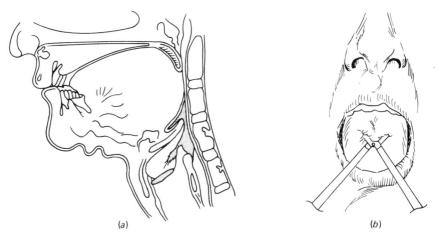

(a)   (b)

Fig. 5-2. Airway management, mandibular fracture. A method of obtaining a patent airway when the base of the tongue has settled posteriorly, obstructing the entrance to the glottis. (a) The tongue occluding the airway because of mandibular fracture. (b) A towel clip in place on the anterior tongue. The tongue is then brought forward, relieving the obstruction.

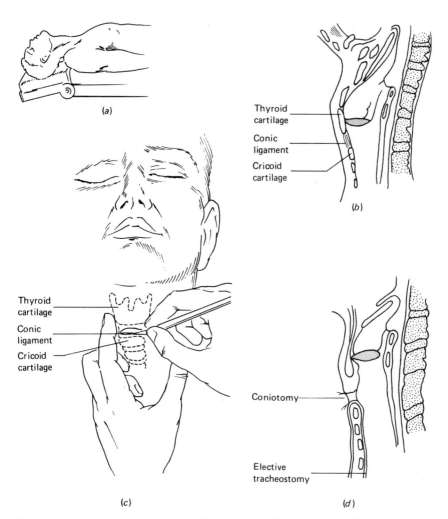

Thyroid
cartilage

Conic
ligament

Cricoid
cartilage

(b)

Thyroid
cartilage

Conic
ligament

Cricoid
cartilage

Coniotomy

Elective
tracheostomy

(a)

(c)

(d)

Fig. 5-3. Coniotomy. A short transverse incision is made just above the cricoid cartilage. One or two stitches hold the edges of the skin back from the wound until an elective tracheostomy can be done. (a) The patient is placed so that his head is extended. (b) Lateral view of the airway showing the thyroid and cricoid cartilages. (c) Coniotomy being performed. (d) Lateral view of the airway with the coniotomy performed with sutures in place, also showing where an elective tracheostomy will be done.

To ascertain mobility and crepitus at the temporomandibular joint, place a finger in each external auditory canal. The examiner should be able to determine the position, shape, movement, and symmetry of the mandibular condyles. Immobility or displacement can be further identified by radiologic study.

"Orbital blow out" occurs when a sudden blow is directed on the closed eye, forcing the globe inward, splintering the orbit's thin floor. There are five (5) cardinal signs of "orbital blow out," any one of which should cause suspicion:

1. Bony deformity with infraorbital or canthal tenderness to palpation
2. Subconjunctival hemorrhage with discoloration of eyelids (palpebral ecchymosis)
3. Infraorbital nerve anesthesia lasting more than 24 hours (numbness of upper lip)
4. Measurably lower position of the center of the pupil on the affected side
5. Early diplopia

Any of these signs dictate surgical exploration; otherwise perforation of the globe may occur from a sharp bone fragment.

Major Coincidental Injuries. Assessment of other major coincidental injuries in maxillofacial injury patients is essential. One special consideration with such patients is immediate assessment for cervical spine, larynx, or tracheal injury. Films should be obtained whenever the possibility exists that these structures have been damaged. Complaints of stiffness, spasm, or pain in the neck are indication enough for further exploration. The patient must be positioned with extreme caution (especially when airway obstruction is evident) until cervical spine injury has been disproved.

The physical examination explained in detail under assessment and priority intervention for general trauma patients, p. 136, is applicable to these patients also.

Shock Syndrome. Bleeding is second only to airway obstruction in causing death in patients with maxillofacial injuries. Hemorrhage is usually controlled by simple compression at the site, even if a major vessel is dissected. Digital pressure is usually effective. Pressure may be applied to pressure points if necessary.

The nurse must also be aware of possible internal bleeding. For example, check the size of the neck for an expanding pharyngeal hematoma, which may potentially obstruct the larynx or trachea.

The patient is not placed in Tredelenburg position for obvious reasons.

The principles involved in treating shock remain the same for maxillofacial injury patients as for general trauma patients. Shock syndrome is covered in detail later in this chapter, under "Assessment and Priority Intervention General Trauma."

Neurologic Assessment. Maxillofacial injury patients should have a thorough neurologic assessment to establish a baseline for future evaluation. Consider the probability of skull fracture and intracranial injury.

Special attention is required when evaluating the eyes, ears, nose, and cranial nerves.

All patients with evidence of maxillofacial injury should have each eye checked carefully for loss of vision. Check the visual quadrants; check for diplopia; check the fundus for vitreous hemorrhage/papilledema, and lens dislocation. A nurse skilled in the use of the ophthalmoscope is invaluable in these circumstances.

With an otoscope, examine the external auditory canal for the presence of blood, clots, cerebrospinal fluid, or rupture of the tympanic membrane. Occasionally a severe blow will drive the mandibular condyles backward, rupturing the wall of the external auditory canal.

Many patients with maxillofacial injuries will have cerebrospinal fluid leaks. The existence of rhinorrhea could probably be established when checking the nose for airway obstruction.

Extracranial injuries to the third, fourth, fifth, sixth, and seventh cranial nerves are commonly found with maxillofacial injuries. The nurse should be alert to: anesthesia of the upper lip and position of the central upper teeth— fifth nerve palsy, suggesting maxillary fracture; facial asymmetry—seventh nerve palsy; diplopia or strabismus—third, fourth, or sixth nerve palsy. Diplopia and strabismus are more commonly due to extraocular muscle palsy due to bony deformities of the orbit. The origin of the extraocular muscles is displaced or trapped in the fracture lines.

Definitive Procedures Maxillofacial Injury

Mandibular Fracture.   The balance of the mandibular arch is maintained by the muscles of mastication. When the mandible is fractured, these powerful muscles readily displace the bony fragments. Therefore, strong methods of fixation as well as longer splinting methods are required when reducing a mandibular fracture. Repair is accomplished by intermaxillary wiring and elastic band fixation or by open reduction and transosseous wiring. The details of the Erich arch bar are shown in Fig. 5-4. Open reduction with transosseous wiring is accomplished by the insertion of small wires through incisions directly into the mandibular fragments.

Dislocation of the Temporomandibular Joint.   This deformity is corrected by manual manipulation and adjustment under local or general anesthesia.

Membranous Bone Fracture.   Membranous bones are lightweight and unite easily. Most nasal fractures can be treated by simple reduction under local anesthesia. A lightly padded nasal elevator, which "snaps" the bone back into alignment, is inserted into the nose. These elevator pads are left in place approximately 4 to 5 days.

For severe comminution of the bridge of the nose, acrylic or lead plates

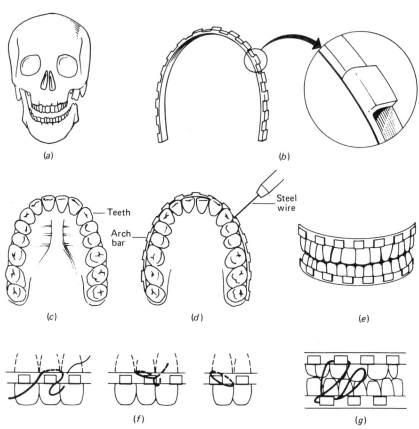

Fig. 5-4. Erich arch bars. (a) A mandibular fracture. (b) The Erich arch bar with enlarged view showing the bar. (c) The lower dental arch without the arch bar. (d) The arch in place on the lower dental arch. The procedure of passing the steel wire about the neck of the molar teeth and about the bar, making the latter secure. (e) The upper and lower arch bars in place. (f) Different methods of applying the wire on canine and incisor teeth. (g) Method of applying traction with rubberband, which is used to bring jaw fragments and teeth into satisfactory occlusion. These details illustrate the method of applying the soft, metallic Erich arch bar to upper and lower jaw to prepare for the use of intermaxillary elastic band fixation of fractured maxillae and mandibles.

are applied to the lateral walls of the nose and wired through the nasal cavity. This type splinting is left in place 10 to 14 days.

Zygomatic Arch Fracture. A fracture of the zygomatic arch is repaired by open reduction and, in some instances, stabilization with a rigid suspension bridge for 10 to 12 days (Fig. 5-5).

Malar Compound Fracture. Malar compound fractures vary greatly; some remain stable with muscular support, while others require open reduction and fixation.

Orbital Bone Fracture.   In the event of "orbital blow out," the globe is forced inward, splintering the thin orbital floor. When it is surgically explored, if large segments of the orbit are badly crushed or missing, they must be replaced. The orbit may be repaired using an iliac autogenous bone graft, Teflon, silicon, or synthetic collagen. This procedure is performed as soon as possible so that repair will not be impeded by edema. If surgery is deferred temporarily, local hypothermia (ice packs) may be somewhat effective.

Middle Face Fractures.   Fractures of the middle face are classified according to LeFort's early-1900 studies (Fig. 5-6). Airway obstruction and hemorrhage must be treated first. Emergency manual reduction of the fractures can usually be done to provide an airway. Hemorrhage is usually severe with maxillary fracture if the internal maxillary or greater palatine arteries are severed. Bleeding may occur through the nose and is controlled with packing and balloon catheters (Fox). These complex fractures are usually treated by

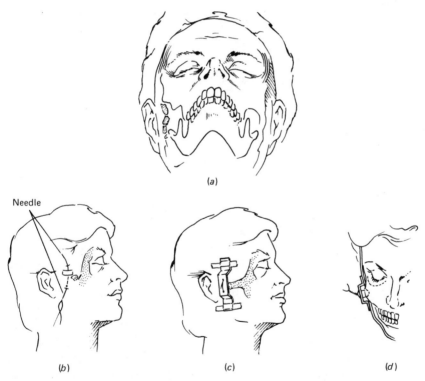

Fig. 5-5. Zygomatic arch fracture fixation. This fracture is reduced by placing an elevator beneath the fracture through a small incision beneath the hairline. (a) Depressed, compound fracture of the right zygomatic arch, inferior view. (b) Needle with a wire being passed beneath the unstable zygomatic arch. (c) Lateral view of rigid bridge support (metal) maintaining restored position of zygomatic arch. (d) Anterior view of same, but illustrating final fixation of wire.

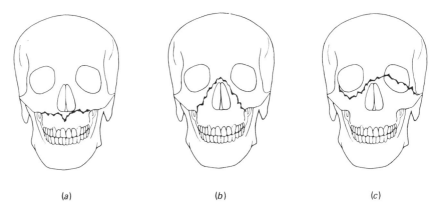

(a)   (b)   (c)

Fig. 5-6. LeFort fractures. Illustration of the three major patterns of fracture lines seen in middle face fractures. (a) Class I LeFort fracture, also called transverse maxillary fracture or a Guerin fracture. (b) Class II LeFort fracture with the nose in the mobile central fragment; also known as pyramidal fracture. (c) Class III LeFort fracture, including both zygomatic compounds in the mobile fragment; also called craniofacial disjunction.

open reduction and interosseous wiring and suspension sling support (Fig. 5-7).

Displaced Frontal Fracture. Displaced frontal fractures are repaired by open reduction and interosseous wiring.

Nursing Objectives Maxillofacial Injury

The postoperative management of patients with maxillofacial injuries parallels that of the patient with head injuries. However, special areas require additional attention.

Ventilation. Bleeding and edema present obstacles for adequate ventilation. The nurse must be vigilant in frequently reevaluating the patient's respiratory status. Restoration and maintenance of a clear airway take priority if the patient is to survive.

Aspiration. If the patient has Erich arch bars with bands or is wired, the nurse will need to observe for symptoms of nausea and vomiting. A suction apparatus should be readily accessible. Anti-emetic drugs may be administered. The patient should be placed in Fowler's position with his head slightly dependent if possible, or in the lateral recumbent position with head to the side. The patient with a tracheostomy should have the cuff inflated immediately if signs of nausea and vomiting are present. Wire cutters should be kept at the bedside for emergency use when absolutely necessary. The nursing objectives and intervention are based on symptomatology and the prevention of aspiration with *minimal damage to the repair work.*

Hygiene. Mouth care must be administered gently and frequently. Whatever procedure and solution are used, the objective is to remove food particles, cleanse the tissue, protect exposed suture lines, and provide an infection-free environment.

Suture Lines. The patient with maxillofacial injuries may have facial lacerations or surgical incisions that require attention. Meticulous cleansing followed by a softening agent will prevent infection and promote wound healing.

Nutrition. The patient requires a high protein, 2000 to 2500 calorie per day diet. Facial fractures, edema, and suture lines may allow the patient to take only fluids orally. Depending on the type of injury, nutrition may have

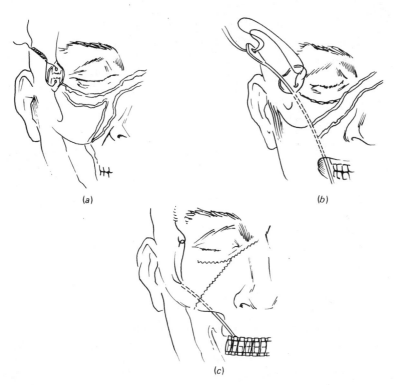

Fig. 5-7. Reduction of LeFort III fracture. (a) The zygomaticofrontal suture line is reunited with steel wire, fixing the zygoma firmly to nonfractured frontal bone. This procedure is performed through a drill hole. (b) A double loop of steel wire is passed through the drill hole and drawn subcutaneously behind the zygoma to emerge in the buccogingival sulcus. Note Erich arch bars in place. (c) The two ends of the suspension wire are passed about the arch bar in an appropriate location to provide strong upward and lateral traction to the central bony fragments of the face.

to be provided by gavage feeding. Sometimes a gastrostomy is done if the patient is unable to swallow for a long period of time.

Pain. The nursing objective is to control and relieve pain. Edema seems to be the primary cause of pain, and mild analgesics usually alleviate it. Medication does not exclude the use of nursing measures providing comfort to the patient.

Conclusion

Maxillofacial injury patients present some unique problems due to the nature of their injuries, affecting respiratory pathways, mastication, sight, hearing, talking, and smelling. The nurse may have to make some personal adjustments before she is able to give care to these patients. The very art of nursing is reflected in accepting the person of the patient disguised in what might be a grotesque appearance. If the nurse cannot overcome this obstacle, she cannot support the patient in sustaining his self-esteem.

Today's society values an aesthetic image, and the patient may be compelled to reassess his own beliefs in this area. The nurse might oblige by offering some thoughts on value clarification. What is the health belief model of the patient? Does life compensate good looks?

Please consider the appearance of the patient to the family. Have they been adequately prepared for the first encounter with the maxillofacial injury patient? Initially the patient and family may be overwhelmed by fear of death. Sooner or later this feeling may be replaced by fear of the patient's not being socially acceptable.

The problem of communication compounds the loss of self-esteem. Every effort should be made to maintain open communication and expression of feelings among the patient, nurse, and family.

Support, guidance, and sense of acceptance are essential components in nursing the patient with maxillofacial injuries.

MECHANISMS OF MASS LESIONS

Intracranial hematomas, as a result of vascular rupture, may occur from head injuries. The critical care nurse must be capable of recognizing and interpreting the signs and symptoms of intracranial bleeds and initiating an immediate course of action. It is probably true that a neurosurgeon's operative mortality on patients with traumatic intracranial bleeds is directly proportionate to the nursing care rendered to these patients.

Intracranial bleeds will be discussed in relation to their anatomical etiology; i.e., epidural, subdural, subarachnoid, and intracerebral. The signs and symptoms, which are similar for some hematomas, will be presented collectively.

Classification of Expanding Lesions

Epidural Hematoma.   A simple concept of trauma is a local bruise that extends from the skin or surface to underlying tissue. An epidural hematoma is such a bruise on the head that is complicated by the presence of a layer of bone between the hematoma and the skin. There results a collection of blood in the abnormally created epidural space. This injury is found in only a very few hospitalized head injury patients and is usually caused by a blunt, low-velocity blow to the head; e.g., an injury suffered in a fall or a fight. The abnormal epidural space is created at the site of impact when the skull moves relative to the dura beneath it, stripping the dura from the bone (shearing stress). Ruptured blood vessels result, which bleed into the epidural space. Epidural bleeds are commonly arterial in origin.

The most frequent areas of impact and the vessels impaired are as follows:

Area of Impact	Vessel Impaired
Parietotemporal	Middle meningeal artery or its branches
Frontal	Anterior ethmoidal artery
Occipital	Transverse or sigmoid sinus
Vertical (vertex)	Sagittal sinus

The patient with an epidural hematoma may be unconscious from the initial injury and then experience a period of alertness before lapsing into stupor and coma. The initial unconsciousness represents concussion incurred at the time of impact; the secondary coma is caused by cerebral displacement and uncal herniation. The presence or absence of the "lucid interval" depends on the initial degree of unconsciousness and the rapidity of the expanding lesion. The significance of deterioration is exactly the same whether or not a lucid interval is present; it is always indicative of cerebral distortion from a complication of injury.

Epidural hematoma is the most serious complication of head injury. The temporal lobe is forced downward and inward, resulting in uncal herniation and eventual death (Fig. 5-8). It carries a high mortality, and requires immediate diagnosis and surgical evacuation.

Subdural Hematoma.   A subdural hematoma is a collection of blood between the dura mater and the arachnoid in the subdural space. Subdural hematomas are classified into acute, subacute, and chronic hematomas, depending on the severity and speed of the progression of symptoms. Only acute subdural hematomas will be dealt with in this chapter. Injury is usually a result of acceleration-deceleration of the skull with rotation of the brain on its atlas and axis. Consequently, the frontal and temporal lobes of the brain are forced against the knifelike sphenoid ridges, the rough orbital bones, and the frontal bone. The resultant cerebral laceration with tear of the arachnoid

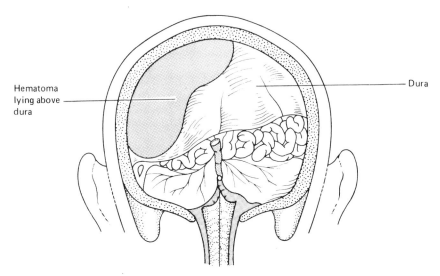

Hematoma
lying above
dura

Dura

Fig. 5-8. Epidural hematoma. A massive epidural hematoma producing tentorial herniation with subsequent brain stem compression.

allows blood (usually venous) and cerebrospinal fluid to escape into the subdural space (Fig.5-9). With acute subdural hematoma the bleed is usually severe enough to produce signs and symptoms within 24 hours post injury. The expanding bleed is a result of primary brain tissue damage as well as a change in the osmotic character of the fluid in the subdural space, which tends to pull water in, thereby increasing the mass.

Subdural hematomas occur in 5% of hospitalized head injury patients. The mortality rate is as high as 70%, owing to the destruction of brain tissue as well as the incidence of cerebral herniation.[8] Early diagnosis and surgical intervention are life-saving.

Subarachnoid Hematoma. A subarachnoid hematoma (from trauma) is caused by injury to a surface vessel lying in the subarachnoid space. The bleed may be immediate or delayed, depending on the size, vasoconstriction, and retraction of the impaired blood vessel.

The effects of subarachnoid hematoma are similar to the symptoms displayed with a ruptured aneurysm. Although the volume of blood is usually insufficient to raise intracranial pressure significantly, the perivascular spaces may secrete excessive amounts of cerebrospinal fluid in response to irritation by the blood, causing a secondary rise in intracranial pressure.

Intracerebral Hematoma. An intracerebral hematoma is a result of surface laceration of the cerebrum and contributes to the development of a sub-

[8]Jackson, Frederick E., "The Pathophysiology of Head Injuries," *Clinical Symposia*, Summit, New Jersey: CIBA Pharmaceutical Co., Vol. 18, No. 3, p. 91.

dural hematoma. It is usually found in the orbital surface or pole of the frontal lobe and in the temporal pole. The hematoma may occur at the lcoation of impact or at some distance from the injury. The bleeding spreads into brain tissue in a few hours or a few days. Increased intracranial pressure results, and focal signs and symptoms present. The results of surgical intervention are poor, owing to existing parenchymal damage.

Signs and Symptoms of Expanding Lesions

Signs and symptoms of expanding lesions include local pressure effects, general pressure effects, or signs of cerebral distortion (see next section).

Local pressure effects. Local or focal pressure produces symptoms as a result of pressure on a local area of the brain or destruction of a brain area. These symptoms indicate a progressively expanding lesion when they develop at an interval post injury: monoplegia, hemiplegia, visual field defects, conjugate deviation of the eyes, sensory loss, and cerebellar signs. These signs are indicative of an expanding lesion appropriate to each part of the brain receiving pressure or being destroyed. The symptoms may be difficult to detect because the patient may be in profound coma.

General Pressure Effects

Headache. Although many patients complain of a headache after a head injury, any increase in severity should suggest a rise in intracranial pressure, even in the absence of other symptoms of increased intracranial pressure.

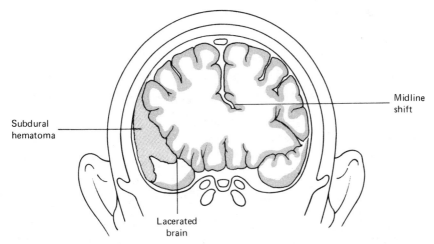

Fig. 5-9. Subdural hematoma. A lacerated brain with a subdural hematoma producing midline shift.

Restlessness. Restlessness and irritability may be indicative of increased pain and increased intracranial pressure in the less than fully conscious patient.

Level of consciousness. Any decrease in the patien't level of consciousness at any interval after injury is an extremely important sign of an expanding lesion.

Vital parameters. When intracerebral pressure rises, the cardiac center is likely to be stimulated. Stimulation of the parasympathetic (vagal) and sympathetic innervation to the heart produces bradycardia and hypertension.

The bradycardia may become severe enough to warrant the administration of atropine. As intracranial pressure rises, eventually the heart compensates with a tachycardia.

The blood pressure is elevated by vasoconstriction. The systolic pressure increases, causing an increase in the pulse pressure. As intracranial pressure rises, this stimulation gives way to depression, producing hypotension.

Although bradycardia and hypertension are quoted as classic signs of increasing intracranial pressure, they may occur only briefly or not at all. If they occur, they are early signs of cardiac center stimulation, and later result in depression of these two vital circulatory centers.

There is also stimulation of the respiratory centers as a result of pressure, which produces an increase in the depth of respirations (increase in tidal volume) with no significant change in rate. Later the rate may increase, but eventually respiratory depression supervenes. The depth may become increasingly shallower, the rate slower (bradypnea); or apneustic gasping and even Cheyne-Stokes respirations may occur.

Papilledema. Papilledema is the last sign of general pressure effects. It may not develop for 8 to 12 hours after a gross increase in intracranial pressure. Papilledema has far more significance in subacute and chronic neurologic lesions.

SIGNS OF CEREBRAL DISTORTION

Signs of cerebral distortion are often the first manifestation of complication of concussion or fracture. These signs are likely to be associated with the syndrome of cortical injury, as well.

There are two major signs of cerebral distortion requiring mention at this time: tentorial herniation (uncal herniation) and cerebellar tonsillar herniation (medullary cone herniation).

Uncal herniation is caused by the medial portion of the temporal lobe slipping across the tentorium into the posterior fossa. This area of temporal lobe is displaced and distorted by the presence of an expanding clot, so that pressure is exerted on the third nerve and ultimately the brain stem. The first signs of cerebral distortion occur from uncal herniation. It is usually manifested by third nerve palsy, pyramidal or upper motor neuron lesion signs, and midbrain signs.

Third nerve palsy is characterized by ipsilateral loss of direct reaction to light, ipsilateral ptosis, ipsilateral loss of medial rectus muscle movement, and contralateral loss of consensual reaction to light. The herniating uncus exerts pressure on the third nerve, or pressure is exerted by blood vessels. In the latter case, the brain stem is pushed downward, carrying the basilar and posterior cerebral arteries, stretching the posterior communicating arteries. Since the posterior communicating arteries pass immediately above the origin of the third nerves, they may compress its upper surface. Since the outer surface of the third nerve contains the parasympathetic pupillo-constrictor fibers, the first effect of pressure may be *stimulation* and hence *constriction* of the pupil. This is a transitory stage often missed as paralysis supervenes and the pupil progressively dilates and becomes fixed. This dilated fixed pupil will almost always be on the side of the lesion. If cerebral distortion is allowed to progress, the contralateral third nerve may also constrict and then dilate. As is true with other symptoms of deterioration, the significance is greatest when the above occurs at an interval after injury.

Signs of injury to the upper motor neuron must be observed for closely. There are six important signs of upper motor neuron involvement. The first sign is motor paralysis affecting functionally related groups of muscles rather than individual muscles. The paralysis is usually partial (paresis), largely transient, and affects mostly the discrete movements of the distal limb segment. The second sign is jackknife spasticity. This is a state of altered tone of skeletal muscle that is elicited most readily when the involved limb is passively moved suddenly. At the beginning of movement there is palpable resistance of the muscle being lengthened; then toward the end of the movement there is an abrupt disappearance of the muscle resistance, and the limb gives readily to the movement. The third sign is hyperactive deep tendon reflexes in the involved limb or limbs. The fourth sign is loss of cutaneous abdominal and cremasteric reflexes on the paretic side. The fifth sign is presence of a Babinski (extensor plantar) response in the foot and leg on the paretic side. Last is the lack of atrophy and fasciculations of involved muscles. All six of these signs may occur in any order and in any combination.

Midbrain signs usually include loss of doll's eyes phenomena, but may progress to a picture of full brain stem lesion: decerebrate rigidity, hyperthermia, and other disturbance of vital function.

The second major sign of cerebral distortion is medullary cone or cerebellar tonsillar herniation, which is caused by the cerebellar tonsil pressing on the medulla. It is often associated with nuchal rigidity, upper motor neuron lesion signs, cerebellar signs, or medullary collapse. The last is characterized by flaccidity and respiratory and/or circulatory collapse. When these signs appear, performance of a lumbar puncture would be life-threatening, as loss of cerebrospinal fluid would give the bleed room to expand, thereby further compressing the cerebellar tonsils on the brain stem. Urea or mannitol might have a similar effect through osmotic diuresis; neurosurgeons rarely gamble with these drugs unless they plan immediate surgical decompression. Surgical intervention for cerebellar tonsillar herniation is not only necessary but usually life-saving.

SYNDROME OF CENTRAL NERVOUS SYSTEM INJURY

Cortical frontal injuries vary widely in clinical presentation. Injury to the anterior portion of the frontal lobes may result in profound behavioral changes, ranging from simple confusion to the use of obscene or profane language, hypersexuality, lack of emotional restraint, impairment of intellectual function, and/or the dulling of certain neurotic traits such as worry and anxiety. As the medial and posterior portions of the frontal lobes become involved, motor paralysis may result. Usually this injury is in the form of upper motor neuron lesion. Frontal lobe injury may also be accompanied by deviation of the patient's eye gaze toward the lesion.

Cortical parietal injuries do not commonly result in sensory loss or visual field defects. Dominant side parietal lesions may present with aphasia, apraxia, alexia, and so forth. It is felt by most clinicians that sensory findings are extremely difficult to observe and interpret.

Temporal injuries can also cause visual field defects; but may be manifested by change in the emotional status of the patient or loss of memory from limbic-related damage.

Occipital lesions commonly result in visual field defects, such as bilateral hemianopsia.

Truncal ataxia, cerebellar tremor, decomposition of movement, and instability of a limb against gravity are common findings in cerebellar injury. Truncal ataxia is manifested by loss of corrdination in the trunk, leaving only the patient's limbs to steady himself. Hence the patient adopts a reeling, staggering legs-wide stance. When the patient is sitting without support to his body, he will assume the "tripod" position of propping on his hands to prevent wavering of his trunk. Cerebellar tremor occurs only when the limb is brought into action. It tends to increase when the target is approached, and so is sometimes called a terminal tremor. Decomposition of movement occurs when the patient loses proper integration of contraction of agonist and synergist muscles with relaxation of the antagonists. The result is that a movement, such as touching the nose, is broken down ("decomposed") into its various components.

In the case of a limb that becomes unstable when attempting to maintain its posture against gravity, the instability can be illustrated by the "pronator test." This is done by having the patient supinate his hands with his arms straight out in front of him with his eyes closed. The affected limb will gradually drift down, and when the arm is paretic, the affected hand will pronate.

Hypothalamic damage commonly occurs with head injuries. It is evidenced by neurogenic hyperpyrexia, hibernation syndrome, and Cushing's ulcers.

In neurogenic hyperpyrexia the patient's ability to lose heat is impaired. Symptoms are increased body temperature (105° to 106° F), dry skin (patient can no longer perspire), pilo-erection (to maintain heat), peripheral vasoconstriction (compensatory to maintain heat), tachypnea (only way to lose heat), and shivering (to produce more heat). This of course must be differentiated from other clinical causes of hyperthermia (infection or hypercapnia). Treatment is aimed at reducing body temperature, a procedure that requires meticulous nursing care. Either hypothermia blankets or iced alcohol baths can be used, the latter being the more effective, especially when a fan is directed on the patient to increase evaporation.

Most patients who suffer from hibernation syndrome are unconscious. Their temperature is extremely low (even less than 80° F), and their vital functions are gravely depressed (heart rate, blood pressure, respiratory frequency). This syndrome is the opposite of neurogenic hyperpyrexia and is characterized by loss or impairment of the heat-saving mechanism. Treatment is to warm the patient carefully.

A Cushing's ulcer is described as a gastric erosion. It is thought to be caused by hypothalamic stimulation of the vagus nerve, which in turn leads to hypersecretion of acid by the stomach. The eventual result is gastric erosion and mucosal sloughing. Symptoms include hematemesis and/or melena. Cushing's ulcer is treated by antacids and discontinuance of steroids when they are in use. The incidence is decreased when gastric aspiration is not employed; placing the patient on a diet as soon as possible may help. In addition cimetidine (Tagemet) is often given for prevention of ulceration.

Injury to the pituitary gland, including severance of the pituitary stalk, is often seen with middle fossa and basilar fracture, especially following acceleration-deceleration forces. When this happens, the pituitary ceases to secrete ADH. The result is diuresis of gross amounts of urine with a persistent specific gravity of less than 1.005. It must be distinguished from other causes of endocrine dysfunction. The problem is corrected by carefully replacing fluid and electrolytes and administering pitressin, with correction usually occurring in a few months. (For further discussion see p. 207.)

Brain stem injuries that are secondary to trauma are often caused by acceleration with resulting hematoma, causing a shift, bruises on the tentorium, tearing or stretching of vascular structures, and avulsion of cranial nerves. Symptoms include altered state of consciousness, neurogenic hyperpyrexia, decortication, decerebration, flaccidity, and the presence of primitive reflexes, i.e., sucking, chewing, snouting, yawning, or teeth grinding. Brain stem signs also include ocular changes such as fluctuating irregular pupils, loss of doll's eyes, loss of upward gaze, and pinpoint pupils in the absence of drugs.

METABOLIC MANIFESTATIONS OF HEAD INJURY

Neuronal Metabolism

The central nervous system is absolutely dependent on an adequate supply of glucose and oxygen.

The neuron utilizes only glucose for energy and has little ability to store glycogen. Any dramatic reduction in serum glucose level will produce disorientation, convulsions, unconsciousness, and coma. These symptoms of cerebral glucose deficiency must be differentiated from symptoms produced by head injury.

The brain itself utilizes 20% of the body's total oxygen uptake. In the absence of an adequate supply of oxygen, there is an interruption of the Kreb's cycle, and anaerobic glycolysis is initiated in an attempt to produce energy. This results in an accumulation of lactic acid and converts the cell to a state of metabolic acidosis. The excess hydrogen ions inhibit normal neuronal function.

The metabolic activity of the brain, though not altered when the organ is at rest, increases 10 to 15% in the presence of fever, a factor that must be considered in controlling the temperature of head injury patients.

The patient may suffer respiratory embarrassment, leading to the retention of carbon dioxide. Respiratory acidosis requires treatment to ensure an adequate oxygen supply to the brain cells and diminish the effects of carbon dioxide narcosis.

The normal cardiovascular and respiratory functions of the body may be impaired as a result of head injury. Damage to vital brain structures will alter the oxygen and glucose supply to the neurons. Every effort must be made to preserve cardiovascular and respiratory function, whether impairment is caused directly by brain damage or secondarily by obstructed airway, inadequate pulmonary ventilation, or shock.

Physiologic Stress

The head injury patient's response to injury is a normal physiologic response to stress. The entire response is attributed to the action of the hypothalamus and hypophysis. Ultimately the clinical picture includes: an increase in the serum glucose level as a result of the action of adrenalin and the glucocorticoid, cortisol; an increase in fluid retention as a result of release of ADH; an increase in sodium retention as a result of the action of the mineral corticoid, aldosterone, which also contributes to the retention of water and alters the serum sodium concentration; and a decrease in serum potassium levels caused by the kidney's inability to reabsorb potassium simultaneously with sodium. When sodium is reabsorbed, potassium is excreted.

In addition, the body is in a state of nitrogen imbalance; there is an increase in protein catabolism, resulting in additional conversion of ammonia to urea by the liver, testing the ability of the kidneys to excrete increasing quantities of nitrogenous wastes.

Fluid and Electrolytes

Head injury patients respond to stress with increased secretion of ADH and consequent water retention for 12 to 36 hours or longer. This fluid imbalance parallels sodium retention after any stress, but the resulting effect is usually more severe after head injury. Increased ADH is released, and sodium retention usually begins on the day of trauma, persisting up to about four days. The severity of the imbalance depends on the status of the patient's extracellular fluid volume before injury, the increased secretion of the mineral corticoid, aldosterone, and the area of the brain injured. For example, patients with lesions of the frontal lobes or the hypothalamus are particularly susceptible to such fluid and electrolyte derangements during this time; the serum sodium level decreases, probably because of dilution from water retention. This sodium aberration is usually followed by a diuretic phase and a return to body fluid equilibrium.

Subsequent to head injury or cerebral surgery, the serum potassium level decreases for several days. This decrease rarely assumes clinical significance unless accompanied by extrarenal loss, such as with vomiting or diarrhea.

Since serum potassium levels can be misleading, the EKG becomes a valuable detector of potassium abnormalities. The following guide may help in assessment of potassium levels:

Abnormality	EKG Changes
Hypokalemia	"U" waves
	Low flat T waves
	Prolonged Q-T interval
	Depressed ST segment
Hyperkalemia	Tall peaked T waves
	Aberrant QRS complexes
	Idioventricular rhythm

Catabolism

The existence of a state of negative nitrogen balance is a common finding in head injury patients. It is a result of nutritional inadequacy in the "NPO" state, and the body's demand for energy in the reparative phase following trauma. The dissolution of body protein occurs at an accelerated rate. The patient assumes a catabolic state, losing approximately 10 grams of nitrogen per day for 7 to 10 days. Severity may increase, with up to 30 grams of loss per day. The excessive amount of urea to be excreted challenges the effectiveness of even normal kidneys. This increase in the production of urea results in an altered osmotic pressure gradient within the tubules, which promotes a marked excretion of water. If it becomes necessary to correct this imbalance, correction is usually accomplished by diet therapy. The administration of a high protein diet (1.5 to 2.0 grams of protein per kilogram of body weight per day) or the parenteral administration of amino acids combined with sufficient calories to meet metabolic requirements (2000 to 2500 calories per day) will restore the nitrogen balance. Occasionally, anabolic steroids are required.

Derangements in Isotonicity of Blood

Hypertonicity or hypotonicity of the blood can cause additional problems for the patient with head injury.

Hypotonicity.   Hypotonic extracellular fluid abnormality (traditionally referred to as cerebral salt wasting) is now described as the syndrome of inappropriate secretion of antidiuretic hormone. There is an oversecretion and release of ADH by the posterior pituitary gland. In patients with head injury, the osmoreceptors that usually control the release of this hormone are probably primarily or secondarily impaired, permitting an excessive production of ADH. At the kidney tubule level water is reabsorbed, expanding extracellular fluid volume.

This volume expansion causes the dilution of body fluids and sodium diuresis. The combination of water retention with salt wasting produces a decrease in the serum sodium level.

Hypotonicity produces symptoms of decreased level of consciousness, delirium, coma, convulsions, and increased cerebrospinal fluid pressure and increased intracranial pressure. These symptoms are attributed to intracellular overhydration and brain swelling.

The treatment of such hypotonicity is directed toward reducing volume. Fluids are restricted to 400 to 500 milliliters per day for a period of three to five days. It may be necessary in the presence of severe symptoms to administer hypertonic intravenous fluids and at the same time cautiously initiate diuretic therapy.

Table 5-2. Hypotonicity and Hypertonicity Summary

HYPOTONICITY	HYPERTONICITY
Syndrome of inappropriate secretion ADH, cerebral salt wasting	Cerebral salt hoarding syndrome
Hyponatremia	Hypernatremia
Normal BUN	Hyperchloremia
Normal creatinine	Hypokalemia
Renal sodium wasting	Hyperglycemia
Specific gravity of urine is greater than 1.003 (Note: 1.003 specific gravity is inappropriately high for hypotonicity)	Specific gravity of urine is greater than 1.018
Absence of edema (water retention usually is less than 3 to 4 liters, most of which moves into cells)	Oliguria
	Absence of edema

Hypertonicity.   Hypertonicity, referred to as cerebral salt hoarding, produces a state of dehydration. Most patients who exhibit its symptoms have suffered closed head trauma, lesions in the frontal lobe or hypothalamus, hypophysectomy, or ruptured anterior cerebral artery aneurysm. The etiology is largely unknown, but attributed to the following series of events: there is a decrease in blood volume; an increase in the secretion of aldosterone; an increase in sodium retention; an increase in water excretion (and often electrolytes); a decrease in urinary volume; an increase in catabolic waste products; and, if it is undiagnosed and untreated, uremia and death.

The therapy for hypertonicity is to replace the patient's blood volume based on urinary specific gravity or osmolarity.

It is important that the nurse be able to conceptualize the effects of hypertonicity and hypotonicity on the patient with head injury. She must be alert to the signs and symptoms of electrolyte imbalances and be accountable for absolutely accurate recordings of the patient's intake and output. A summary of hypotonicity and hypertonicity effects may be found in Table 5-2.

CEREBRAL EDEMA AND HEAD INJURY

The subject of cerebral edema is further presented in Chapter 7. The purpose of this section is to relate cerebral edema to head injury.

For many decades physiologists, neurologists, and neurosurgeons have debated the occurrence and clinical significance of cerebral edema. The criteria used in studies as well as the conclusions vary greatly. One well-known authority feels "safe" in concluding that cerebral edema is a frequent, if not inevitable, sequela to severe craniocerebral trauma. He further maintains that failure to recognize its presence is probably attributed to undue reliance on cerebrospinal fluid pressure measurements as a precise reflection of intracranial pressure. Langfitt, as well as other authorities, stresses the importance of continuous intracranial pressure monitoring for evaluating intracranial dynamics after head injury. The symptoms of cerebral edema include general pressure effects as well as signs of cerebral distortion.

The general principles of treatment may be summarized as follows:

1. Correct those conditions most likely to kill the patient.
   (a) Ensure adequate airway and ventilation (normal $PaCO_2$ and PaO_2).
   (b) Control external hemorrhage.
2. Rule out space-occupying lesion early, or correct it if present. Hyperventilation with high inspired fractions of oxygen which may rapidly reduce intracranial tension may be attempted.
3. Administer hypertonic intravenous solutions (urea, mannitol) which reduce brain bulk rapidly.
4. Administer corticosteroids (see p. 265).
5. External decompression: the neurosurgeon leaves an opening in dura and skull for decompression. Although it may be life-saving, there is risk of severe brain damage.

Cerebral edema is, or appears to be, a significant part of the pathophysiology of head injury. It is probably the most common cause of death in those patients who survive initial injury and do not develop expanding lesions.

The nurse's responsibilities include preparing the patient for therapy, continual reassessment of the patient's neurologic status, ensuring adequate blood–gas exchange, and the safe administration of chemotherapeutic agents.

ASSESSMENT AND PRIORITY INTERVENTION
GENERAL TRAUMA

Emergency Stabilization and Evaluation

Ventilation. Priorities vary little in the emergency department in dealing with trauma: AIRWAY is always of primary importance. In terms of head injuries, there are two basic concerns of airway management: the assurance and preservation of appropriate gas exchange and the establishment of a mechanical airway. The assurance and preservation of appropriate gas exchange has absolute priorty on a patient with a head injury because of the detrimental effect of hypoxia and hypercapnia on cerebral vasculature and neuronal metabolism. The frequent analysis and interpretation of arterial blood gases is the most accurate way to determine if the oxygen and carbon dioxide levels are appropriate.

Hypoxia causes altered permeability of cell membranes promoting exudation of fluid into the tissues, which leads to cerebral edema and increased intracranial pressure. Life is made possible by the continuing production of energy by living cells, which requires oxygen. Energy cannot be piped from a site of production to a site of utilization; it must be generated by each cell for its own use. In hypoxia the brain energy sources are lacking, a situation that leads to rapid, irreversible anaerobic changes.

Hypercapnia also has its effects on cerebral circulation. Carbon dioxide is an extremely potent vasodilator; dilatation of cerebral blood vessels and increased blood flow consequently contribute to cerebral edema and increased intracranial pressure. Severe hypercapnia narcotizes the respiratory center in the medulla, and the combination of hypoxia and hypercapnia is clearly a major threat to the integrity of the organism. Therefore assurance and preservation of ventilation require vigilant observation, monitoring of arterial blood gases, and the recording of respiratory patterns by the nurse.

The establishment of a mechanical airway deserves serious consideration. In reaching a decision, thought should be given to the following questions:

1. Is the patient's own airway adequate to maintain proper physiological ventilation; e.g., is his airway obstruction-free?

2. Is the patient's position adequate for ventilation? For example, make sure the patient is not supine; make sure the head of the bed is up and the patient is in the lateral recumbent position.

3. Where are the patient's dentures? Make sure they are not in his mouth.

4. Is the patient's level of consciousness consistent with #1? Can the patient maintain a proper position without nursing assistance? Do not leave the unconscious patient unattended for any length of time.

5. Has the patient sustained severe maxillofacial injuries that could potentially obstruct the airway? (Refer to p. 113.)

6. Has the patient sustained a cervical spine injury? ASSUME HE HAS UNLESS IT IS PROVED OTHERWISE. (Refer to p. 154.)

In relation to the responses to these questions, a decision may be made to insert a mechanical airway. Generally, the first choice of airway assistance is oral or nasal endotracheal tube. While this may prove safe and efficient for some patients, it may be a poor choice for patients with particular neurologic injuries. For example, the most common reason for not using oral endotracheal tube is cervical spine injury. Hyperextension of the neck, which is needed to facilitate intubation, could easily be disastrous to the spinal cord of a patient with a cervical spine fracture. For this reason it must always be assumed that the patient with head injury has suffered cervical spine injury until it is proved otherwise. When the judgment has been made that cervical spine injury does not exist, careful orotracheal intubation may be carried out, preferably by an anesthesiologist. If cervical spine fracture does exist, anticipate a tracheostomy to be done when an airway is needed; this is often performed by a neurosurgeon rather than by a general surgeon. Tracheostomy or coniotomy is also the preferred airway for patients who have severe maxillofacial injury making intubation impossible. Following tracheostomy ensure that the tracheostomy ties are not secured too tightly as they can easily impede venous return in the jugular veins, increasing intracranial pressure. If the patient has severe facial fractures, cerebrospinal fluid and cortex leaks, avoid cannulation of the airway or esophagus with plastic suction devices, unless overseen by a neurosurgeon. Too easily a suction catheter could find its way through fracture lines, fractured sinuses, and/or torn dura, resulting in disaster.

Major Coincidental Injuries.   A search for unsuspected distant injuries should be initiated early. A complete physical examination will not only discover a complicating injury but also provide data for future use.

Examine the chest thoroughly for anything interrupting respiratory function.

A thorough evaluation of the back is necessary, especially in relation to cervical spine injuries and determining the mobility of the patient to be permitted during the physical examination.

The upper abdomen may incur injury in automobile injuries. The presence of a ruptured spleen or liver may be the cause of hemorrhage and shock.

The insertion of a urethral catheter would be helpful in diagnosing injury to the bladder and also in permitting accurate monitoring of the urinary output.

Examine the patient's extremities for lacerations and signs of fracture. Any suspected fracture should be splinted immediately.

Shock Syndrome.   Soon after the airway is established, symptoms of bleeding must be assessed and shock controlled. If shock syndrome is present, look for a cause other than head injury. Head injuries rarely cause hemorrhagic (hypovolemic) shock. However, neurogenic shock can occur with head injuries; it is caused by activation of the brain stem vasomotor centers.

This neurogenic or vasogenic shock is seen as simple syncope, such as following exposure to unpleasant sights or sudden pain. These stimuli appear to increase vagal influence on the heart, causing bradycardia and decreased cardiac output. Atropine will block these stimuli. The clinical picture of neurogenic shock varies greatly from that of hypovolemic shock. Although the blood pressure may be low, the heart rate is usually slow. The skin is warm, even flushed, owing to the normovolemic state of the patient. Blood is pooled into capillaries, however, and arterioles, venules, and peripheral veins are full. The urine output is normal, and the patient is alert. Treatment is usually not necessary.

Chest, abdominal, and pelvic injuries and long bone fractures are common traumatic causes of hypovolemic shock syndrome. When head injury is present, the treatment employed here does not vary from the classical treatment of shock symdrome. Therefore the shock must be treated quickly and efficiently by standard means. The first priority would be to expand blood volume by increasing colloidal pressure, which does not have a detrimental effect on intracranial pressure. On occasion, massive blood loss from the scalp in adults or subgaleal hematoma in infants results in hypovolemic shock syndrome.

Neurologic Assessment. The performance of a careful, detailed, baseline neurologic evaluation becomes the next priority. If possible obtain a careful medical history from anyone available to give it. There are several questions to consider if the patient has suffered trauma before the nurse performs the examination:

1. Did the patient lose consciousness?
2. Was the patient moving all four extremities at the scene of injury? In what manner was he moving them?
3. If the patient was transferred by fire aid vehicle or ambulance, what assessments were made by paramedical personnel? For example: Did the patient's pupils respond to light? What was the patient's level of consciousness immediately after injury? Has there been any deterioration in the status of the patient during, or since, extrication and transportation? How much time has elapsed from injury, extrication, and admission to the emergency department? Was extrication particularly difficult?
4. Does the patient have any bony deformities, discolorations, or drainage from the head?
5. Does the patient have any drainage from the eyes, or nose? Is the drainage serous or sanguinous?

These questions may be asked of relatives, bystanders, paramedical personnel, law enforcement officers, or, in part, of the patient himself. However they are asked, the answers become not only pertinent diagnostic clues, but important early determinants of management. The questions will be considered again, this time to examine the answers:

1. Did the patient lose consciousness? If he did, it must be assumed that the patient HAS suffered injury to the brain. This patient must certainly be evalu-

ated in the emergency department. Remember: the amount of damage is directly proportionate to the duration of unconsciousness, which can be, in part, predicted by the amount of retrograde amnesia. If he has not lost consciousness, do *not* assume his brain is free of injury. Depending on the severity of the accident, the patient must still be evaluated for further injury or at least warned of sequelae to closed head trauma.

2. Was the patient moving all four extremities at the scene of injury? Motor response is an important neurologic baseline evaluation. Decortication or decerebration could imply extensive intracranial damage and might partially dictate treatment. Motor response is also an important factor in determining cervical spine injury.

3. If the patient was transported by fire aid vehicle or ambulance, what assessments were made by paramedical personnel? This information is frequently overlooked and must be stressed as highly important in the priorities of neurologic trauma assessment. If a third nerve palsy is detected in the emergency department, whether or not that pupil responded *originally* takes on paramount importance. If a third nerve lesion was originally missed in the neurologic assessment, expanding lesion might be excluded in diagnostic logic, and the lesion would be considered static as a result of the initial head injury until more blatant deteriorative signs appeared. The earlier the diagnosis is made, the earlier surgical intervention can be executed, early diagnosis is always a factor in a better patient prognosis. The same applies to deterioration of any neurologic findings prior to admission, especially if a fair amount of time has elapsed. The ease with which extrication occurs corresponds to time lost or gained prior to admission. This could influence proportion of blood lost, time hypoxia was tolerated, and many other critical factors including spinal cord status following cervical spine injury.

4. Does the patient have any bony deformities, discolorations, or drainage from the head? The first consideration would be to control hemorrhage. Discolarations, i.e., Battle's sign, may be suggestive if not pathognomonious of skull fracture.

5. Does the patient have drainage from eyes, ears, or nose? Pay particular attention to drainage from the ears and nose. It may be cerebrospinal fluid or even cortex otorrhea or rhinorrhea (cerebrospinal fluid orbitorrhea can occur, though rarely). Cerebrospinal leaks as otorrhea or rhinorrhea are commonly due to frontal or basilar skull fractures. The traditional rule is not to clean the ear for examination. However, most neurosurgeons will, being careful to use sterile technique. If they are familiar with the procedure, it may be requested of the professional nursing staff. Cerebrospinal fluid in the middle ear is difficult at best to detect; it often escapes into the eustachean tubes and presents as rhinorrhea. If rhinorrhea or otorrhea is suspected, the head of the bed should be elevated 15° to 20° to facilitate drainage. If it is difficult to ascertain the presence of cerebrospinal fluid, one of two methods may be util-

ized. First, if the drainage is *clear*, presence of cerebrospinal fluid may be confirmed by the positive action its reducing sugars have on the glucose test tapes commercially available. The sugars in blood always render sanguinous drainage a "false" positive; therefore, do not test serosanguinous drainage for glucose reaction. If the fluid is bloody, however, one can confirm the presence of cerebrospinal fluid by the clear halo of moisture that cerebrospinal fluid will create around a focus of pigmented blood stain on a clean piece of tissue or other porous paper. There is probably not a "name" for such a test, but it is used widely and is clinically accurate. If a patient does have rhinorrhea, avoid nasotracheal suctioning, avoid inserting a nasogastric tube, and do not allow the patient to blow his nose (this can dislodge cortex). It is wise to explain the reason for this prohibition to the patient, since he is less likely to cooperate if he does not understand. Blowing the nose is a social behavior, and any patient would have difficulty if asked to adhere to an unreasonable, unexplained, and hastily made rule.

Now the careful neurologic examination of the nervous system is performed and recorded. It may take time, but it proves worthwhile. *It must be done as soon as possible.*

Other considerations in conjunction with the neurologic examination are:

1. Careful examination of the entire patient is necessary. The head injury patient may have other major coincidental injuries that have gone unnoticed.

2. Frustration may be encountered when examining a patient who is intoxicated. Do as much as possible, and consider that most neurosurgeons wait, watch, and examine later. Neurologic signs can be misleading at best following depression of the central nervous system with ethanol. The patient's cooperation, or more likely lack of cooperation, may prevent careful or accurate evaluation.

3. For the most part we all labor under the illusion that a lumbar puncture is a useful diagnostic procedure, but in some circumstances it may be dangerous and harmful, allowing brain stem herniation. Do not anticipate a lumbar puncture being done if symptoms suggest the presence of an expanding lesion. This also applies to the use of osmotic diuretics. As previously explained, these drugs are not likely to be used if expanding lesion is suspected unless surgical decompression is soon planned.

Admission to Intensive Care Unit

The patient should be transferred to the intensive care unit when stabilized. Surgical intervention may precede this transfer. Following his admission to the intensive care unit, the nurse responsible for the patient should consider the following (the order and performance of which may vary, acording to the seriousness of the patient's condition):

1. Assess airway, oxygenation, and ventilation. Connect to ventilator as indicated. Carefully observe for increased restlessness, color changes, or other changes suggestive of respiratory distress or changes specific to an expanding lesion. Be prepared to relieve airway obstruction or apnea.

2. Assess vital parameters; heart rate, respiratory frequency, blood pressure, temperature, and EKG. Connect the patient to necessary monitoring equipment and observe serial readings. EKG monitoring is highly recommended as a useful guide in the evaluation of the head injury patient.

3. Do a baseline neurologic examination to determine the current clinical status of the patient.

4. Has pharmacological therapy been initiated? Did it include the administration of tetanus prophylaxis?

5. Address yourself to the psychological needs of the patient and family. Concern for the family and conscious support of their effort to adjust to the situation presented is a major aspect of nursing care planning. Arrange for the family to see the patient as soon as possible to allay fears; explain what is being done; if necessary, clarify the physician's explanation; get telephone numbers and record them in a convenient place for emergency use. Have the family decide on one person who is readily available to be the contact person and spokesman for the group. Should the patient deteriorate, nursing care is expedited by the necessity of one telephone call only.

6. Is the patient's religion known? If so, has pastoral care been notified when appropriate?

7. Make sure proper admission permits are signed. In the event of emergency surgical intervention, most neurosurgeons and hospitals require additional written permission. These permits must be readily available, and the procedure for completion of these documents must be well understood.

8. Craniotomy usually requires a type and crossmatch. If type and crossmatch has not been ordered, it may expedite matters greatly to obtain a venous clot (commonly placed in a "red top" tube), label it carefully, and either store it in the intensive care unit refrigerator or send it as a "hold" to the blood bank. This saves precious time when emergency surgery is scheduled and a type and crossmatch ordered.

9. Have emergency equipment nearby and ready for use: emergency respiratory equipment—suction apparatus, oxygen, endotracheal tube with laryngoscope, coniotomy or tracheostomy tray, and a respirator; emergency decompression equipment—clippers for hair removal, twist drill tray (Steinman pin tray can suffice); emergency drug tray.

10. Always know precisely where the attending neurologist or neurosurgeon is so he may be reached in an emergency.

INTERVENTION GENERAL TRAUMA: MODALITIES OF THERAPY

Nonoperative Management

The first priorities of management are establishing an airway, the support of shock, and the neurologic assessment. Careful and vigilant observation of the vital parameters and neurologic signs is of utmost importance and is therefore mentioned and emphasized again.

Cerebral edema may follow impact as a result of cellular and vascular trauma as metabolic toxins are released in lacerated and necrotic brain substance. Certainly hypoxia and hypercapnia complicate this vicious cycle. Cerebral edema is often difficult to treat; despite even vigorous therapy it often leads rapidly to death. Treatment includes preservation of adequate ventilation as first priority. Intracranial space-occupying lesion as well as large areas of necrotic brain tissue should be evacuated or debrided. Hypothermia, although once used, has been found to be of little value. If space-occupying lesion is not present and dynamic lesion is thought to be presenting, osmotic diuretics may be life-saving. Remember that in the presence of intracranial hemorrhage, shrinkage of the brain permits rapid expansion of the hemorrhage. The use of glucocorticosteriods, e.g., dexamethasone, has been found by most authorities to be valuable. Usually large doses are employed— dexamethasone 10 mg $\bar{q}$ 4 to 6 hours for 24 hours, then taper off in 10 days. If the patient is on steroid therapy, be alert for gastric bleeding; antacids may help reduce gastric irritation. Dehydration is not advised by most authorities. Intravenous therapy may be used two to three days. After this time, tube feeding is advisable for nutritional maintenance. Frequent determinations of electrolytes and serum osmolality are necessary to warn of hypotonicity or hypertonicity and other metabolic disturbances. Urinary output, urinary specific gravity, and daily weights are used as clues to hydration. Be alert for the development of diabetes insipidus and other water and electrolyte disturbances.

The incidence of seizures following head injury is extremely low. They are commonly caused by subarachnoid hemorrhage, intraventricular hemorrhage, cerebral concussion or contusion, laceration, or mass lesions. Focal seizures suggest discrete cerebral lesion; if not reported and promptly treated, they tend to become generalized. The use of anticonvulsive drugs, diphenylhydantoin (Dilantin) and phenobarbital, may be indicated. If the patient is having continuous seizures which may simulate status epilepticus, IV medication may include phenobarbital, thiopental, diazepam, or amobarbital.

Vomiting occurs uncommonly in patients with head injury. The milder the injury, the more common vomiting is. It is rare in severe head injury. It may occur as the patient regains consciousness or be associated with attacks of vertigo that accompany vestibular trauma. Aspiration must be prevented by placing the patient in the prone position with the face to one side or by using a nasogastric tube and aspirating gastric contents.

The safety and security of the patient are important. Elevate the head of the bed 15° to 45°, frequently turn the patient from side to side, and avoid the supine position, particularly if the patient's level of consciousness is depressed. Early and constant attention to proper positioning is necessary to prevent contractures.

Surgical Management

All operative procedures for trauma may be divided into three main groups: trephinations, exploration for elevation of depressed fractures, and exploration for debridement of the brain. Most intracranial hematomas can be evacuated through trephinal openings, and although the trephines are routinely enlarged, it is rarely necessary to turn craniotomy flaps. Surgical intervention of bleeds can be further discussed considering their anatomical location: epidural, subdural, or intracerebral.

Epidural exploration is carried out using trephine openings, usually made in the subtemporal, frontal coronal, and posterior parietal areas. These trephinations may be performed in the emergency department, ICU, or the operating room. In extremely grave situations, trephines can be performed in ICU using a twist drill. This small twist drill (Burton-Blacker) with a bit less than one-half inch is used infrequently because of the danger of missing significant collections of blood unable to pass through needles. Since an intraventricular tap may be done through the drill holes, patients with suspected massive intraventricular hemorrhage may be candidates for such drilling. When the burr holes are drilled, using the larger burr drill to facilitate better visual contact with the operative field, the skin and muscle (where applicable) are first incised, the skull is opened near the fracture line, and the opening is enlarged to about the size of a silver dollar (Fig. 5-10). After the clot is removed, the bleeding point can be identified and either ligated or electrocauterized. The dura is then generally opened so that the subdural space can be inspected for hematoma and cerebral injury. After closure the dura is tented to the bone. Commonly epidural drains are left in place for 24 hours or so.

Subdural hematoma must be similarly evacuated. However, the type of procedure depends usually on the status of the clot (liquid in first two days, solid thereafter). Trephine openings are placed in the skull, usually two that are spaced apart, and the clot is then washed out, using a rubber catheter and sterile isotonic saline. Subdural drains are often left in the space and connected to sterile flasks (such as empty IV containers) for 24 to 48 hours. If appropriate the subdural drain may be connected via a stopcock to a manometer or more sophisticated monitoring device. (See Chapter 3, under "Intracranial Pressure Monitoring.")

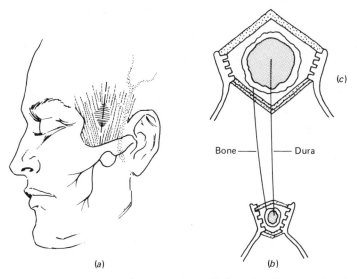

Fig. 5-10. Trephination. The method of performing trepine openings for evacuation of subdural and/or epidural hematoma. (a) Location of temporal trephine opening under the temporalis muscle. (b) A small (approximately 1.5 cm) trephine opening. The skin is retracted with small mastoid retractors. (c) The opening rongeured to the size of a silver dollar (approximately 5 cm).

Open depressed skull fractures require operative intervention to prevent infection, remove foreign bodies, remove necrotic material, remove complicating hematomas, and minimize post-injury sequelae. After opening of the scalp, fragments of fractured bone are carefully removed, leaving a well-defined bony defect that can be repaired months later. If fragments are not extremely comminuted and contamination is minimal, many surgeons save the fragments to form a bony cranioplasty. This practice apparently works well. Since the inner layer of the skull usually shows more damage than the outer layer, a small burr hole is frequently made adjacent to the fracture in order to gain acess to remove bone. Bone fragments that are deeply penetrating are removed under direct vision so as not to damage cerebral tissue. If a major dural sinus is lacerated, careful manipulation is required. The earlier-performed wide bony defect permits control of hemorrhage that is bound to follow and allows the surgeon to repair the torn dura. When the dura is torn, underlying cortex is observed and debrided when necessary by gentle suction; nonviable dura is removed. Dural lacerations are repaired, and grafts are used to replace and repair defects. Penetrating wounds are debrided and excised early and carefully; complications are managed as described above. If bone or metal fragments are allowed to remain in the brain, abscess and infection may occur. Massive intracranial hemorrhage may occur with low- or high-velocity missile wounds. High-velocity missiles usually cause extensive cerebral destruction; often debridement is all that can be offered to these patients. In some cases in fact the fragments must be left in place to prevent additional brain damage from cranial incision and exploration. Injuries to the dural sinuses usually involve the sagittal and transverse sinuses. With depressed fractures, bleeding rarely occurs until the wound is debrided and the bone fragment removed that was tamponading the tear. Therefore, the neurosurgeon must be ready for rapid, severe hemorrhage. The sagittal sinus is occasionally ligated (only, however, in the anterior portion) without resulting profound neurologic deficit. Tears are repaired by suturing or grafting. Tears of transverse and lateral sinuses are usually doubly ligated.

NURSING OBJECTIVES GENERAL TRAUMA

Care of the patient in ICU revolves around the following guidelines:

1. Maintain airway, and attend to pulmonary toilet to prevent further complications.

2. Assess, evaluate, and manage vital parameters; blood pressure, heart rate, EKG, respiratory pattern, and temperature (maintain normothermia).

3. Establish a baseline neurologic examination, and record data on return from operating room.

4. Make neurologic checks a minimum of every 15 to 30 minutes to observe for complicating cerebral edema or increasing intracranial pressure from other sources. Neurologic assessment will vary somewhat according to the patient's condition, level of consciousness, and nature of injury. It is always best discussed with the operating surgeon immediately after return of the patient from the operating room or emergency department.

5. Monitor hourly urine output and specific gravity when indicated. Pay attention to fluid balance, state of hydration, nutrition, and electrolyte status.

6. Maintain a comfortable, safe, and therapeutic environment for the patient. Elevate the head of the bed; position frequently, if indicated; apply ice bags to orbital region; administer analgesics when appropriate to maintain comfort as long as it does not conflict with other objectives.

7. Ensure patency of other tubes. Note color, consistency, amount, and pH of nasogastric drainage.

8. Provide preventive measures for further bodily complications. This includes active and passive range of motion exercises for prevention of deep leg thrombosis, prevention of infection, and preservation of the patient's physiological defenses.

9. Be prepared to observe and manage seizures.

AFFECTIVE REALM

The Nurse

The intensive care nurse commonly deals with a variety of trauma. Patients involved in attempted suicide or homicide may interfere with her moral statutes beyond compromise. Until this personal conflict is resolved, offering psychological support to the patient would be detrimental.

The patient with head injury may appear revolting, ugly, and deformed. The nurse may consciously have to focus on the person beneath the devastating body image in order to function effectively. Meaningful communication must be established with the patient in a manner that reflects acceptance and respect for the individual and his reactions and concerns.

The patient's behavior may be expressing anger, fear, grief, or frustration. He may be irritable, forgetful, or anxious. The nurse may have to call forth all of her resources to remain stable in dealing with this patient in severe crisis. A psychological assessment of the patient's strengths will place the interaction on a more positive level and assist the patient and nurse in reaching a degree of adjustment in their relationship.

The nurse–patient relationship in the intensive care unit may not be long-term, but certainly attitudes developed by the patient at this time can be the beginning of necessary change on his long road to recovery.

The Patient

Consider the absence of normal physiological functions the patient with trauma encounters. He may not be able to chew, hear, see, talk, or smell. The contours of his face, jaw, and skull may all be abnormal.

The loss of functional capabilities and his destroyed self-image may provoke feelings of helplessness and hopelessness.

The Interactive Process

The nurse–patient relationship having been established, let us look at the interactive process.

People customarily deal cognitively in interpersonal relationships. We give and receive factual information in response to queries, and are thus protected from involvement; facts are safe and comfortable. Nurses, trained in a scientific discipline, approach patients on a cognitive level. Patients, void of their usual defense mechanisms, are often apprehensive, fearful, and hurting. These are feelings in the affective domain, which are sometimes positively overwhelming for the patient. A practitioner, skilled in active listening, is often able to discover clues that reveal the patient's present state of emotions.

Remember—*you cannot solve an emotional problem on an intellectual level.*

The literature suggests several techniques for offering psychological support to the injured patient: establish an accepting, caring relationship; begin where the patient is, i.e., in the here and now, full of anxiety, anger, and frustrations; allow the patient to ventilate his feelings, experiencing them to the fullest; reflect his feelings with empathy. All of these suggestions are worth consideration by the individual nurse. Whatever skills are utilized, they become integrated in the person, a result that is possible only if the nurse is comfortable using the techniques she has adopted.

Occasionally it becomes necessary to assist the patient in developing new coping mechanisms. His self-concept may be destroyed, and he may believe his self-image to be unredeemable. Sometimes a program in value clarification becomes necessary for the patient whose life-style and appearance have been altered by injury.

There will come a time when problem solving and decision making become purposeful. One way to reactivate the patient's adaptive process is to reestablish his sense of control. The patient has the right to be part of the decision-making process, which involves setting goals for his rehabilitation.

A good resource person to generate ideas and foster viable alternatives is invaluable to the patient.

The Family

The trauma patient does not enter the hospital alone. His ecosystem requires the inclusion of the family with regard to information, condition, and therapy. Often the family perceives destruction and inevitable death in a serious crisis. The nurse can make herself available to the family, identifying their stress level and evaluating their support systems.

Society

The trauma patient returns to social interaction even while in the intensive care unit. How do other patients perceive his injury and disfigurement? Do friends visit or avoid him? All of these things must be considered through the acute phase, as well as when the patient begins the long road to rehabilitation. His functional limitations may prohibit his return to his occupation.

The nurse is well advised to seek the professional psychological support of available consultants. It is this author's experience that the help of such a consultant greatly benefits patients, relatives, nursing staff, and neurosurgeons. In the years spent in a neurosurgical trauma ICU, an experienced psychiatric nurse joined the staff and was heavily relied upon for advice, counseling, and patient care (for patients, families, and staff). The resulting difference in morale, professional attitude, and quality of services rendered left an impression deep enough to warrant urging of all ICU staffs to seek the same assistance. Coping with the mortality in a neurosurgical ICU is in itself sufficient reason to seek additional counseling. The rewards of having such a person on the team are bountiful. Mental health is preserved for all.

CONCLUSION

We have explained the pathophysiology and symptomatology of head injuries for the purpose of giving the nurse an understanding of the problems that may develop for the patient. The nursing assessment of the situation becomes vital in setting priorities. The scope of intervention encompasses a multidisciplinary team effort if the patient is going to survive or adapt to a high level of wellness. The head injury patient needs to feel as much "in control" of his life as possible. The nurse–patient relationship will become a vehicle for evaluating progress toward mutual goals. Nursing care plans will necessarily become modified as wounds heal and coping mechanisms strengthen.

The critical care nurse can assist the trauma patient who is striving to live his life to the fullest within such limitations as may be imposed by disease.

BIBLIOGRAPHY

Ballinger, W., Robert B. Rutherford, and George Zuidema, eds., *The Mangement of Trauma*, Philadelphia: W.B. Saunders Co., 1973.

Chusid, Joseph G., *Correlative Neuroanatomy and Functional Neurology*, 5th ed., Los Altos, California: Lange Med. Pub. Co., 1973.

Elliot, Frank S., *Clinical Neurology*, 2nd ed., Philadelphia: W. B. Saunders Co., 1973.

Gardner, Ernest, Donald Gray, and Ronan O'Rahilly, *Anatomy*, Philadelphia: W. B. Saunders Co., 1974.

"Glossary on Head Injury," Prepared by a Committee of the Congress of Neurosurgeons, *Clin. Neurosurgery*, 12, Spring 1966.

Gurdjian, E. S., V. R. Hodgson, L. M. Thomas, and L. M. Patrice, "Significance of Relative Movements of Scalp, Skull, and Intracranial Contents during Impact Injury of the Head," *Journal of Nerosurgery*, 29:70, 1968.

Gurdjian, E. S., and L. M. Thomas, "Surgical Management of the Patient With Head Injury," *Clin. Neurosurgery*, 12:56–73, 1965.

Guyton, Arthur, *Textbook of Medical Physiology*, 5th ed., Philadelphia: W. B. Saunders Co., 1976.

Jackson, Frederick E., "The Pathophysiology of Head Injuries," *Clinical Symposia*, Summit New Jersey: CIBA Pharmaceutical Co., Vol. 18, No. 3, 1967.

Jackson, Frederick E., "The Treatment of Head Injuries," *Clinical Symposia*, Summit, New Jersey: CIBA Pharmaceutical Co., Vol. 19, No. 1, 1966.

Jamieson, Kenneth G., *A First Notebook of Head Injury*, 2nd ed., Boston: Butterworth Pub., 1971.

Kahn, E. A., et al., *Correlative Neurosurgery*, 7th ed., Springfield, Ill.: Charles C. Thomas, 1969.

Lopez-Antunez, Luis, *Atlas of Human Anatomy*, Philadelphia: W. B. Saunders Co., 1971.

Luckmann, Joan, and Karen Sorensen, *Medical-Surgical Nursing*, Philadelphia: W. B. Saunders Co., 1974.

Miller, Benjamin F., and Claire Brackman Keane, *Encyclopedia and Dictionary of Medicine and Nursing*, Philadelphia: W. B. Saunders Co., 1972.

Plum, F., and J. B. Posner, *The Diagnosis of Stupor and Coma*, Philadelphia: F. A. Davis Co., 1966.

Warwick, Roger, and Peter L. Williams, *Gray's Anatomy*, Philadelphia: W. B. Saunders Co., 1975.

Youmans, Julian R., *Neurological Surgery*, Vols. 1, 2, and 3, Philadelphia: W. B. Saunders Co., 1973.

6
SPINAL CORD INJURY

INTRODUCTION

Interruption of the spinal column and its contents inflicts such severe limitations on bodily structural design that few nonfatal injuries equal its devastating physical and psychological disability. No other traumatic insult can result in such clinical devastation in proportion to the extent of injured tissue; these lesions are not only adversely unique but also truly pernicious. Accurate statistics reflecting the incidence of spinal column injury in the United States are unavailable; neither are there figures reflecting the percent of people who develop neurologic dysfunctions after spinal column trauma. It has been *estimated* that approximately 10,000 people become victims of severe spinal cord injury every year; 50% of these patients become quadriplegics, and 50% become paraplegics.[1]

Nurses attending patients with spinal cord injury have a very difficult but extremely satisfying role. The most critical period post injury for these patients is the first 24 hours. Emergency room nurses and critical care nurses become primary patient advocates during this time when damage to the cord may be prevented, arrested, or reversed. The philosophy of preservation and restoration of optimum level of functioning must be sustained throughout the episodic and distributive phases in the care and management of patients with injury to the spinal cord.

DYNAMIC MECHANISMS OF INJURY

Spinal column trauma may be classified simply as closed or open injuries. An example of the former would be an automobile accident or fall, and an example of the latter would be a penetrating missile wound. Obviously, the critical factor in both closed and open injuries is the resultant damage to, or interruption of, the neural contents of the spinal column. Therapy must be aimed at achieving a delicate balance between mobility and stability of the neck and trunk, as well as protection of the spinal nerve roots and the cord. Management of these patients is influenced by the mechanics of each injury as well as the extent of injuries.

---

[1]Crigler, Lee, "Sexual Concerns of the Spinal Cord–Injured," *Nursing Clinics of North America,* 9 (No. 4):pp. 703–715, December 1974.

Closed Injuries

Unfortunately, the areas of the vertebral volumn that allow the greatest mobility are relatively unstable because the muscular and articular supports are inadequate when resisting violent forces. These areas of greatest vulnerability are: the junctional region between the lower three cervical vertebrae; the junctional region between the thoracic and lumbar spine; and the junctional region between the lumbar and sacral spine.

Hyperflexion injuries. Extreme flexion injuries are the most common type of severe spinal cord trauma (Fig. 6-1). Flexion injuries occur when direct or indirect violence produces extreme movement of a portion of the spine beyond its normal range of motion. Two common illustrations of this type of injury are provided by: the person who suddenly decelerates in a head-on vehicular collision; and the person who inadvertently dives into shallow water. In flexion injuries there is a wedging force on the adjacent vertebra which often crushes it, driving bony fragments posteriorly into the spinal canal. The fracture may be dislocated forward onto the lower vertebrae; this occurs when the posterior longitudinal ligaments or the articular ligaments are torn. The severity of flexion injuries is primarily determined by the suddenness and force of impact. The degree of damage to the spinal cord is determined by the extent of encroachment by the dislocated or fractured vertebrae.

Hyperextension injuries. When the cervical spine is extended to the extreme, the spinal cord is stretched against the ligamenta flava, which may contuse the dorsal columns or even cause posterior dislocation of the vertebrae (Fig. 6-1). The elderly are particularly prone to hyperextension injuries in accidents, such as when they fall striking the chin. Gerontologists have discovered the problem of the narrowing of the spinal column by osteoarthritic spurs, as well as a thickening of the ligamenta flava reducing its elasticity and threatening the integrity of the cord blood supply. The main stress in injuries of this nature is tolerated in the central portion of the spinal cord, causing acute central cervical cord injury syndrome. This syndrome is attributed to cord compression as well as an interruption of the cervical cord blood supply. Hence both contusion and ischemia may produce severe cord damage *even* in the absence of a fractured or dislocated vertebra.

Subluxation injuries. Subluxation (complete or incomplete dislocation) deformities usually occur with vertebral fractures. When bony fragments are subluxed into the spinal column, injury to the spinal cord may or may not occur; the spinal cord occupies only one-half of the spinal column and may occasionally be spared.

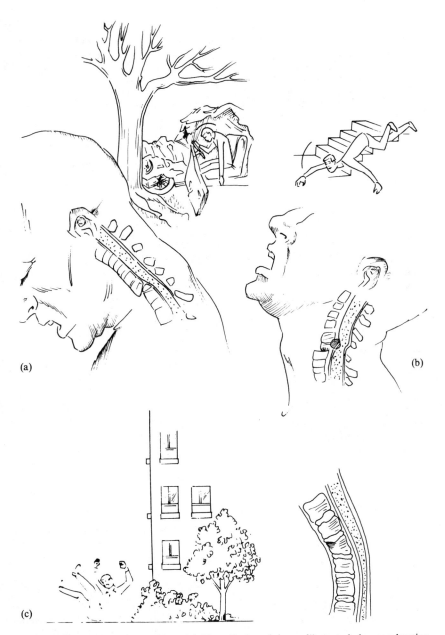

Fig. 6-1. Mechanisms of injury. (a) Hyperflexion injury; illustrated by acceleration-deceleration. (b) Hyperextension injury; illustrated by a fall in which victim lands on head. (c) Compression injury; illustrated by a fall in which the victim lands on buttocks.

Acceleration injuries. Cervical cord injury may occur when the head suddenly accelerates relative to the trunk. The result is the common "whiplash" injury associated with rear-end automobile collisions. The mechanism of injury to the cord is the hyperextension that occurs as the neck recoils. Most people who sustain an injury of this nature suffer noncomplicated muscle strain; but nerve root injury, subluxation, or fracture of the vertebrae may occur.

Compression injuries. This type of injury may occur as a person falls from some distance landing on the feet or buttocks (Fig. 6-1). There is a compression of the lower thoracic and lumbar vertebrae which may be severe enough to produce a fracture. The muscular and ligament supports of these vertebrae are a bit stronger and less mobile in comparison to cervical vertebrae and are, therefore, protected from subluxation.

Special fractures. Two special fractures will be mentioned: "tear-drop" fracture and "hangman's" fracture.

"Tear-drop" fracture. A "tear-drop" fracture is one in which the anterior corner of the vertebra is separated from the rest of the vertebral body. This fracture usually occurs as a result of severe flexion or hyperextension injuries and is usually associated with the protuberance of disc material and subsequent neurologic deficits. This type of injury, therefore, requires early aggressive management.

"Hangman's" fracture. This injury occurs when there is a fracture through the lamina of the axis and, commonly, subluxation of the second cervical vertebra onto the third cervical vertebra. This cervical spine fracture is similar to the injury incurred in judicial hangings, hence the name "hangman's" fracture.

Open Injuries

Open injuries to the spinal column may be caused by missile wounds or stab wounds. Both types of injury usually cause compound fractures of the vertebrae, which are usually stable and do not require fusion procedures.

Missile wounds. Severe cord injury, including transection, occurs commonly when a foreign object directly penetrates the spinal column. Explosive blasts or high-velocity bullets may bypass the spinal column but leave a pressure shock wave that causes injury to the cord. The transection injuries of missile wounds are extremely serious; the prognosis is doubtful for the patient who is immediately rendered quadriplegic or paraplegic by a gunshot wound.

Stab wounds. Knife wounds of the cervical and thoracic spine are common injuries, producing cerebrospinal fluid leakage and a clinical picture of hemisection (partial transection) of the cord called the Brown-Séguard syndrome. (See next section.)

MANIFESTATIONS OF SPINAL CORD INJURIES

The patients with spinal cord injuries who require admission to the intensive care unit have suffered injury at the midthoracic level or above. These patients, unlike patients with other spinal cord injuries, demand intensive care primarily for cardiovascular and respiratory support. The majority of these patients will present with symptoms suggesting one of the following syndromes: spinal shock syndrome, Brown-Séguard syndrome, central cervical or anterior cord injury syndrome.

Spinal Shock Syndrome

The complete and sudden transection of the spinal cord results in spinal shock. The following symptoms develop *at* or *below* the segmental level of the lesion:

1. Complete flaccid paralysis of all skeletal musculature
2. Absence of all spinal reflexes
3. Absence of all cutaneous sensation
4. Absence of all proprioceptive sensation
5. Transient urinary retention
6. Transient fecal retention

The complete transection of the cord at or above the third cervical vertebra is incompatible with life. The vital functions impaired in this situation are respiratory control, cardiovascular control, and body temperature regulation. Although transection of the cord below the second thoracic vertebra spares the upper extremities, the loss of autonomic function still results in vasomotor instability such as orthostatic hypotension.

Spinal shock generally persists in survivors for one to six weeks with progressive recovery in six to twelve months. The sequence of symptoms in the recovery phase is summarized in Table 6-1.

The recovery phase of a patient with a cord transection from flaccid paralysis to extensor or flexor rigidity is explained on the basis of "spinal automatisms," which are automatic spinal reflex activities that eventually function after transection when the brain no longer influences movements. These spinal automatisms are primitive spinal mechanisms normally inhibited by higher centers and now released from cerebral control. Examples of spinal automatisms are: flexor spasms invoked by cutaneous stimulation, reflex emptying of the bladder and bowel, and reflex priapism or ejaculation in the male invoked by cutaneous stimulation. (See Table 6-1.)

Brown-Séguard Syndrome

Brown-Séguard syndrome occurs after a transverse hemisection of the spinal cord interrupting the lateral half of the cord (on either side) above the level of the lumbar segments. The result is homolateral (symptoms occurring on the same side of the body as the lesion) upper motor neuron paralysis, vasomotor paralysis, and loss of position and vibratory sensation below the level of the lesion. There are contralateral (symptoms occurring on the opposite side of the body as the lesion) loss of pain and temperature sensation below the level of the lesion. This syndrome rarely appears in pure clinical form; therefore, the essential feature is considered to be the presence of homolateral spastic weakness with loss of contralateral sensation (pain and temperature). Myelography is generally done for precise lesion location, as sensory loss on the trunk has been shown to be an unreliable indicator of lesion location.

Central Cervical Cord Injury Syndrome

This syndrome may occur with hyperextension injuries or interruption of the blood supply to the spinal cord. Also called central cord syndrome, it is characterized by a disproportionately greater weakness in the upper extremities than the lower extremities, possibly because the arm and hand fibers of the upper motor neuron lie more centrally in the cord than the leg fibers. Since it is usually central edema and/or hemorrhage exerting pressure on the anterior horn cells (upper motor neuron) that causes symptoms, recovery of these cells is to be expected without surgical intervention.

Anterior Cord Injury Syndrome

This syndrome may result from acute anterior spinal cord compression (e.g., bone fragments or disc) or mechanical destruction of the anterior cord (e.g., anterior spinal artery occlusion). Anterior cord injury syndrome is characterized by immediate, complete paralysis, hypesthesia, and hypalgesia below the level of the lesion with preservation of the posterior column sensations of touch, motion, position, and vibration. Myelography followed by a decompressive laminectomy is usually performed.

ASSESSMENT AND PRIORITY INTERVENTION
Emergency Stabilization and Evaluation

Recognition of injury. Certain observations can be made when examining a patient suspected of spinal cord injury. These clues will assist the examiner in discovering the nature and extent of injury.

Table 6-1. Progressive Recovery Symptoms

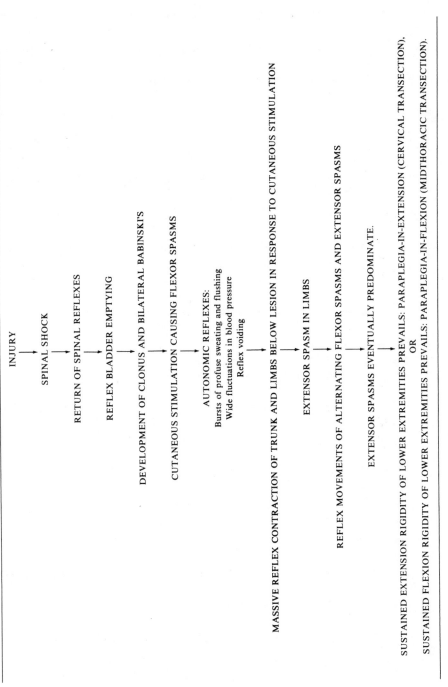

INJURY

→ SPINAL SHOCK

→ RETURN OF SPINAL REFLEXES

→ REFLEX BLADDER EMPTYING

→ DEVELOPMENT OF CLONUS AND BILATERAL BABINSKI'S

→ CUTANEOUS STIMULATION CAUSING FLEXOR SPASMS

→ AUTONOMIC REFLEXES:
Bursts of profuse sweating and flushing
Wide fluctuations in blood pressure
Reflex voiding

→ MASSIVE REFLEX CONTRACTION OF TRUNK AND LIMBS BELOW LESION IN RESPONSE TO CUTANEOUS STIMULATION

→ EXTENSOR SPASM IN LIMBS

→ REFLEX MOVEMENTS OF ALTERNATING FLEXOR SPASMS AND EXTENSOR SPASMS

→ EXTENSOR SPASMS EVENTUALLY PREDOMINATE.

SUSTAINED EXTENSION RIGIDITY OF LOWER EXTREMITIES PREVAILS: PARAPLEGIA-IN-EXTENSION (CERVICAL TRANSECTION),
OR
SUSTAINED FLEXION RIGIDITY OF LOWER EXTREMITIES PREVAILS: PARAPLEGIA-IN-FLEXION (MIDTHORACIC TRANSECTION).

1. Does the patient have difficulty moving the lower extremities upon command?
2. Does the patient have difficulty moving the upper extremities upon command?
3. Can the presence of a sensory level by pinprick be determined?
4. Does the patient complain of pain in the neck or back?
5. Is there gross deformity present or any tenderness to palpation?
6. Is the patient unconscious?
7. Is the patient unconscious with forehead lacerations or abrasions?
8. Is there a penetrating object in view?

Special precautions. Everyone ministering care to the spinal cord injury patient must exercise sound judgment during this period of stabilization and evaluation.

1. Continually evaluate the patient's airway.
2. Prevent any further movement of the spine.
3. Support the patient's head and neck at all times.
4. Sandbag both sides of the head to prevent rotation.
5. Maintain firm, manual, longitudinal head traction when moving the patient; log-roll the patient to ensure spinal alignment at all times.
6. Keep the patient on a fracture board.
7. Keep the patient in the supine position.
8. Do not allow the patient to sit up.

Initial assessment and Priority Intervention. After initial resuscitation the following areas should be assessed and appropriate action taken.

Ventilation. Determine the adequacy of the patient's respiratory status. Provide for an adequate airway, suctioning when necessary. Extreme caution is employed with intubating the patient or when a tracheostomy is performed until the integrity of the cervical cord is ensured.

Major coincidental injuries. A rapid evaluation of the total situation is done for the purpose of establishing the presence of other major injuries. Intervention is based on the presence of life-threatening problems at this time in the emergency room. Secondary problems will be reassessed and appropriate intervention initiated when the patient is admitted to the intensive care unit for more definitive treatment.

Shock syndrome. Assess the patient for cardiovascular problems that may present as the shock syndrome. Hypotension may be present in the spinal cord injury patient because of loss of sympathetic vasomotor tone; it is usually corrected by elevating the patient's legs.

Neurologic assessment. A rapid neurologic assessment should be performed (see page 77). In addition to data collection, if the patient is paraplegic or quadriplegic, an indwelling urinary catheter is inserted to prevent damage from an overdistended, flaccid, urinary bladder.

If at all possible, the critical care nurse should be present in the emergency room during the emergency stabilization and evaluation of the spinal cord injury patient. The information obtained at this time will become the baseline for future assessment when the patient is admitted to the intensive care unit. In addition, the critical care nurse may be able to interact with the patient and the family at a very critical point in this traumatic episode.

Admission to the Intensive Care Unit

The patient will be admitted to the intensive care unit when: the vital processes are stable, immobilization is accomplished, and diagnostic and radiographic procedures have been completed. The patient will require a more complete assessment at this time (see page 140). A complete respiratory, cardiovascular, and neurologic assessment is important. The respiratory assessment of the patient with spinal cord injury requires special mention, depending, of course, on the level of cord injury. The following questions may be used as guides for gathering essential information:

1. Does the patient have an adequate airway, and, if so, is the air exchange sufficient? Is the patient alert and oriented?
2. Have arterial blood gases been drawn? What are the results, and are they appropriate for the patient's age and general health status?
3. Is the patient's color reflective of adequate alveolar ventilation, or is he dusky, cyanotic, or flushed?
4. Is the patient restless? Are there any indications of respiratory distress such as flaring nares?
5. Does the patient feel as though he is getting enough air?
6. Does the paralysis include the diaphragmatic and/or the intercostal muscles?
7. Does auscultation of the lungs reveal clear, deep ventilation? Are breath sounds equal bilaterally? Are there any adventitous sounds?
8. What is the respiratory rate, depth, and rhythm?

Discuss pertinent findings with the neurosurgeon and assist with procedures when respiratory assistance is required.

If the patient is already intubated or has a tracheostomy, answer the following questions:

1. Is the patient assisting with ventilation? What is his spontaneous frequency?

2. What is the patient's spontaneous tidal volume and minute volume? Are they appropriate for his age and general health status?
3. Are the arterial blood gases adequate?
4. Does the patient require suctioning?
5. Is the ventilator set up appropriately? Discuss the appropriate mechanical assistance with the anesthesiologist or respiratory therapist.

INTERVENTION: MODALITIES OF THERAPY

Skeletal Traction

The application of skeletal traction for the patient with a cervical spine injury warrants explanation. This procedure will be presented in outline form for clarity and simplicity.

Equipment

1. Stryker frame, Foster frame, or Circ Olectric bed with fresh linen.
2. Vinke tongs preferred, or substitute: Crutchfield tongs, Cone, Gardner-Wells Skull Calipers.
3. Sterile tray containing drill. A special drill is part of Vinke equipment.
4. Local anesthetic of choice; e.g., 1% lidocaine.
5. Surgical antiseptic of choice; e.g., betadine.
6. Razor and/or clippers.
7. Variety of needles for anesthesia.
8. Syringe.
9. Scalpel with blade #15 or #21.
10. Suture material for scalp closure.
11. Dressings.
12. Surgical gloves.
13. Surgical light.
14. Mayo stand.
15. Traction apparatus set up on bed or frame with 5-pound weights.

Procedure

1. The patient must be placed on the frame of choice prior to the procedure. Carefully connect and arrange tubes (such as respirator, nasogastric and urinary catheters) for convenience and patency. Connect the patient cable to the cardiac monitor.
2. Shave and prepare bilateral areas of the scalp: above the thin area of the temporal bone and along an imaginary line between the external auditory meatus and the transverse process of the cervical vertebrae.
3. The physician will then infiltrate these areas with a local anesthetic.

4. A scalpel is used to incise the scalp, and then the Vinke drill is used to penetrate the outer table of the skull.

5. The Vinke tong points are then inserted through the holes and fastened into the skull by the opening of a small flange between the inner and outer tables of the skull. This flange prevents the tongs from dislodging or slipping through the outer table. Vinke tongs are preferred primarily for this feature.

6. The skin is sutured closed around the tongs, and dressings are applied.

7. Ropes connected to the tongs, placed over pulleys, now receive the 5-pound weights, producing traction.

8. The neurosurgeon applies the traction initially, using the following guidelines:

Nondisplaced fracture: 5–10 pounds
Dislocated fracture: 10–15 pounds
Additional traction is applied as necessary up to 45–50 pounds.

The patient may be placed in a position of hyperextension to provide the fullest benefit of the traction. This will be determined by the neurosurgeon.

Nursing implications:

1. *Turning and positioning:* Patients with Vinke tongs or any other cervical traction device must be turned and repositioned at least every two hours. The purpose, of course, is to allay the hazards of immobility. This includes turning the patient from side to side as well as anterior-posterior if the patient is on the Circ Olectric bed or Stryker frame. For details concerning the manipulation of these beds or frames, the nurse should consult procedure books and survey the manufacturer's product literature. It should be stressed that the patient in skeletal traction on such a frame must be turned by *at least two* critical care nurses. This practice is deemed necessary for the purpose of: reassuring the anxious patient, adjusting and caring for the "inevitable tubes" during turning, maintaining traction, and checking the bolts and other mechanical devices. It is a catastrophe to have tongs slip or to have half of the frame fall off during the turning procedure. Such a thing occurs infrequently, but to have it happen just once is a disaster. A rigid procedure should be established for two nurses to turn the patient, checking and double-checking the bolts to ensure patient safety and security.

2. *Patient and family education:* The patient and the family should both be totally familiar with the traction device, bed, or frame. They should be clearly aware that sudden movements by the patient should be avoided to prevent the interruption of callus formation.

3. Preservation and restoration of physiologic function and goal setting for these patients are considered on page 162.

Lumbar Puncture

A lumbar puncture is performed as soon as the site of spinal injury has been stabilized. The patient is placed in the prone position after the application of traction. Primarily, the procedure is done to determine the presence of a cerebrospinal fluid block, which suggests cord compression. A Queckenstedt test is done (see page 90). If there is no associated rise in spinal fluid pressure, manual abdominal compression is performed. This technique rules out a manometric block. A positive Queckenstedt test indicates a spinal column blockage and necessitates a myelogram and surgical intervention.

Operative Management

The operative management of patients with spinal cord injury consists of decompression, fusion, or debridement. Any presence of shock syndrome or respiratory distress will influence the mortality rate of these operative procedures. Patients with cervical injuries will have skeletal traction maintained *before, during,* and *after* surgery. Procedures are performed while the patient remains on the frame or Circ Olectric bed. If intubation is required, it will be done cautiously, avoiding manipulation of the head and neck.

Decompression. The surgical procedure of decompression is performed when there is evidence of mechanical compression of the spinal cord or its nerve roots. It is usually warranted when: progressive neurologic deficit is present; manometric (Queckenstedt) or myelographic block is present; bony fragments are projecting into the spinal canal; or there is injury to the conus medullaris or the cauda equina.

Fusion. A fusion is performed to provide internal operative stabilization of a fracture; however, external stabilization with skeletal traction *alone* will result in a spontaneous fusion within six to eight weeks. Therefore, operative fusion is indicated selectively for comminuted fractures and "tear-drop" cervical fractures. These two types of fracture tend to heal by a fibrous union that poses a risk of instability and cord compression in future months or years. Fusion may also be employed for patients with a cervical fracture that is rapidly reduced with skeletal traction, indicating considerable ligamentous disruption. Although fusion offers the physical and psychological advantage of early mobilization, the patient still requires some form of *external* stabilization for six to eight weeks postoperatively. This can be accomplished by the continued use of tongs or a halo fixation. The latter permits sitting and ambulation.

Debridement. Debridement for retained foreign bodies is performed by doing a laminectomy, which tends to offset the development of scar tissue.

Left alone, this scar tissue may produce pain and increase the neuronal damage.

New Therapeutic Approaches

Several new therapies are being investigated in the treatment of spinal cord injuries: corticosteroids, local hypothermia, osmotic diuretics, anti–norepinephrine synthesis drugs (norepinephrine is thought to produce hemorrhagic necrosis at the site of injury through local accumulation), and hyperbaric oxygenation. Corticosteroids and local hypothermia are currently being utilized in humans and will be discussed here.

Corticosteroids. It has been suggested that an anti-inflammatory effect can be derived from the administration of steroids (see page 265) for one to two weeks. The disadvantage is the depressing effect of steroids on the secretion of mucoprotein, thereby increasing the risk of stress ulceration.

Local Hypothermia. This therapy is initiated after the cord is surgically exposed in the operating room. The operative wound, with exposed dura or cord, serves as a reservoir for ice-cold saline at 2° to 3° C. The saline is pumped in by a perfusion circuit at 100–500 milliliters per minute. The procedure continues for about three hours, after which the perfusate is removed and routine closure of the wound follows. Early studies indicate that this technique may reduce the degree of cord injury incurred.

BIOPSYCHOSOCIAL PROCESS

It has been said that tragedy and sorrow never leave us where they find us. The paraplegic or quadriplegic patient presents a complex nursing challenge: the critical care nurse becomes a tool for his biological, mental, and social redevelopment. Effective teaching in the cognitive, psychomotor, and affective domains is extremely important if the patient is going to lead a useful, personally rewarding life. The entire health team must focus on a common objective: the restoration of the patient to an optimum adjustment to life in spite of his paralysis.

Affective Realm

The affective realm is a difficult area for the nurse to deal with. The critical care nurse is compelled to deal with technology for the preservation of life. This orientation does not readily lend itself to the psychological needs of the patient, and it will take a conscious effort for the nurse to focus on the patient's feeling level. Some feelings that may be present in the patient's agony of need are: hostility, depression, withdrawal, fear, insecurity, frustration, and/or hopelessness. The patient has a distinct need to know that someone understands how he feels. He may go through several phases simultaneously and/or repetitively, causing him conflict and confusion about how he does feel. Various defense mechanisms will be employed, protecting his ego system.

The patient may have to learn new methods of coping with his feelings about his immobility, the medical regimen, and the medical personnel. There may be a period of time in which he is working through the grief process, owing to the loss of self-image, self-direction, and his independence. The idea of immobilization is probably a new one that will require a maximum adjustment from him. He may perceive interaction with the environment as being totally beyond his control.

The nurse must understand the feelings of the paraplegic or quadriplegic patient and be prepared to offer psychological support. Often referral to social services or the mental health department is a beneficial option to pursue.

Preservation and Restoration of Physiologic Function

In a hierarchy of needs, once the overwhelming need for emotional support has been met, the patient may now participate in preserving and restoring his bodily functions. The professional nurse becomes the primary instrument in assisting him in his progress toward this objective. It is not the purpose of this text to discuss long-term rehabilitation, but it is recognized that certain activities, essential for the patient's recovery, should be instituted in the critical care setting.

Systems.   A review of the physiologic systems which may alert the nurse to potential problems affecting rehabilitation will be presented.

Cardiovascular.   Interruption of sympathetic innervation frequently produces vasodilatation and hypotension. Observe the patient for orthostatic hypotension when turning him on the Circ Olectric bed. Elevation of the legs may correct this problem; however, the trendelenberg position is not recommended, for it may lead to respiratory embarrassment. This same dilatation contributes to venous stasis in the lower extremities, increasing the risk of thrombus and embolus. Prevention entails the use of antiembolic hose, passive exercises, and the elevation of legs on a pillow.

Respiratory.   Oxygen administration in the early phase post injury may be of some benefit in reducing hypoxic changes in the injured cord. Arterial blood gases should be drawn routinely to establish the adequacy of ventilation. The nurse should be alert for signs of respiratory failure—a frequent sequela of cervical cord injury. The development of hypostatic pneumonia is also of prime concern. A respirator, IPPB therapy, blow bottles, and frequent turning may prevent its occurrence. Perhaps a respiratory assessment flow sheet would be valuable for recording the following: PaO_2; $PaCO_2$; pH; HCO_3^-; color; pertinent auscultatory findings; respiratory frequency; level of consciousness; and irritability or restlessness.

Nutrition and metabolism. During the acute phase of injury the patient may exhibit a state of marked negative nitrogen balance as well as a significant urinary loss of calcium. The patient's serum protein level and hematologic values may deviate from the norm. Frequent blood chemistries, and hematologic values must be obtained and reported for appropriate action. The loss of protein plays an important role in the susceptibility of the paraplegic or quadriplegic to urinary tract infection and the development of decubitus ulcers. A reasonable therapeutic diet would include 3500 calories, a minimum of 125 grams of protein, and supplemental vitamins. Fluid intake should approach 4000 milliliters per day to promote "irrigation" of the urinary tract and to contribute to gastrointestinal tract motility.

Spinal cord injury may trigger a neurohumoral mechanism resulting in gastric erosion. This stress ulcer may hemorrhage or perforate. Characteristic symptoms may not include pain or distress, but the patient's condition may suddenly deteriorate. Hematemesis or melena may be present. Prophylactic measures consist of an ulcer regimen; administration of antacids; use of cimetidine, a histamine H_2 receptor antagonist; routine guaiacs; and routine pH determination.

Musculoskeletal. Spinal automatisms (see page 153) are reflex mechanisms released by transection of the cord. These reflexes are no longer under the control of the higher centers, and may occur in one to six weeks as the patient recovers from spinal shock. Spinal automatisms elicit responses in the patient that he may perceive as puzzling, frightening, or (inappropriately) encouraging. For example, cutaneous stimulation of the lower abdomen or thigh may provoke reflex micturition or reflex ejaculation. The understanding nurse will avoid areas known to elicit responses, and when they occur, will adopt an unembarrassed, accepting attitude.

Mass flexor or extensor spasms may present serious problems. The uninformed patient and perhaps the family may believe motor function is returning. For example, when a limb is stimulated, mass flexion of the upper and lower limbs is produced. The interpretation of this response may falsely encourage the patient. How do you withdraw hope? The nurse who is a critical thinker may foresee the development of this problem and introduce the patient to the concept of mass flexion and extension before it occurs. A pre-occurrence, cognitive explanation may, or may not, combat the excitement and idea of returning motor function when the response is actually exhibited.

Immobility contributes to tendon contractures, joint ankylosis, and muscle shortening. The following preventive program may be instituted 48–72 hours after injury if the physician agrees:

1. Position the patient every two hours.
2. Maintain proper body alignment at all times.
3. Provide a footboard when the patient is supine.
4. Adjust the linen so it is not in contact with the feet when the patient is supine.
5. Maintain 15° flexion of the knees when the patient is supine.
6. Perform passive range of motion exercises every two hours while the patient is awake.
7. Have the patient perform active range of motion exercises when indicated every two hours while he is awake.
8. Physiotherapy, such as massage and electrical stimulation, may be initiated while the patient is in the intensive care unit.
9. Splints may be necessary to prevent wrist and foot drop.

Elimination. In the presence of normal bowel activity (meaning the absence of a paralytic ileus, which may occur in spinal cord injury patients one to four days post injury) a training program must begin in the critical care unit. A delay in initiating a program may hinder any future success at bowel continence. Bowel training can be achieved in approximately 80% of paraplegics and quadriplegics. The patient's participation in the program is essential. Patient commitment may be achieved if he realizes that attaining continence may later determine his vocational future and will certainly affect his self-confidence. The following nursing measures are directed toward the ultimate goal of bowel continence:

1. Prevent, detect, or treat constipation.
2. Encourage fluid intake.
3. Adjust diet to establish a routine pattern of bowel elimination.
4. Use suppositories as necessary. Avoid enemas which increase dependency on evacuation procedures.
5. Utilize conditioned reflex activity to reestablish habitual bowel evacuation.
6. Maintain an accurate intake and elimination record.

The presence of an atonic bladder may persist from weeks to months. Bladder retraining is not usually initiated in the acute phase. Attention is directed toward care of a patient with an indwelling catheter. Reflex micturition may not return if the bladder has been overdistended or in the presence of a bladder infection. The following measures are implemented in the intensive care unit:

1. Routinely check for bladder distention.
2. Ensure catheter patency.
3. Encourage fluids to 4000 ml/day.
4. Maintain an accurate intake and output record.
5. Administer medications as ordered.
6. Maintain aseptic technique when performing routine catheter care.
7. Observe genitals for drainage or discharge.
8. Monitor lab work for signs of infection.

These patients may ultimately suffer the effects of immobility on the renal system: renal calculi, pyelonephritis, and/or urinary tract infection.

Integumentary. Decubitus ulcers are indeed a dreadful complication for the paraplegic or quadriplegic. There is a lack of circulation to the denervated tissue and a lack of sensation. The patient cannot perceive pain or pressure that ordinarily prompts a change in position. The following regimen is immediately initiated in the intensive care unit.

1. Turn and position the patient every two hours.
2. Minister skin care every two hours.
3. Carefully examine and treat the vulnerable skin sites for breakdown every two hours.
4. Perform a total body massage as frequently as possible to promote circulation.
5. Maintain clean, dry skin with special attention to the perineal area.
6. Ensure the presence of clean, dry linen.
7. Avoid linen contact with skin whenever possible.
8. Employ the use of a pneumatic mattress whenever possible.
9. Perform foot and nail care as necessary to prevent nails from rubbing or cutting the skin.
10. Avoid the administration of IM medications below the level of the lesion where capillary circulation is diminished.

Selected Concepts. Three selected concepts will be discussed: pain, immobility, and sexuality.

Pain. Spinal cord injury patients may have pain present at the level of injury in the area of nerve root distribution. The discomfort may be a result of nerve root irritation or the development of scar tissue. Mild analgesics usually produce relief. Later, pain may occur with spasticity, usually in the lower extremities. Opiates, sedatives, and/or antispasmodics may be administered to alleviate the pain and spasms. If relief is not attained, neurosurgical intervention such as a neurectomy or a cordotomy may be indicated.

The use of learning principles for the purpose of changing behavior may be initiated in the intensive care unit. The application of a reinforcement theory such as operant conditioning may prove valuable for the patient. The object is to condition the patient's response in relation to pain. Brammer states that "emphasis is upon removing inhibiting behavior, not symptoms, through environmental change."[2]

Immobility. The anticipated effects of immobility have been considered in relation to most of the bodily systems previously reviewed; however, a great deal of emphasis should be placed on its psychological impact. The patient's total dependence upon others for even basic need satisfaction and experience of daily living certainly disrupts his psyche. The loss of motor and/or sensory perception may, unmeaningly, place him in total isolation. Communication must be established and maintained, based on an all-encompassing sense of trust to combat his sense of helplessness and loneliness. Interaction with people and his environment is essential to preserve his self-esteem as a social being. Very early after injury, spontaneous decision-making by the patient, minor though it may be, should be encouraged and sustained. This will assure him of at least a "quasi" sense of control over his destiny. This positive approach toward independence will be invaluable in the long process of rehabilitation toward becoming an autonomous being.

Sexuality. The spinal cord injury patient may harbor doubts and fears concerning his sexual being, depending on the level of injury. He may, or may not, express his feelings regarding his sexual identity, sexual functioning, or fear of social rejection. The nurse, however, should be alert to overt and covert clues indicating his need to resolve those feelings. Often, in the intensive care unit, an active listener is more important than a person with explanations regarding return of sexual function. The "how-to techniques" may be introduced later in his recovery phase. Patients should be referred to the growing specialty of sexual counselors for guidance in learning unconventional techniques for sexual satisfaction, for both the normal and the impaired partner.

Goal Setting for Paraplegics and Quadriplegics

Ultimately the entire health team, in mutual agreement with the patient, should be progressing toward the identified goal of considerable biopsycho-

---

[2]Brammer, Lawrence M. and Everett Shostrom, *Therapeutic Psychology,* Englewood Cliffs, New Jersey: Prentice-Hall, Inc., 1968, p. 54.

social independence for the patient. He may need assistance in adopting an attitude of sufficient emotional acceptance of his disability to function adequately. He will need to relearn psychomotor skills for locomotion, depending on the degree of impairment to the neuromuscular system. In addition to independent mobility, a knowledge of the steps necessary for social reintegration is important for the disabled person.

These goals may not require or even deserve primary emphasis in the intensive care unit, but certainly, depending on the patient's readiness to learn, some of the concepts can be introduced. Definitely, the intensive care nurse needs to be aware of the total restorative process even if her role is designed toward intervention in the acute phase of the spinal cord injury patient.

CONCLUSION

The patient with spinal cord injury has entered a new world of disability. It may take some time for the realization to be integrated into his personality that his life-style will be altered considerably. His home, his family, his occupation, all will come under scrutiny for readjustment in his attempt to become a functioning, productive, social, autonomous being. The nurse in the critical care unit, brief and transient though her relationship with him may be, can be instrumental in guiding the spinal cord injury patient toward a satisfying new life.

BIBLIOGRAPHY

Carini, Esta, and Guy Owens, *Neurological and Neurosurgical Nursing*, 6th ed., St. Louis: The C. V. Mosby Co., 1974.

Crigler, Lee, "Sexual Concerns of the Spinal Cord–Injured," *Nursing Clinics of North America*, 9 (No. 4):703–715, December 1974.

Hall, Calvin S., and Gardner Lindzey, *Theories of Personality*, 2nd ed., New York: John Wiley & Sons, Inc., 1957, pp. 490–502.

Luckman, Joan, and Karen Sorenson, *Medical-Surgical Nursing: A Psychophysiologic Approach*, Philadelphia: W. B. Saunders Co., 1974, pp. 442–463.

Moidel, Harriet, et al., eds., *Nursing Care of the Patient with Medical-Surgical Disorders*, New York: McGraw-Hill Co., 1971, pp. 1021–1051.

Olson, Edith V., "Hazards of Immobility," *American Journal of Nursing*, April 1967, pp. 780–796.

Redman, Barbara K., *The Process of Patient Teaching in Nursing*, 3rd ed., St. Louis: The C. V. Mosby Co., 1976.

Taylor, Ann, "Autonomic Dysreflexia in the Spinal Cord Injury Patient," *Nursing Clinics of North America*, 9 (No. 4):717–725, December 1974.

7
INTRACEREBRAL TUMORS

INTRODUCTION

The critical care nurse will frequently encounter patients with central nervous system tumors. The impact of their disease makes the management of their care worthy of serious consideration. Purposeful assessment and interpretative judgment are based on an understanding of the classification, clinical manifestations, diagnostic measures, and treatment modalities of intracranial tumors.

Predilection

Tumors of the brain may occur at any age. There tends to be a rising increase in frequency during the first seven years of life, at which time the rate declines until puberty; a second rise in frequency begins at puberty, and the incidence peaks in the fifth and sixth decades of life. The majority of tumors that occur in childhood are found in the posterior fossa; the majority in adult life in the cerebral hemispheres. No age is immune from brain tumor pathology. Males show a slight increase in incidence over females for most brain tumors. Race, occupation, or history of trauma have not been established as predisposing factors of occurrence. The general incidence of all intracranial tumors has been estimated to be between 4.2 and 5.4 per 100,000 persons.[1]

Prognosis

It has been estimated that 40% of people with brain tumors are restored to a useful life; 30% acquire palliation.[2] There are several factors to be considered in discussing the prognosis of the patients: the degree of anaplasia of each tumor; the aggressiveness of the tumor cellular components; the location of the lesion; and the quality of surviving life. Consider the degree of anaplasia: there are a variety of tumors that affect the cerebrum, and each type of tumor varies in its degree of destructiveness of normal brain tissue. Necrotic neurons do not regenerate. Consider the aggressiveness of the tumor: all expanding mass lesions are eventually fatal if untreated, for there is little room

---

[1]Youmans, Julian R., ed, *Neurological Surgery*, Vol. III, Philadelphia: W. B. Saunders Co., 1973, p. 1320.
[2]Rubin, Philip, *Clinical Oncology for Medical Students and Physicians, A Multidisciplinary Approach*, 4th ed., The American Cancer Society, 1974, p. 354.

for volume extension within the skull. The tumor ultimately exerts lethal pressure on vital brain centers. The aggressiveness of the cellular components of the tumor determines the rapidity and seriousness of its invasive properties. Consider the strategic significance of the tumor's architectural location: a tumor discovered in the tip of the right frontal lobe may be surgically excised; a tumor of the hypothalamus may not. The quality of surviving life must be examined: with a prognosis of a certain number of years, a description should be included of the quality of long-term survival the patient and family can plan on.

CLASSIFICATION OF TUMORS

Intracranial tumors may be classified in several different ways: supratentorial versus infratentorial, intrinsic versus extrinsic, anterior fossa versus posterior fossa. We have selected an intracerebral versus extracerebral classification, the former for discussion in this chapter and the latter for discussion in Chapter 8. The intracerebral tumors (those within the brain substance, generally within the cerebral hemispheres) are further divided into primary tumors (gliomas) and secondary tumors (metastatic carcinomas and sarcomas).

Primary Tumors

Gliomas account for nearly all of the primary intracerebral tumors. They are ectodermal in origin and may develop in any glial cell of the brain connective tissue. All gliomas are regarded as malignant lesions. There is a subclassification determined by the type of glial cell the tumor arises from: astrocytoma, ependymoma, medulloblastoma, or oligodendroglioma.

Astrocytoma. This type of glioma arises from the glial cell, the astrocyte. Astrocytomas are graded by their degree of malignancy; although all levels of malignancy may be found in one astrocytoma, they are graded by the highest degree of malignancy they contain—Grade I being the least and Grade IV the most malignant. All grades are invasive—some subtly, some conspicuously; they may increase in malignancy within a given time frame. The more benign forms of astrocytomas are usually found in children; the more malignant in adults.

Grade I astrocytoma. This tumor may also be called a fibrillary or protoplasmic astrocytoma. Grade I astrocytomas account for one-third of all gliomas and may occur anywhere in the brain; they are usually found in children. This is a slow-growing tumor, which may run a course of years. The infiltrative character and lack of encapsulation contribute to the tumor's classification as a Grade I malignancy rather than as benign. The local invasion of the tumor produces symptoms of an expanding lesion, which usually cause the patient to seek medical advice. Surgical resection is the treatment of choice for these tumors. In the operating room the presence of the tumor may be detected by a slight pallor of the brain tissue (which may be difficult to distinguish from normal brain white matter), widening of the cerebral convolutions, and a palpable increase in the firmness of brain tissue. Prognosis after surgical intervention for a Grade I astrocytoma is generally measured in terms of a few years.

Grade II astrocytoma.   This tumor may also be called astroblastoma. It is quite rare, occasionally being found in children although more commonly found in young adults. Grade II astrocytoma differs from a Grade I in a quantitative way only: the cells are more abundant and contain multiple nuclei. Active proliferation to blood vessels is suggested, but the tumor itself lacks hemorrhage and necrosis. Surgical resection is the treatment of choice, with subsequent irradiation for residual tumor. Prognosis after surgical intervention for a Grade II astrocytoma is generally measured in terms of a few years.

Grade III and IV astrocytoma.   These tumors are usually called glioblastoma multiforme. They are the most common tumors of all gliomas and are usually found in adults, occurring almost exclusively in the cerebral hemispheres. They grow rapidly, attaining an incredible size, and, unrestrained, they are probably the most ominous of all tumors. They produce a multicolored, ragged, vicious appearance. Often cystic, they actively proliferate into blood vessels and present with local hemorrhage, necrosis, and serious edema. The cysts are filled with clear, amber, proteinacious fluid that readily accumulates after withdrawal. When the fluid becomes turbid, it suggests necrosis within the cyst wall. This tumor can rarely be surgically excised, therefore, conjunctive irradiation is used. The prognosis of the glioblastoma multiforme patient is generally measured in a few months.

Ependymoma.   This tumor is derived from the ependymal cell of the lining of the ventricle and occurs along the ventricular pathway. Ependymomas are the second most common gliomas. They originate from glial cells; therefore, they are intrinsic (within brain substance) in nature, but 70% of them occur in the fourth ventricle.[3] They are mentioned here for classification with gliomas, though they do not often occur intracerebrally; they are discussed in more detail in Chapter 8, which includes extracerebral and posterior fossa tumors.

[3]Robbins, Stanley L., *Pathologic Basis of Disease*, Philadelphia: W. B. Saunders Co., 1974, p. 1519.

Medulloblastoma. This tumor is of glial origin in the cerebellum. Intrinsic in nature and found in the infratentorial compartment, it will be further discussed in Chapter 8.

Oligodendroglioma. This tumor is the third most common glioma and arises from the oligodendroglia. It is usually found in middle-aged adults and has a slow progressive course, being in the lower range of malignancy. It is usually confined to the white matter in the cerebrum and presents as a gray, fleshy, soft mass, sometimes cystic and hemorrhagic. The oligodendroglioma often contains sufficient calcium deposited in the periphery to permit X-ray visualization. It is usually deep in brain tissue and by nature invasive, making total surgical removal impossible. Life may be extended by even partial excision, but surgery also seems to accelerate the tumor growth; serious consideration is given before surgical intervention is proposed.

Secondary Tumors

Metastatic tumors are relatively common, representing approximately one-third of all brain tumors. The most common tumor found to metastasize to the brain is bronchogenic carcinoma, followed in frequency by tumors of the gastrointestinal tract and urinary tract. All carcinomas and sarcomas in the body have the capacity for intracranial metastases. The secondary tumor may produce symptoms before there is any evidence of a primary tumor. All parts of the brain are susceptible to the highly invasive, destructive growth of metastatic cancer. Since metastasis rarely occurs as a single tumor entity, surgical excision is uncommon; irradiation is the treatment of choice. The prognosis for metastatic tumor patients is poor.

Malignant metastatic melanoma is a relatively common tumor of the cerebral hemispheres. The origin of the tumor is disputed: some oncologists believe the primary lesion to be carcinoma of the skin with metastasis to the brain; others believe it may occur as a primary lesion of the central nervous system with metastasis to the skin. In the brain the tumor presents with a soft, friable, necrotic, hemorrhagic appearance with a black pigment throughout the tumor substance. The course of the tumor is unpredictable; death may not approach as inevitably as with other metastatic tumors.

CLINICAL MANIFESTATIONS

The patient with a brain tumor may have a history of onset of symptoms followed by a symptom-free period. Generally, after careful exploration it is discovered that there has been an inexorable progression of symptoms from the time of initial onset to the time when the patient seeks medical advice. Symptoms produced may occur from general pressure effects of increasing intracranial pressure or local pressure effects of a tumor in a specific area of the brain.

General Pressure Effects

A space-occupying lesion produces general pressure effects by increasing intracranial pressure. There are multiple factors involved: by nature the tumor is expanding in *volume* taking up space; the tumor provokes *cerebral edema* in surrounding brain tissue; the tumor has a capacity for *obstructing the circulation and absorption of cerebrospinal fluid*; the tumor has a compressive effect *impeding cerebrovascular circulation.* Singly or in combination, these multiple factors consequently produce general pressure effects and the following associated clinical manifestations.

Headache. The presence of a tumor may produce pressure or stress on structures that are sensitive to pain, such as the dura, blood vessels, and cranial nerves. The patient may experience dull, intermittent, diffuse pain in the frontal or occipital areas or sharply localized pain on the right or left side of the head. It may be aggravated by activities that increase intracranial pressure: walking, coughing, stooping, and so forth. The sensation is thought to be mediated through the trigeminal nerve from deflection of the falx and tentorium. Typically the patient complains of severe headache upon arising in the morning; indeed, the headache pain wakens the patient. The prolonged recumbent position at night increases venous pressure, leading to vascular congestion in and around the tumor, which distorts the falx and tentorium, producing intense headache that awakens him.

Nausea and vomiting. These symptoms are a result of direct irritation of the medullary emetic center by the tumor or indirect reflex stimulation due to increased intracranial pressure. Forceful or projectile vomiting often occurs in the absence of associated nausea. This singular symptom of projectile vomiting (which may not always occur) is not the basis for a differential diagnosis of cerebral disease. The vomiting may be viewed as the body's physiologic response to increased intracranial pressure; indeed, the dehydrating effect reduces cerebral edema and diminishes intracranial pressure. Symptoms caused by general pressure effects (especially headache) may thus be relieved.

Altered mental status. An early (but sometimes late) effect of increased intracranial pressure is a change in the mental faculties of the patient. There may be subtle personality changes that escape the notice of the patient and those close to him. Emotionally, there may be a flattening of affect; intellectually, there may be confusion in the thought process; diminished ability to think abstractly, dulling or blunting of recent and/or remote memory, impaired judgment, shortened attention span, and/or episodes of bizarre behavior. As pressure on the cerebral hemispheres and reticular activating system increases, the patient may progress from a state of lethargy to drowsiness, stupor, and finally coma.

Seizures. Seizures may be a result of general pressure effects, discussed in this section, or local pressure effects (see below). Seizures may occur initially or as a symptom at any time in the course of the illness. They include classic grand mal seizures and may present with either no aura or an unidentifiable aura that is of no value for localization. It is generally assumed that in the absence of any other pathology the onset of seizures in the adult is indicative of cerebral neoplasm.

Vital parameters and autonomic changes. When there is a rise in intracranial pressure, the vital centers—cardiac, respiratory, and vasomotor—in the medulla are stimulated and subsequently depressed. The ultimate results of interference within these centers are respectively: bradycardia progressing to cardiac arrest; bradypnea progressing to apnea; hypertension progressing to hypotension. Hypothalamic disturbances may produce hyperthermia in the absence of other infectious processes, and it is not uncommon prior to death. Interference of the autonomic pathways may result in disturbances of sweating and the presence of a Cushing's ulcer. Vagal stimulation increases the secretion of hydrochloric acid, causing erosion of the gastric mucosa.

Papilledema. This condition is a result of an obstruction of venous return from the retina. It may develop early or late in the disease process, depending on the rapidity of the intracranial pressure increase and the height the pressure attains. The existence of papilledema is quite variable; e.g., children develop the symptom more rapidly than adults, and in the elderly it may not be present at all. Visual acuity may not be lost until very late. Occasionally papilledema appears in one eye before the other. Tumor compression may produce uniocular optic atrophy on the side of the tumor and contralateral papilledema (Foster-Kennedy syndrome).

Local Pressure Effects

Cortical region symptoms. See Fig. 7-1.

Selected symptoms. Three common local symptoms produced by intracerebral mass lesions are selected for further discussion.

Visual impairment. Hemianopsia may result from tumor disturbance of visual pathways. The symptom elicited is determined by the location of the

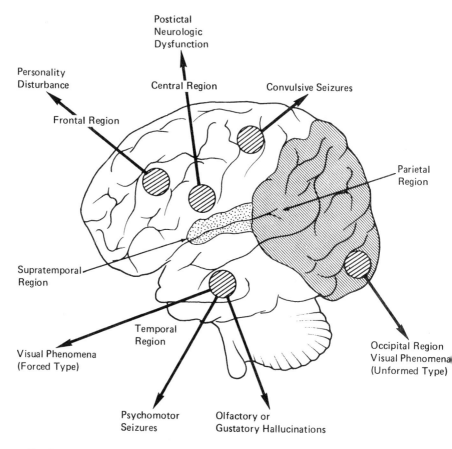

Fig. 7-1. Cerebral lesion sites and examples of their respective localizing manifestations.

lesion: optic chiasma—bitemporal hemianopsia; optic tract, optic radiation, or occipital cortex—contralateral homonymous hemianopsia; temporal pole—contralateral homonymous superior quadrantopsia (pie in the sky defect). (See Fig. 7-2.)

Motor and sensory impairment.   The occurrence of focal motor or sensory seizures usually indicates the cortical area of tumor involvement. Temporal lobe seizures include a complex variety of symptoms. Referred to as psychomotor seizures, these attacks may include feelings of unreality, anger, fear, detachment, déjà vu, and vertigo. The symptoms of a psychomotor seizure may be very difficult to distinguish from outbursts of immature or psychotic behavior. Posterior frontal region involvement produces symptoms of motor interference affecting the hand, arm, and face. When a tumor is situated behind the fissure of Rolando, sensory impairment of an arm or leg is characteristic. Invasion of the parietal sensory cortex affects sensory localization, two-point discrimination, graphesthesia, stereognosis, and position sense. Contralateral spastic hemiparesis and contralateral hemisensory defects are encountered with hemispheric lesions as well. Lesions of the thalamus produce sensory impairment of touch, pain, temperature, and proprioception.

Aphasias.   Various forms of aphasia are produced by dominant cerebral hemisphere lesions. The development of aphasia is usually insidious and commonly overlooked by the patient. Some tumors produce apraxia and agnosia as the initial symptom. Speech defects contribute little to the localization of the lesion, other than attributing expressive aphasia to the anterior frontoparietotemporal region and receptive aphasia to a region situated more posteriorly in the same area.

DIAGNOSTIC MEASURES

That the neurologic history and the neurologic examination can be utilized as diagnostic tools in determining the *presence* of cerebral lesions is beyond dispute. However, the data obtained only provide the basis for a provisional diagnosis. Other techniques of investigation are necessarily employed for *localization* of the cerebral lesion. These diagnostic measures, which are discussed in depth in Chapter 4, are considered here with pertinent information specific to intracerebral tumors.

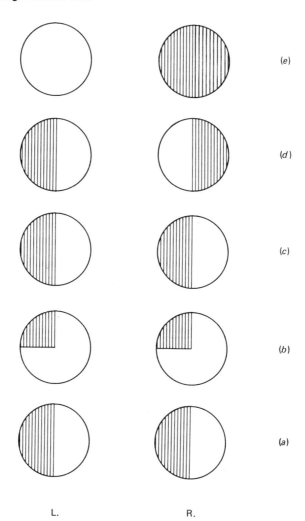

L.   R.

Fig. 7-2. Visual field defects. Illustration of anopsia in the right eye (R) and the left eye (L). (A) Left homonymous hemianopsia (right optic radiation). (B) Left homonymous superior quadrantopsia (bilateral temporal poles or optic radiation, partial). (C) Left homonymous hemianopsia (right optic tract). (D) Bitemporal hemianopsia (optic chiasma). (E) Right anopsia (right optic nerve).

Neuroradiologic Procedures

Skull and chest films.   Skull films are obtained to determine the position of the usually calcified pineal gland; a shift indicates the presence of a hemispheric space-occupying lesion. A cerebral mass may also displace the glomus, a calcified round structure of the choroid plexus in the lateral ventricle. Some tumors (astrocytomas and oligodendrogliomas) become calcified, permitting X-ray visualization. Tumors may erode the cranial vault, showing a hammered effect of the inner table of the skull. Chest films (PA and lateral views) are routinely done on patients with suspected cerebral lesion in search of primary bronchogenic or mammary carcinoma. These primary lesions are frequently metastatic invaders of the cerebral hemispheres.

Brain scans.   Radionuclide imaging study has become the procedure of choice for screening of suspected brain tumors. The presence of the radioactive tracer in brain tissue suggests a pathological disruption of the blood-brain barrier. It is useful in diagnosing the presence of a lesion, but does not indicate its pathological process. EMI scans are used for tumor localization. The tomographic views permit visualization of X-ray–dense cranial contents.

Cerebral angiography.   This technique is widely employed, revealing information regarding the vasculature of the tumor and its relationship to adjacent blood vessels. It is particularly successful in determining tumors of the anterior two-thirds of the cerebrum.

Encephalography.   Air studies visualizing cerebrospinal fluid circulation (pneumoencephalogram and ventriculogram) may be used as diagnostic aids for cerebral tumors. They are extremely accurate in predicting the presence and the location of the lesion.

Neurodiagnostic Procedures

Cerebrospinal fluid examination.   A lumbar puncture is contraindicated when there is obvious evidence of increased intracranial pressure. It becomes detrimental under these circumstances, increasing the risk of herniation of the brain structures into the foramen magnum. The test is useful in the determination of increased intracranial pressure. The spinal fluid is analyzed for protein elevation (may be indicative of intracranial tumor) and the presence of tumor cells.

Electroencephalography.   The EEG is useful in determining brain wave abnormalities, but yields little information revealing localization of the tumor. Neither does it reflect the pathological process (tumor versus infarct) in the presence of the abnormalities.

Echoencephalography.   The use of ultrasound is somewhat limited to the determination of a midline shift. It is not predictive in outlining cavities or encapsulated tumors.

INTERVENTION: MODALITIES OF THERAPY

The treatment of intracerebral tumors is based on the following objectives:

1. Tumor excision to effect a permanent cure.
2. Preservation of vital brain tissue from treatment-induced damage.
3. Palliative therapy to provide relief of symptoms, patient comfort, and support during remaining life.
4. Efforts directed toward prolonging life span when location of tumor prevents its removal.

Generally a tumor requires surgical exploration to establish its pathological nature, gross tissue characteristics, extensiveness, and, naturally, position. The pathology report precedes the determination of the protocol of treatment to be employed. Treatment generally consists of one, or a combination, of the following: surgery, radiotherapy, chemotherapy, immunotherapy.

Surgery

The operative risk of patients undergoing intracranial surgery has been reduced by the introduction of several artificially induced states: hypothermia, hypotension, dehydration. The goal of therapy is to reduce the tumor effects on cerebral function.

Tumor excision.   Complete or partial removal of an intracerebral tumor is accomplished by means of a supratentorial craniotomy (Fig. 7-3). The patient is positioned, draped, and anesthetized. A series of burr holes (trephine) (Fig. 7-4) is made, and the bone between the holes is cut with a special saw to remove a large bone flap, usually behind the hair line on the anterior two-thirds of the head. The removal of this bone flap permits visualization and maneuvering within the skull. The bone flap is preserved and replaced or left out entirely. It may be used as a mold set for a prosthesis of acrylic, which is wired in place at a later time. An incision is made in the meninges, exposing brain tissue for inspection. A biopsy of the tumor is obtained for frozen section and permanent paraffin section.

After the histology report is received, the physician is in a position to determine the extent of surgical removal of the tumor: partial or complete resection.

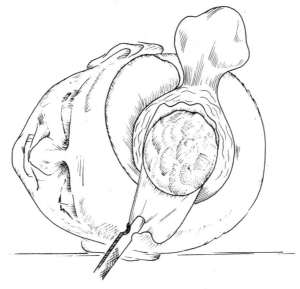

Fig. 7-3. Supratentorial craniotomy. Visualization of the cerebrum following removal of large frontal bone flap.

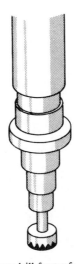

Fig. 7-4. Trephine. Illustration of a burr drill for performing trephination.

The tumor shell may be left intact by removing only the diseased tissue, thereby protecting the surrounding brain from operative trauma, or the complete radical resection of tumor tissue and capsule may be attempted. Naturally, the goal is to provide the patient with the best chance for survival and functional restoration. If the tumor is positioned in such a way that resection is impossible, the surgeon may place metal clips along the borders of the lesion for identification and definition for subsequent radiotherapy. Hemostasis, wound closure, and dressing complete the procedure.

Decompression.   If the tumor is not amenable to total resection, the neurosurgeon attempts some form of decompression to permit the expansion of brain tissue. Internal decompression consists of removal of tissue not invaded by the tumor, allowing room for a volume increase. External decompression consists of removing the bone flap or not replacing it and closing the scalp only, thereby relieving intracranial pressure.

Cerebrospinal fluid diversion.   Tumors in the region of the third ventricle are the only intracerebral tumors likely to cause internal hydrocephalus. If the tumor cannot be removed, obstruction of the flow of cerebrospinal fluid can be relieved by a shunt. Cerebrospinal fluid can be diverted in several ways: lateral ventricle to cisterna magna (Torkildsen), ventriculoperitoneal, or ventriculospinal. Each of these techniques has advantages and disadvantages to be weighed by the surgeon when considering each patient's individual problem.

Radiotherapy

Treatment of tumors is inevitably multi-modal. Radiotherapy may be initiated as primary therapy, palliative treatment, or an adjunct to other therapies. X-rays disrupt the cellular DNA pattern and cause radiation-induced cellular death. The goal of therapy is to deliver a massive concentrated dose of radiation to the intracerebral tumor and a minimal dose to surrounding normal brain tissue. The indiscriminate destruction of brain tissue is controlled by consideration of several factors: the type of tumor, the radioresponsiveness of the identified type of tumor, the anatomical location of the tumor, the extent of tumor invasiveness, and the patient's level of toleration to the therapy, including his age.

Radiation therapy is initiated postoperatively for most malignant intracerebral tumors—primary and metastatic. There is little documentation of the effectiveness of preoperative versus postoperative radiation. However, the institution of postoperative radiation has the advantage of histological proof of type of tumor, which facilitates the decision-making process regarding the treatment plan.

Radiotherapy generally adds to the patient's longevity and may allay symptoms. A favorable radiation reaction response would be a gradual reduction of symptoms, whereas an unfavorable radiation response would be radiation edema and radionecrosis. The nursing implications would be to support the patient before, during, and after treatment. The discussion of symptoms, objective assessment, and treatment of untoward reactions to therapy are of paramount importance in assisting the patient through the therapy and providing the physician with essential data influencing the course of treatment.

Chemotherapy

The investigation of chemotherapy for the treatment of brain tumors has not provided clear evidence of benefits. The agents currently in use are not specific for gliomas, and the side effects and toxicity preclude general adoption. Drugs being used are BCNU (carmustine), vincristine, and methotrexate. The nursing responsibilities in chemotherapy are similar to those of radiotherapy. The sequence of events from initial administration to period of remission and relative toxicity become a major concern for the patient as well as the nurse. Again, her knowledge, relationship with the patient, and interpretation of data will be important factors in the course of therapy.

Immunotherapy

Immunotherapy is currently being investigated in the treatment of neoplastic tumors. Active specific therapy involves the administration of BCG, a live bacillus, which causes the immune system to respond aggressively to foreign cells. Vaccines are being developed to control tumor growth by increasing the cell-mediated immunity response. Passive therapy involves the injection of gamma globulin with antibodies from blood of patients who have recovered from hepatitis. These antibodies play a role in the patient's immune process, attacking cells and tumor growth. Perhaps the research will prove beneficial in the treatment of intracerebral tumors. It certainly opens an area of exploration for health services personnel.

BIOPSYCHOSOCIAL PROCESS

Preoperative Nursing Management

The preparation of the patient and family for craniotomy involves setting priorities, planning intervention, and patient teaching.

Biological preparation.   The patient with an intracerebral tumor may present with neurologic deficits. The nurse is obliged to support and assist a patient who is immobile, one who has visual defects, one who is aphasic, and so on. A neurologic history and examination will provide the intensive care nurse with valuable information for integration into the preoperative and postoperative nursing care plan. The baseline neurologic assessment will be viewed for comparison in the extension of the present problem or as a contrast to the postoperative neurologic assessment.

The physical preparation of the head usually requires shampoo and shaving. Customarily the hair is saved for the patient in the event that it would be suitable for a hair piece. Medications may be administered preoperatively to diurese the patient and to provide analgesia. It is the nurse's responsibility to accurately validate a narcotic order with the physician. All narcotics depress cerebral function and should be used judiciously. Morphine is rarely ordered because of its depressing effect on the respiratory center. Elimination is encouraged—both bowel and bladder. The patient is instructed to refrain from straining, which has a tendency to increase intracranial pressure. Laxatives, stool softeners, and enemas are given *only* as directed. The patient is requested to void (when physically able to do so), and an indwelling catheter is inserted. Intravenous fluids are administered as ordered. Surgical permits must be explained and signed by the patient if possible. Preoperative teaching of postoperative positioning and breathing exercises is a necessity.

Psychological preparation. The patient with an intracerebral tumor needs considerable emotional support. There may be overt and covert clues indicating the degree of anxiety; the nurse must be extremely perceptive. A thorough explanation of diagnostic procedures and surgical intervention may allay his apprehension. An existing confident relationship will be the vehicle for emotional support. A description of his postoperative appearance and a discussion of postoperative expectations may diminish the anxiety-inspired resistance commonly found in the confusion after surgery. Explanations for patient consent forms are deemed necessary, but the critical care nurse moves beyond these requirements by providing additional quantities of time in a comfortable atmosphere for the patient to express his needs and his fears.

Social preparation. The family needs are to be considered in preparing the patient for a craniotomy. Cancer-phobia may be openly discussed with the nurse who is willing to listen attentively. The patient has undoubtedly experienced symptoms that the family has witnessed and interpreted. Surgery may be viewed as a last resort or as a miraculous circumstance culminating in a cure for the patient. Either extreme carries with it overwhelming emotions. Remember, you cannot meet an emotional problem on an intellectual level. Experiencing the affective realm with the family and then proceeding to rational explanations, in a language they are capable of comprehending, seems to be the most effective method. Do not fail to prepare them for the initial postoperative visit, portray to them realistic expectations for the patient, and open avenues for future problem solving.

PRESERVATION AND RESTORATION OF PHYSIOLOGIC FUNCTION FOR SUPRATENTORIAL CRANIOTOMY

Immediate Assessment

In the immediate postoperative period the supratentorial craniotomy patient requires assiduous nursing care. Nursing actions evolve around the detection and treatment of surgical complications and the preservation and restoration of the patient's physiologic functions. The nurse, in maintaining meaningful communication with the patient and family, will have discovered specific areas of strengths and needs. An extreme amount of skilled ministration will enhance the patient's progress toward restoration and well-being.

A great deal of emphasis is placed on the nurse's ability to assess and evaluate the patient's present clinical status, and many tools have been devised for the purpose of guiding the nurse through a systematic assessment. We have selected a bodily-system approach by priority. This method allows the incorporation of immediate areas of attention, a focus on surgical complications, and a consideration of long-term goals. The nursing process concept is the hallmark of professional nursing care.

Airway. Intracranial surgery may interfere with the respiratory center or the cranial nerves controlling gag and swallow reflexes, or render the patient unconscious. An adequate airway must be established and maintained. The patient may have excessive secretions that he is unable to expel. Position the patient to facilitate drainage and prevent obstruction or aspiration. The patient is encouraged to deep-breathe, but vigorous coughing is prohibited because of its effect on intracranial pressure. Cautious pharyngotracheal suctioning may be employed. An adequate air exchange is important, for both hypoxia and hypercarbia increase cerebral edema. Oxygen may be administered to maintain normal PaO_2 levels. Signs of restlessness may be due to an inadequate air exchange.

Neurologic assessment. A thorough neurologic examination is essential. The critical care nurse must discuss the details of the neurologic examination with the neurosurgeon so that he may relate specific areas of concern. The nurse must continually reassess the patient's level of consciousness. A state of mental confusion and restlessness may be symptoms of increasing cerebral edema or increasing intracranial pressure. The neurologic check will also include assessment of cranial nerve function with particular attention to pupillary response and extraocular movements. Palsies of the third, fourth, and sixth cranial nerves are often indicative of increasing intracranial pressure. Pathological reflexes, such as Babinski's and clonus, must be observed for and reported. Seizures may occur which increase bleeding and cerebral edema; medications may be ordered prophylactically. It may be necessary to ensure the patient's safety and security during seizures with side rails and bed padding. Evaluate the patient's motor ability, including spontaneous activity, and make frequent evaluation of the pronator test so that paresis or paralysis may be discovered early. The craniotomy patient may have an interference with the temperature control mechanism in the hypothalamus. The patient should be maintained in a normothermic state. Hyperthermia increases the brain's metabolic demands; nursing measures should be employed for temperature reduction.

Dressings and edema.   Dressings should be checked frequently for hemorrhage or cerebrospinal fluid drainage. A catheter may be placed in a cerebral ventricle and attached to a closed drainage system, with the entire system kept at the level of the ventricle. The neurosurgeon should inform the nurse about what to expect in terms of quantity and quality of drainage and how to deal with it. The wound for supratentorial craniotomy is usually behind the hair line on the anterior two-thirds of the head. After suture removal (approximately three days) hydrogen peroxide may be used to remove any crusting or drainage. Observe the incision frequently for any swelling (intracranial pressure, fluid accumulation, or infection). Following a craniotomy the patient may have periocular edema, which may be relieved with light cold compresses or ice packs. Eye care may include cleansing and application of petrolatum to eyelids or instillation of artificial tears (methyl cellulose).

Position and activity.   Positioning of the patient postoperatively is of major importance. Several goals may be achieved simultaneously by proper positioning. The patient may be placed in a lateral position on the unaffected side to assist the removal of secretions and prevent aspiration. If a large tumor has been removed, it is inadvisable to place the patient laterally on the operative side, particularly if the bone flap has not been replaced; this position may cause gravity displacement of brain structures. The lateral position with the head elevated 45° and a pillow placed under head and shoulders is recommended. The effect is to minimize cerebral edema and decrease intracranial pressure. In addition, it would decrease hemorrhage, increase cerebrospinal fluid circulation, and promote cerebral venous return. The patient is usually limited in activity, requiring nursing assistance for total care. A quiet atmosphere is maintained.

Pain.   The patient may have a headache postoperatively. He may be able to communicate this pain verbally or may have symptoms of restlessness. In either case the pain should be treated with the prescribed medications. Nursing measures would include: positioning; maintaining a quiet, dimly lit environment; eliminating any excessive noise; restricting unnecessary activity; and preventing any sudden movements.

Surgical Complications

The postoperative supratentorial craniotomy patient faces the same surgical risks as other surgery patients. In addition, specific neurologic complications may occur, such as cerebral edema, causing increased intracranial pressure, and the development of a surgical hematoma. The nurse should be alert to neurologic deterioration and be prepared for emergency intervention when necessary.

Cerebral edema/increased intracranial pressure. Cerebral edema usually exists to some degree in the presence of a tumor. Operative manipulation simply aggravates the condition until the degree is severe enough to cause increased intracranial pressure. Neurologic deficits progressively deteriorate, and emergency intervention is required. Severe cerebral edema may lead to cerebral distortion or herniation, resulting in irreparable neural damage and death. Cerebral angiography may be necessary to differentiate diffuse edema from intracranial hemorrhage. Undifferentiated diagnosis dictates immediate surgical exploration. The following factors are worthy of consideration in the nonoperative management of edema:

1. Ventilation and perfusion must be adequate to sustain arterial blood gases within normal range. Recall that retention of carbon dioxide enhances tissue permeability and also causes vasodilation contributing to cerebral edema.

2. The patient should be placed in a semi-Fowler's position to support venous return from the brain as well as cerebrospinal fluid circulation.

3. Eliminate, when possible, any additional stress that increases intracranial pressure, such as straining, coughing, hiccoughing, vomiting, and so forth.

4. Refrain from administering respiratory depressant drugs.

5. If the patient is on a ventilator, the automatic cycle should have a small negative phase to avoid the deleterious affects of an exclusively positive-pressure, artificial inflation; this maintains the negative intrathoracic pressure of inspiration, which normally aids venous return from the head.

6. Osmotic diuretics may be ordered. Observe for symptoms of severe dehydration. Accurately record intake and output. Weigh the patient when possible.

7. Hypothermia may be employed for severe cerebral edema. This is usually accomplished by total body cooling to a core temperature of 30°C. Note: The amount of osmotic diuretics required to reduce intracranial pressure under hypothermic states is less than that required for a normothermic patient.

8. Adrenocorticosteroids have proved valuable in controlling cerebral edema. The drug of choice is usually dexamethasone (page 265). Patients on steroid therapy commonly receive oral antacids to prevent gastric erosion.

Surgical Hematoma. The alert nurse will assess the patient for signs and symptoms of a surgical hematoma:

1. The development of or increase in cranial pain or headache.
2. The development of or progression of neurologic deficits corresponding to the operative site.
3. Alteration of or deterioration in the patient's level of consciousness.
4. Signs or symptoms of herniation or cerebral distortion: pupillary signs of third cranial nerve compression, changes in respiratory pattern, extraocular muscle palsy, homolateral upper motor neuron dysfunction, visual field defects, decorticate or decerebrate posturing.

The clinical picture is usually a progressive, unrelenting deterioration in the patient's neurologic status. A change in the patient's level of consciousness is the most significant observation. Intracranial pressure monitoring will reveal ominous, dynamic changes of intracranial contents. Postoperative cerebral angiography will confirm the pathological process of the complication. A surgical hematoma represents a life-threatening crisis, and surgical evacuation is performed immediately.

Respiratory Status

Respiratory assessment. Vigilant observation of the patient's respiratory status is necessary. Immediate postoperative management of the airway has been discussed on page 183. Reassessment and evaluation may alert the nurse to insidious problems.

Respiratory complications. The common causes of respiratory obstruction are improper positioning of the unconscious patient, aspiration, and the presence of a mucous plug. The critical care nurse is certainly capable of determining the existence of an obstruction and initiating action. Any suctioning procedure should be accompanied by EKG monitoring and the administration of oxygen. Periodic determination of arterial blood gases should be performed to ensure adequate ventilation.

Pneumonia. Inflammation and infection of the lung is probably the single most common respiratory complication of neurosurgery. It is believed that the major pathophysiologic mechanism for pneumonia in neurosurgical patients is aspiration. Management of pneumonia may include the administration of antibiotics and steroids and the utilization of mechanical measures. Nursing responsibilities include: obtaining cultures for bacterial identification initially and serially as ordered; administering medications as ordered; performing frequent tracheobronchial suctioning with sterile technique; turning the patient regularly; encouraging the patient to deep-breathe and cough with moderate effort; patient teaching whenever possible regarding respiratory hygiene; and employing effective hand-washing technique along with other appropriate measures to prevent cross contamination.

Atelectasis.   Atelectasis is the second most common respiratory complication of neurosurgery: hypoventilation, aspiration, and neural paresis are all contributing factors to the development of atelectasis. The following symptoms are fairly reliable indications of a problem: apprehension, respiratory distress, elevated temperature, increased heart rate, deviation of the trachea, decreased chest expansion, flatness to percussion, and decreased breath sounds on auscultation. A chest X-ray usually confirms the diagnosis. Prompt, direct, and vigorous management is aimed at reinflation of the collapsed lung.

Bronchospasm.   This condition may be associated with asthmatic attack or COPD; it may be precipitated by suctioning or accompanied by an allergic reaction. Bronchospasm can usually be managed by: the administration of bronchodilators, steroids, and antibiotics; the humidification of inspired air; and the control of pH imbalances.

Pulmonary edema.   The existence of pulmonary edema in the neurosurgical patient may be of primary neural origin from a lesion in the medulla or hypothalamus. However, it is more commonly produced by the development of left ventricular heart failure in association with fluid overload or respiratory tree obstruction. CVP or PAWP monitoring and cardiac monitoring are especially recommended for patients particularly vulnerable to vascular overload. Any abnormal elevation is indicative of ensuing heart failure. Treatment of pulmonary edema includes control of fluids, rotating tourniquets, the administration of oxygen, digitalization, and IPPB. IPPB impedes venous return to the thorax and is effective in treating pulmonary edema; but it may also aggravate intracranial vascular congestion and is therefore used with discretion.

Cardiovascular Status

Cardiovascular assessment.   Because the cardiovascular system assessment is so totally integrated with neurologic and respiratory assessment, the nurse is automatically collecting data as she monitors the immediately postoperative patient. She should assess particularly the indices of peripheral circulation: neck vein distention, color and temperature of extremities, peripheral pulse, and so on. The existence of hypotension may be due to hypovolemia (page 136), atelectasis, myocardial infarction, pulmonary emboli, sepsis, transfusion reaction, gastric distention, or the administration of opiates. Treatment goals are determined primarily by the etiology of the hypotension.

Cardiovascular complications. The most common arrhythmia post neurosurgery is supraventricular tachycardia. A cardiologist usually manages the problem with electric synchronized cardioversion. If a ventricular arrhythmia occurs, hypoxemia or digitalis intoxication must be considered. These death-producing arrhythmias must be promptly identified and treated immediately.

Fluid and Electrolyte Status

Fluid and electrolyte assessment. The patient with postoperative hypovolemia commonly presents with cool extremities, faint peripheral pulse, narrow pulse pressure, oliguria, hypotension, restlessness, and thirst. Treatment is aimed at the replacement of fluid volume.

Fluid and electrolyte complications. The postoperative patient may inherit a state of dehydration induced intraoperatively by the administration of osmotic diuretics. The usual pattern of dehydration encountered is water loss in excess of electrolyte loss—hypertonic dehydration. This is corrected by administering D 5½ S to return the balance. Occasionally there is an electrolyte loss in excess of water—hypotonic dehydration, which may be encountered in patients who have adrenocortical insufficiency. The balance is regained with the administration of electrolyte solutions.

Clinical measures of patients with fluid and electrolyte imbalances include: measuring body weight daily, urinary output and specific gravity hourly, and serum osmolality and serum sodium concentration levels as indicated; and maintaining accurate intake and output records. The prevention of urinary infection through routine catheter care and the establishment of an adequate sterile drainage system is important.

Psychosocial Status

Generally this category is considered at the end of the health maintenance continuum because of the critical biological condition of the patient in the intensive care unit. We have chosen to consider it fifth in priority as we set goals for the preservation of the patient's defenses and his restoration to function. In the hierarchy of setting objectives the patient's psychosocial status must be interrelated and dealt with concurrently with his biological needs. Recognition of the patient's ecosystem encompasses directing our attention to the family as well as the patient.

The patient.   The impact of illness on the postoperative neurosurgical patient may be quite severe. There has probably been minimal time for him to adapt to the sick role model, and all of his coping mechanisms may be directed toward survival. The need for reciprocal relationships may be temporarily diminished, but nevertheless still present. If a nurse–patient therapeutic relationship has been established, it certainly can contribute to the patient's orientation and adaptation to the physical environment of the intensive care unit. Fear may be an overriding emotion in the face of the multiple electronic systems sustaining his life. Sensory deprivation effected by immobility and absence of family and friends, and/or sensory overload effected by intensive medical attention and equipment, are contributing factors to the environmental stress placed on the patient's psychosocial system. Nursing goals are directed toward assisting the patient in maintaining a state of equilibrium.

The family.   Preoperatively, the family may be a valuable asset to the nurse, providing information regarding the patient's usual behavior, perception, and coping mechanisms. This kind of information, identifying strengths and weaknesses, will be beneficial in assessing the patient's present status and in planning outcome criteria. Postoperatively, however, the family may be in a position of dire need, requiring nursing assistance and supportive measures. Primary fear and secondary anxiety are usually the overwhelming emotions experienced by the family. Some problems can be eliminated if the nurse establishes time periods for family communication. This dialogue might include cognitive explanations of what surgery has been performed, reinforcing the physician's medical explanations. It is imperative for the family to communicate with the patient; therefore, a descriptive illustration of his appearance will minimize the shock of the first visit. In time, the family should be aware of some of the patient's limitations; he may be unconscious, aphasic, and/or immobile with no head turning or twisting, and so on. Long-term goals set with the patient should be shared with the family. The successful achievement of these goals may depend on the family's problem-solving abilities rather than the patient's. Open communication is recommended in light of the patient's possible temporary or permanent physical or mental limitations.

Nutritional and Metabolic Status

Nutritional and metabolic assessment.   The postoperative neurosurgical patient is kept NPO until there is gag and swallow reflex evident. An NG tube may be inserted to prevent aspiration and may be used for gavage. Whenever possible the tracheostomy should be removed prior to the institution of nasogastric feedings. If this is not feasible, the tracheostomy cuff should be inflated during feeding and for 30 minutes thereafter. The head of the bed should be elevated, and there should be no tracheal suctioning carried out during the feeding. Exercise caution to prevent abdominal distention. When the patient is able to eat, a diet progressing to regular may be ordered. Feeding the patient, at least early postoperatively, may help eliminate some fatigue.

Nutritional and Metabolic Complications. The patient will be utilizing energy reserves and may be in a state of negative nitrogen balance (page 132). Gastric ulcerations may occur and perforate or hemorrhage. Elimination may become a problem, and stool softeners are ordered to prevent effects of immobility and gastrointestinal tract disturbances.

Musculoskeletal Status

Musculoskeletal assessment. Data collected in a systematic fashion provide information regarding several systems. It would appear that this system should be evaluated conjointly with the neurologic examination and the fluid and electrolyte status.

Musculoskeletal complications. Patients with an electrolyte imbalance will develop notable muscle symptoms such as weakness, flaccidity, and/or twitching. When the imbalance is corrected, the symptoms diminish. Immobility contributes to muscle weakness and atrophy. Rigid turning schedules with the patient assisting and active/passive range of motion exercises will prevent contractures, preserve the integrity of the skin, and promote circulation.

CONCLUSION

The patient with an intracerebral tumor has a system of health beliefs that have been indoctrinated and integrated throughout his life. Does he believe in high level wellness? Will he take his physical and mental potential and adjust his behavior accordingly after diagnosis and treatment? The nurse is pledged to consider the impact of this illness on his well-being and assess his remaining strengths and weaknesses. The entire health team will conjointly aim at restoration of the person to home and society.

The patient with a minimum quality of life remaining will need a great deal of support. The nurse is confronted with "comfort versus recovery" issues. As a health professional dedicated to intervene and "cure," she may find that there are times when minimal intervention is more realistic. Philosophies of nursing will be reexamined and conflict resolved by the individual nurse. Can nursing minister comfort to the body and allow peace to the soul? Death and dying concepts will need to be evaluated and employed for the nurse, the patient, and the family.

BIBLIOGRAPHY

"Anxiety, Recognition and Intervention," A Programmed Text, *American Journal of Nursing,* 65 (No. 9):130–152, September 1965.

Beeson, Paul B., and Walsh McDermott, eds., *Textbook of Medicine,* Vol. 1, 14th ed., Philadelphia: W. B. Saunders Co., 1975.

Elliott, Carolyn St. John, "Radiation Therapy: How You Can Help," *Nursing 76,* September, pp. 34–41.

Elliott, Frank A., *Clinical Neurology,* Philadelphia: W. B. Saunders Co., 1971.

Kintzel, Ray Corman, ed., *Advanced Concepts in Clinical Nursing,* 2nd ed., Philadelphia: J. B. Lippincott Co., 1977.

Luckman, Joan, and Karen Sorensen, *Medical-Surgical Nursing: A Psychophysiologic Approach,* Philadelphia: W. B. Sanders Co., 1974.

Robbins, Stanley L., *Pathologic Basis of Disease,* Philadelphia: W. B. Saunders Co., 1974.

Rubin, Philip, *Clinical Oncology for Medical Students and Physicians, A Multidisciplinary Approach,* 4th ed., New York: The American Cancer Society, 1974.

Shafer, Kathleen, et al., *Medical-Surgical Nursing,* St. Louis: The C. V. Mosby Co., 1975.

Youmans, Julian R., ed., *Neurological Surgery,* Philadelphia: W. B. Saunders Co., 1973.

8
EXTRACEREBRAL TUMORS

INTRODUCTION

Tumors of the central nervous system can be divided according to two distinct anatomical locations: intracranial tumors, which are inside the brain substance, chiefly found within the cerebral hemisphere—*intracerebral* tumors (Chapter 7); and those found outside brain substance and below the tentorium—*extracerebral* tumors. The extracerebral tumors for presentation in this chapter include tumors of the meninges, the cranial nerves, posterior fossa, and the sellar and parasellar region. The chapter has been divided into two sections: Section I, discussing the grouping of extracerebral tumors including the nursing intervention for patients having infratentorial craniotomies; Section II, presenting some specific information on sellar and parasellar tumors including nursing intervention peculiar to patients who have had a hypophysectomy.

SECTION I: EXTRACEREBRAL TUMORS

Classification

Meningeal Tumors. A tumor of the meninges may be of primary or secondary origin. The most common primary tumor of the meninges is the meningioma, constituting 15% of all brain tumors.[1] It is generally agreed that these tumors arise from the arachnoid granulation. They are grayish-white nodular tumors which appear discrete and encapsulated, are slow-growing, contain arachnoid fibroblasts, and are usually attached to the dura mater, compressing but not invading brain substance. Calcification is common, allowing visualization on skull roentgenogram. Often meningiomas occur in the sagittal sinus, fissure of Rolando (central fissure), fissure of Sylvius (lateral fissure), sphenoid ridge, olfactory groove, sella turcica, or cerebellopontine angle. The tumor is somewhat more common in females than males and adults rather than children; average age of occurrence is 50 years. Malignant changes may occur in a meningioma as indicated by anaplasia, mitosis, and tumor giant cells. The prognosis for a patient with a meningioma is excellent following surgical extirpation.

---

[1]Youmans, Julian, R., ed., *Neurological Surgery*, Vol. III, Philadelphia: W. B. Saunders Co., 1973, p. 1389.

Clinical manifestations. Meningiomas produce signs and symptoms indistinguishable from those of other intracranial tumors in the same location. However, there are special features that favor a differential diagnosis of meningioma, depending on the *site* of the mass, which will be presented here.

There is a strong possibility that a tumor may prove to be a meningioma when a mass is localized to the sagittal region, the sphenoid ridge, the olfactory groove, or the diaphragma sellae. Positive pathological identification is seldom made with any certainty until the mass has been explored and biopsied.

A mass in the sagittal region may produce a local swelling of the skull, bony hard to palpation, with indefinite margins. As with other intracranial lesions, dementia, focal epilepsy, and spastic weakness of the legs may occur.

A tumor of the medial sphenoid ridge commonly produces the Foster-Kennedy syndrome (page 173). When a tumor exists in the roof or lateral orbital wall and outer one-third of the sphenoid ridge extending to the orbit, proptosis results. This is a forward displacement and bulging of the eye and usually represents a meningioma.

An olfactory groove meningioma produces bilateral or unilateral anosmia. Meningiomas of the diaphragma sellae produce optic chiasmal compression and result in temporal or bitemporal visual field defects. The combination of anosmia and chiasmal compression is more characteristic of a meningioma than any other lesion.

Diagnostic measures. Plain X-rays of the skull may reveal the site of a meningioma. Stereographic or tomographic views often show the center of the tumor's attachment. The EEG is usually normal with meningiomas, since the neuronal activity of the brain remains relatively undisturbed. A radioisotope brain scan generally shows the tumor's precise location. A lumbar puncture provides little relative information in diagnosing meningioma and is used discriminately because of the danger of precipitating cerebellar tonsillar herniation. An echoencephalogram is likely to show only evidence of a midline shift. Angiography may be used to determine tumor location by indication of blood vessel displacement. Air encephalography studies may be used as diagnostic aids, usually demonstrating meningiomas successfully, since these tumors are extrinsic to brain tissue.

Treatment modalities. Meningiomas that have symptomatically declared their presence are surgically explored: to confirm the diagnosis; to determine the extent of the lesion; and to evaluate surgical extirpation. The placement of incision and bone flaps varies according to tumor location; usually a wide flap is provided for greater exposure (Fig. 7-3). Dural defects are repaired with fascia lata, temporalis fascia, or pericranium grafts. Occasionally tumors, such as cavernous sinus tumors or medial sphenoid ridge tumors, are situated in such a way as to prevent surgical removal. In these circumstances, external decompression and partial tumor removal is attempted. The role of radiotherapy and chemotherapy is refutable in treating benign meningiomas.

Cranial Nerve Tumors.   Neuromas originate from the root of a nerve; the majority occur on the eighth cranial nerve and are called acoustic neuromas. It is thought that they originate from the vestibular rather than the auditory portion of the eighth cranial nerve. Acoustic neuromas comprise a small percentage of all brain tumors and are generally located in the cerebellopontine angle. They are encapsulated tumors that distort and compress rather than invade brain substance. They characteristically dilate and erode the internal auditory meatus. Slow-growing, they usually compress the fifth and seventh cranial nerve and eventually the pons and medulla, ultimately obstructing cerebrospinal fluid flow. Although acoustic neuromas are benign, they are often difficult to remove and may carry a high mortality rate.

Clinical manifestations.   Acoustic neuromas usually produce a hearing loss of gradual onset, often associated with tinnitus. This hearing loss and tinnitus are ipsilateral, and the hearing loss may be partial or complete. Episodes of true vertigo may occur. Nystagmus is generally a neurologic finding, and there are symptoms of seventh cranial nerve compression (ipsilateral or bilateral facial paralysis). As the tumor becomes large, the fifth cranial nerve is affected so that the corneal response is lost ipsilateral to the tumor; the patient may notice paresthesia and numbness of the face.

Diagnostic measures.   The vestibular test (ice weater calorics) is an essential component of the neurologic workup when an acoustic neuroma is suspected. Loss of or decrease in the response on the ipsilateral side is usually present. Special auditory tests (other than pure-tone audiometry) have been developed for gross differentiation between conductive and sensorineural hearing loss. These tests do not indicate that a person has an acoustic neuroma, but rather that the hearing loss is from a lesion located in the cochlea versus the eighth cranial nerve. Plain skull films often demonstrate acoustic neuromas. Tomography of the petrous pyramids has become a useful screening test for acoustic neuromas, since it illustrates the internal auditory canals and thus any erosion or asymmetry on the affected side. Positive contrast cisternography may be beneficial. For this procedure iophendylate (Pantopaque) is injected into the cerebello-pontine angle cistern under fluoroscopy, and the patient's head is tilted and manipulated to fill the internal auditory canal. Various selective views of the canal are then obtained. The possibility of an acoustic neuroma is illustrated in a vertebral angiogram by the displacement of surrounding vessels. When tomography is used during a pneumoencephalogram, cerebello-pontine angle tumors can be readily diagnosed. If the tumor is confined within the internal auditory canal, it will not be seen.

Treatment modalities. Acoustic neuromas are treated surgically. The tumor is removed by a posterior fossa (suboccipital), transmeatal approach. A microsurgical dissection of the internal auditory canal under the binocular operating microscope is performed. The hazard of this surgery is damage to the vessels supplying the brain stem or direct damage to the brain stem itself while the tumor is being dissected.

Posterior Fossa Tumors. Two tumors commonly occur in the posterior fossa: the ependymoma and the medulloblastoma.

The ependymoma is a glioma derived from the ependymal cell lining the ventricles, and occurs along ventricular pathways. Although they may occur anywhere in the ventricular system, ependymomas are usually found in the fourth ventricle. Found most commonly in children and young adults, they represent the second most common glioma. The tumor, which has a gray fleshy appearance, differs in appearance from an astrocytoma. Cystic degeneration occurs, but necrosis and hemorrhage are rare. Ependymomas are graded in four categories of malignancy similar to those for astrocytomas. In fact, some Grade IV astrocytomas (glioblastoma multiforme) may begin as ependymomas. The prognosis for a patient with an ependymoma is not much better than for one with an astrocytoma. Postoperatively, survival depends on the grade of malignancy and generally compares to survival for comparable grades of astrocytomas.

Medulloblastoma is a glioma peculiar to the infratentorial compartment. The cell of origin of this glioma remains in pathologic controversy; it may arise from the cells of the external granular layer of the cerebellum. This layer is present in the infant in well-developed form and may contribute to the neuronal and glial population of the infant's developing cerebellum. Despite the unknown origin, medulloblastomas are always found in the cerebellum, nearly always occurring in children or young adults. In children they are located principally in the midline, and in older groups in the lateral lobes of the cerebellum. The tumor appears as a nonnecrotic, nonhemorrhagic, gray fleshy mass. It is connected to the cerebellum and hangs down into the fourth ventricle. More than any other glioma it has a habit of seeding through the subarachnoid space, creating a frosted appearance of the brain and cord. The extreme malignancy of a medulloblastoma produces a grim prognosis, and total recovery is rarely achieved. Radiation and surgery occasionally delay the final act of the tragedy for several years.

Clinical manifestations. Patients with posterior fossa tumors generally complain of pain (headache) and neurologic dysfunction. The headache is usually localized behind the ear or in the suboccipital region, being most marked on the side of the tumor. The patient may carry his head rotated toward the side of the tumor. When headache is severe and localized to the subocciput, traction on the upper cervical nerve roots may be present from herniated cerebellar tonsils. The patient thus may be in danger of medullary collapse with resultant respiratory and vascular collapse. In addition, the headache is insidious in onset, steady in progression, often worse in the morning, and often relieved by vomiting. Neurologic dysfunction is usually related to direct pressure or invasion of neural structures within the posterior fossa, or hydrocephalus from obstruction of cerebrospinal fluid flow. These problems may cause cranial nerve palsy or cerebellar signs such as ipsilateral ataxia, intention tremor, a staggering gait, and dysmetria and hypotonia. Nystagmus is commonly present.

Diagnostic measures. The diagnostic aids used to determine the presence of posterior fossa tumors are essentially the same as those for intracerebral lesions (page 176–178).

Treatment modalities. Posterior fossa tumors are treated when possible by surgical extirpation. A suboccipital craniotomy using a midline incision is usually employed, extending from C-6 to an inch or so above the external occipital protuberance and from mastoid to mastoid. The atlas is partially removed and the vertebral spine and lamina if the cerebellar tonsils are suspected to be as low as C-2. A microscope is often used for dissection of the tumor away from the brain stem's blood supply and the cranial nerves. (See Fig. 8-1 for infratentorial craniotomy illustration.)

Occasionally a patient suffering from posterior fossa tumor enters the hospital ill enough to require temporary control of hydrocephalus prior to treatment of the lesion. Either a ventriculo-atrial shunt or a procedure with an external ventriculostomy with Holter-type valve attached is performed. When the wound is clearly healing satisfactorily, irradiation may be initiated. Radiotherapy is considered absolutely essential by most authorities in treating a medulloblastoma. Although chemotherapy of all malignant brain tumors is still in its infancy, medulloblastomas may be responsive to some oncolytic agents, especially intrathecal methotrexate and intravenous vincristine.

Nursing Intervention for Infratentorial Craniotomy

The surgical manipulation of the brain stem and the cerebellum during posterior fossa surgery predisposes the patient to a greater degree of danger than surgery in the cerebral hemispheres. This is due to the architectural position of anatomical structures and the location of the vital centers. General

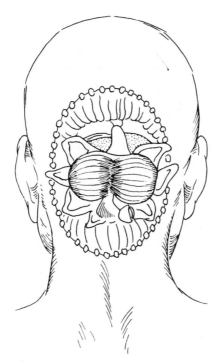

Fig. 8-1. Infratentorial craniotomy. Illustration of an infratentorial craniotomy as the cerebellum is exposed.

considerations for care of the patient having an infratentorial craniotomy will be discussed here.

Respiratory Status. A thorough respiratory assessment of the postoperative patient is essential. Any patient who has had posterior fossa surgery may be in real danger from damage to the ninth and tenth cranial nerves. Impairment of these nerves, which supply the muscles of the pharynx and larynx, may cause paralysis of the vocal cords and the muscles necessary for swallowing and coughing. The patient may be in danger of aspiration with resultant pneumonia. Observe carefully for symptoms of dysphagia and/or lack of secretion control. Be certain the gag and swallow reflex is present before feeding the patient. A patient with tenth cranial nerve damage may require a tracheostomy and/or a gastrostomy because of his inability to swallow or cough effectively. Use your assessment skills and implement your plan of care accordingly.

Neurologic Status. In addition to the standard neurologic assessment, direct your attention to the problem of cerebral edema and its effect on the structures in the posterior fossa. Cerebral edema in the posterior fossa is likely to produce cerebellar tonsillar herniation with resultant respiratory and cardiovascular crisis. The risk of cerebral edema may be minimized by administering an osmotic diuretic and steroids, ensuring adequate ventilation, and monitoring and controlling fluid balance. Many surgeons prefer that these patients remain flat for 24 hours to reduce the possibility of herniation. Remain alert and knowledgeable about your patient at all times.

Occasionally a brain stem infarction occurs postoperatively, probably due to vasospasm. It may develop in patients who appear quite well and seem to be progressing. Exercise caution in the prevention of any situation that might induce hypotension, such as leaving the patient in a sitting position unattended. Such hypotension is believed to be a contributing factor in brain stem infarct.

Another special neurologic problem with patients who have had posterior fossa surgery (especially surgery in the cerebello-pontine angle) is loss of function of one or more cranial nerves. If there is a loss of function of the fifth cranial nerve, careful prevention of drying and protection of the face from local trauma may be all that is necessary until function returns. Methyl cellulose drops and an eye patch may be beneficial. Eye patches may also help if the patient is suffering from diplopia from damage to the third, fourth, or sixth cranial nerves. If damage to any of the cranial nerves is severe, reparative surgery may be necessary.

Gastrointestinal Status. Gastrointestinal hemorrhage in the form of a Cushing's ulcer is more likely to occur following posterior fossa surgery than after supratentorial surgery, especially when the surgery involves manipulation of the floor of the fourth ventricle. In addition to the usual observations, monitor the patient's nasogastric drainage and stools for guaiac. Autonomic fibers from the vagus nerve affect the gastrointestinal tract, and impairment may contribute to a paralytic ileus. Be aware of this possibility and also the problem of constipation; intervene when appropriate. Impairment of the ninth, tenth, and twelfth cranial nerves may cause difficulty in swallowing, and the type of diet offered the patient may have to be regulated in quantity and adjusted in consistency until function returns.

Psychosocial Status. The goals for a patient who has had posterior fossa surgery are directed toward mobility and independence. These patients sometimes have crippling defects in coordination, but may show a remarkable capacity for recovery in time. The goal of working toward autonomy must be introduced very early in the rehabilitation program and sustained throughout its course.

There is another matter in the psychosocial aspect of the patient to be considered: there may be damage to the brain stem mechanisms that subserve consciousness and/or emotions (reticular activating system). Prolonged coma (akinetic mutism) may exist and lead to death from complications of stasis. However, many patients suffering this complication may return to a state of full mental functioning. Occasionally emotional states such as euphoria or severe depression follow brain stem damage. Care may become a real challenge as the nurse deals with the emotional behavior of the patient until he gains control of his feelings.

Immobility may contribute to sensory deprivation, and the critical care nurse will need to take measures to provide stimulation. Whenever possible encourage visitors, provide reading material, provide a telephone, clock, and radio, and eliminate monotony and routines in the environment.

The period of waiting for determination of what function will return may cause overwhelming anxiety. Psychological support from the nurse and the patient's family is extremely important. As we have mentioned so often, the added assistance of the resources available to the patient in the intensive care unit is invaluable. This is not to imply that the nurse is relieved of any responsibility, but to confirm the advantages of a team concept in patient care through the utilization of representatives of other health care disciplines, such as social service people, mental health counselors, and other specialists.

SECTION II: SELLAR AND PARASELLAR TUMORS

Pituitary Anatomy and Physiology

A review of pituitary anatomy and physiology is essential for comprehension of tumor classification, clinical manifestations, diagnostic measures, intervention, and nursing objectives for patients with these problems.

The pituitary or hypophysis cerebri is located at the base of the brain in the sella turcica of the sphenoid bone. The optic chiasma lies just above the anterior portion of the diaphragma sellae; this structural relationship is highly significant in identifying symptoms and determining intervention for sellar and parasellar tumors. The pituitary, while continually monitoring the internal environment, is controlled by neurosecretory substances, or releasing factors, of the hypothalamus. The pituitary is divided into two lobes of differing embryonic origin: the anterior pituitary or adenohypophysis, a glandular structure, is embryologically formed from the roof of the mouth; the posterior pituitary or neurohypophysis is of neural origin, embryologically developed from the nervous tissue of the brain.

The adenohypophysis synthesizes and releases seven hormones which control the activity of the thyroid, adrenal cortex, gonads, and mammary glands. The synthesis and release of these hormones to their target glands is

Table 8-1. Pituitary Hormones

ANTERIOR PITUITARY

Name	Releasing Factor	Target Cells	Response	Increased Level	Decreased Level
STH	STH-releasing factor	Bone, muscle	Stimulates growth; promotes active transport of a.a. into cell and influences lipid, CHO, and calcium metabolism	Child: gigantism (prior to epiphyseal closure) patient grows very tall adult: acromegaly (after epiphyseal closure) bones increase in thickness and increase in soft tissue growth	Child: dwarfism adult: lethargy, increased weight, loss of reproductive function, premature aging
ACTH	ACTH-releasing factor	Adrenal cortex	Stimulates adrenal gland secretion of mineralocorticoids and glucocorticoids	Cushing's disease: increased amounts of cortisol and aldosterone	Addison's disease: decreased cortisol and aldosterone, increased MSH
TSH	TSH-releasing factor (depends on quantity of thyroid hormones available to tissues)	Thyroid	Stimulates thyroid to increased secretion of thyroxine (controls rate of most chemical reactions in the body)	Goiter, increased BMR, decreased weight, increased cardiac output, HR and BP, increased cerebration, fine muscle tremors	Reduced thyroid activity, decreased BMR, increased weight, decreased cardiac output, HR, BP, and cerebration, somnolence
LTH	LTH-releasing factor	Breast	Stimulates breast to lactate	Too much milk	Too little milk

FSH	FSH-releasing factor	Ovaries, testes	Stimulates growth of ovaries and sperm	Early puberty	Late puberty
LH—F ICSH—M	LH-releasing factor	Ovaries, testes	Growth of follicles and increased secretion of estrogen and progesterone; ICSH—increased secondary male sex characteristics	Excess progesterone, excess testosterone, menstrual cycle disturbance	Amenorrhea, diminished progesterone and testosterone
MSH	MSH-releasing factor	Skin	Regulates skin pigments	Increased pigmentation	Decreased pigmentation

POSTERIOR PITUITARY

| oxytoxin | Childbirth, sucking | Uterus, breasts | Stimulates uterus to contract at childbirth; stimulates lactation | Precipitate childbirth, excess milk | Prolonged childbirth, diminished milk |
| ADH (vasopressin) | Dehydration | Arterioles, distal renal tubule | Vasoconstriction of arterioles to increase arterial pressure; increased water reabsorption in distal tubules, stimulates smooth muscle of GI tract | Increased BP, decreased UA output, edema | Diabetes insipidus, dilute urine, increased urinary volume |

controlled by neurosecretory substances secreted within the hypothalamus. The hormones of the adenohypophysis are:

TSH	Thyroid stimulating hormone	Thyrotropin
ACTH	Adrenocorticotropic hormone	Corticotropin
STH	Growth hormone	Somatotropin
FSH	Follicle stimulating hormone	Gonadotropin
LH	Luteinizing stimulating hormone, "female"	Gonadotropin
ICSH	Interstitial cell-stimulating hormone, "male"	
LTH	Luteotropic	Gonadotropin
MSH	Melanocytic-stimulating hormone	

Tumors of the anterior pituitary directly affect the synthesis and release of these hormones by increasing or decreasing their availability.

The neurohypophysis stores and releases two hormones which are manufactured by the hypothalamus: antidiuretic hormone (ADH) and oxytoxin.

The neurohypophysis is rarely invaded by tumors; but when it is diseased or surgically removed, the hormone levels of ADH and oxytoxin may not be altered because they continue to be manufactured by the hypothalamus.

A summary of the pituitary hormones may be found in Table 8-1.

Classification of Tumors

The common sellar and parasellar tumors are pituitary adenomas (anterior pituitary tumors) and craniopharyngiomas.

Pituitary Adenoma. Only a few intracranial tumors are pituitary tumors. They are discovered more frequently in young and middle-aged adults. The anterior pituitary is comprised of three basic cell types: eosinophils (almost 40% of all cells), basophils (about 10% of all cells), and chromophobes (about 50% of all cells). Benign pituitary adenomas are the result of hyperplasia of one of the three cell types. These cells differ in their affinity for hematoxylin and eosin staining and, therefore, offer a time-honored classification of tumors based upon staining properties.

Chromophobe Tumor. This tumor, with no affinity for staining, is the most common benign pituitary adenoma. It accounts for at least 50% of all pituitary tumors. The chromophobe tumor may, or may not, be hormone-secreting. It may produce a state of hyperpituitarism with an increase in ACTH and growth hormone. More commonly it is a nonfunctional, non-secreting, slow-growing tumor that exerts progressive pressure on the remaining normal pituitary gland. Atrophy of the residual gland results in a state of hypopituitarism.

Eosinophilic Tumor.   This tumor, with an affinity for eosin staining, is
the second most common benign pituitary adenoma. It is a hormone-secreting
tumor, producing excessive amounts of STH (growth hormone; somatotropin) and LTH (leuteotropic hormone; prolactin), causing a state of
hyperpituitarism.

Basophilic Tumor.   This tumor, with an affinity for hematoxylin staining, is the least common benign pituitary adenoma. It is a hormone-secreting
tumor that excretes excessive amounts of several hormones, but typically an
oversecretion of ACTH (adrenocorticotropic hormone; corticotropin). The
resultant effect of this hyperpituitary state is Cushing's syndrome.

All pituitary adenomas are benign, slow-growing, encapsulated lesions.
They are spherical, soft, and red-brown in color, varying in size from microscopic to a diameter of over 10 centimeters. They may spread beyond the
sella turcica invading the cavernous sinus and paranasal sinuses, and may
even erode the nasopharynx. The prognosis for a patient with a pituitary
adenoma is variable; although the tumor may be "cured," the abnormal
effects on the human body may be longlasting.

Craniopharyngioma.   This tumor is the second most common hypophyseal tumor, found primarily in children and young adults. It is usually
benign; but, rarely, malignant changes do occur. The tumor may develop
anywhere along the craniopharyngeal canal; thus it may be within the sella
turcica or external to it, usually lying above the sella. The tumor is usually
well encapsulated and has multilocular cysts containing turbid fluid. Occasionally the slow-growing tumor attains a considerable size of up to 10 centimeters in diameter. Symptoms develop as a result of the expanding mass
compressing the anterior pituitary (hypopituitarism) and invading the hypothalamus (mental disturbances).

Clinical Manifestations

Sellar and parasellar tumors present signs and symptoms as a result of local
pressure on surrounding brain structures and as a result of the endocrine effect
of the tumor.

Local Symptoms.   These symptoms are a result of tumor pressure on
anatomically related brain structures.

Visual disturbances.   The optic chiasma lies just above the anterior portion of the diaphragma sellae. Compression of the optic chiasma by a sellar or
parasellar tumor occurs before the fibers cross over and results in bitemporal
hemianopsia (lateral half of each visual field is lost). This disturbance may
occur very slowly and often goes unnoticed by the patient; however, as the
nasal half of the macula is involved, the patient rapidly loses visual acuity.

The optic discs are usually found to be normal or atrophic; papilledema is distinctly rare, but may occur with very large tumors.

Headache. Headache is a frequent symptom of patients suffering from sellar and parasellar tumors. It is probably due to traction on the pain-sensitive dura of the diaphragma sellae rather than increased intracranial pressure.

Endocrinopathy. Endocrinopathy is quite common in some form in patients with sellar or parasellar tumors. Negative endocrinopathy or hypopituitarism is a deficiency of one or more of the anterior pituitary hormones, while positive endocrinopathy or hyperpituitarism is an excess of one or more of the anterior pituitary hormones.

Hypopituitarism. Severe deficiency of anterior pituitary hormones produces symptoms that are attributed to a decrease in the level of each of the hormones (see Table 8-1).

A decrease in the circulating levels of the gonadotropins (FSH, LH-ISCH, and LTH) results in a decrease of the secondary sex characteristics, sterility, and diminished sex drive. In the adult male decreased libido, loss of facial and body hair, diminished spermatogenesis, and testicular atrophy occur. In the adult female decreased libido, infertility, and amenorrhea occur.

A decrease in the level of ACTH results in a decrease of the hormones produced by the cortex of the adrenal gland, resulting in Addison's disease.

A decrease in the level of STH, or the growth hormone, results in severely stunted growth—dwarfism. It occurs prior to epiphyseal closure of long limb bones.

Hyperpituitarism. The increase of anterior pituitary hormones produces symptoms related to an increase in the level of each of the hormones.

An increase in the levels of gonadotropins (FSH, LH-ISCH, and LTH) results in early puberty, an excess of progesterone and testosterone, and menstrual cycle disturbances.

An increase in the levels of TSH results in an increase in the production and secretion of thyroxin in the thyroid gland.

An increase in the levels of ACTH results in an increase in the adrenal cortex hormones, resulting in Cushing's syndrome.

An increase in the levels of MSH results in increased skin pigmentation.

An increase in the levels of STH in children before the ephiphyses of the long limb bones are closed results in gigantism. These individuals may grow as tall as eight or nine feet. If there is an increase of STH in the adult, there is a characteristic largeness of all of the extremities, producing an appositional enlargement called acromegaly.

Diagnostic Measures

Laboratory Studies. Sellar and parasellar tumors which involve anterior pituitary hormone secretions may be diagnosed by assessing the individual's circulating hypophyseal hormone levels (radiobioimmunoassay).

Radiographic Studies. Neoplasms near or in the sella may be diagnosed by plain skull films. The tumor usually thins the posterior clinoid process and widens the sella cavity.

Contrast Studies. These studies are important for differential diagnosis (e.g., to rule out parasellar aneurysm) and to demonstrate tumor extensiveness.

Intervention: Modalities of Therapy

There are several approaches to the treatment of sellar and parasellar tumors. Obviously the physician will determine the treatment of choice based on the individual and the extent of the tumor involvement. However, the nurse should be familiar with the mode of treatment selected to enable her to answer any inquiries the patient may have regarding his care.

Radiotherapy. Some physicians utilize internal (yttrium-90 implantation) or external irradiation initially in the treatment of pituitary adenomas that present classical symptoms indicating accurate diagnosis. There are divergent views on the positive and negative value of radiotherapy as a primary or secondary treatment of pituitary tumors. The hazard of radiation edema, radionecrosis, and deleterious long-term effects is being investigated.

Craniotomy. Surgery is indicated for pituitary tumors in the following situations: when the diagnosis is doubtful (an exploratory craniotomy is done); when there is more than 50% visual field loss; when severe general pressure symptoms exist; when there is tumor involvement of the cavernous sinus; and when severe symptoms of endocrinopathy are present. The fairly recent development of adequate hormonal replacement therapy (e.g., corticosteroids) has reduced the operative risk. The total or partial removal of the pituitary gland may be accomplished through a low frontal craniotomy (see page 178).

Transphenoidal Microsurgery. The use of microscopes in the operating room has made possible new approaches to the cranial vault and its internal structures. This procedure involves entry into the sellar region through the sphenoid sinus, approached through the nasal septum. This technique may be used to remove the pituitary gland if the tumor does not have significant extension or intracranial attachments.

Stereotaxic Surgery. This surgery is frequently employed for precise positioning of a given site, in this instance the pituitary gland. The concept of locating a site in space by identifying three reference points corresponding to the *X, Y,* and *Z* axes in three-dimensional graphic plotting is used. In this manner a variety of stereotaxic instruments can be accurately guided to reach a precisely calculated site within the brain. Destruction of the pituitary can be accomplished by: the introduction of an electrode (electrolysis); the introduction of refrigerants through a cannula (cryosurgery); induction heating produced by high frequency current; coagulation with radiofrequency; the creation of a true surgical lesion with a leukotome; instillation of corrosive or sclerosing fluids; and the use of ultrasound. These stereotaxic procedures have the advantage of minimizing intracranial operative disruption, but the disadvantage of allowing the physician very limited control over the amount of tissue destroyed.

Nursing Intervention for Hypophysectomy

Preoperative Care. The preoperative care of patients scheduled for a hypophysectomy is similar to that of patients undergoing any other cranial surgery (pages 181–182).

It is pertinent to remind the intensive care nurse that she may encounter patients who are having pituitary destruction or removal for reasons other than pituitary tumors. An ablative hypophysectomy may be performed for: growth retardation of endocrine-dependent carcinomas of the breast and ovaries, retardation of metastatic cancer, and retardation of progressive diabetic retinopathy. Surgery of the last type diminishes the secretion of several anterior hypophyseal hormones that exert a diabetogenic effect.

Medications may be administered preoperatively, including dexamethasone for prevention of cerebral edema and hormonal therapy, depending on the patient's particular problem.

The advantages of a preoperative neurologic assessment cannot be overemphasized. The baseline information may be used postoperatively to determine any change in the status of the patient. It is highly significant in evaluating the patient's neurologic system prior to and immediately after the surgery.

Postoperative Care

Neurologic status. A thorough neurologic assessment is necessary with these patients as well as any other neurosurgical patients. Observations for evidence of cerebral edema, increasing intracranial pressure, and postoperative meningitis are important so that early management may be instituted. The patient who has had transphenoidal microsurgery will return to the unit with nasal packs. Observe for a clear nasal drip or constant swallowing, indicating a cerebrospinal fluid leak. The packs are usually removed in 2 to 12 days.

Endocrine status. Postoperative management of a patient who has had a hypophysectomy is usually predicated on the assumption that no pituitary function exists whatever. Cortisone, thyroid, and gonadotropic and growth hormones are usually replaced postoperatively.

Cortisone administration is initiated preoperatively in a specified dose and then tapered by the tenth postoperative day. After the patient's surgical recovery, pituitary and adrenal function may be reevaluated and glucocorticoid supplements given as indicated. "Hypothalamic storm" may occur postoperatively when patients have been inadequately prepared with glucocorticoids. The clinical manifestations are hyperthermia, restlessness, hypertension, and seizures. It may be controlled by hypothermia measures and the administration of chlorpromazine and promethazine. These patients must have electrolytes checked closely and any abnormalities promptly corrected. Excessive sodium retention may occur and, in fact, be quite persistent. Body weight is an excellent guide to the patient's fluid status. Particularly in children, twice-daily body weight determination as compared to an accurate preoperative weight is extremely useful in order to follow sodium retention with its attendant water excess.

A deficiency in thyrotropic hormone is usually not seen until about three weeks after surgery. It is treated with desiccated thyroid or its equivalent, which maintains linear growth and a normal basal metabolism.

Nearly all patients who have craniopharyngiomas removed show gonadotropic hormone deficiency as manifested by failure to mature sexually. Long-term management of this problem is effected with the administration of estrogens, progesterone, and testosterone.

Even when all other hormones are lacking, STH (growth hormone) may be produced by a very small residual portion of viable anterior pituitary tissue, thus ensuring the progress of skeletal growth. However, when necessary, growth may be stimulated by commercially available STH.

Diabetes insipidus may occur as the posterior pituitary fails to secrete ADH. The body begins to lose volumes of fluid; careful observation and recording of intake and output and urine specific gravity, both on an hourly basis, are extremely important in the first 48–72 hours postoperatively. If pitressin (extract of the posterior pituitary) is used to treat this condition, the aqueous form may be ordered rather than pitressin in oil. The latter may produce water intoxication from excessive ADH and subsequent aggravation of cerebral edema. If pitressin preparations are used, several nursing precautions are advised:

1. Warm the medication to room temperature.
2. Mix the contents well by shaking the container, which ensures adequate suspension of the hormone in solution.
3. Use fresh stock of medication.
4. Avoid injecting the medication into scar tissue, since excessive body deposits may build up that may require days for release and may confuse dosage and lead to water intoxication.

During pitressin administration the patient's fluid and electrolyte balance must be assessed frequently. The drug may produce water intoxication (complicating the treatment of cerebral edema), renal failure, decrease in the patient's level of consciousness, and seizures. When diabetes insipidus occurs following hypophysectomy, it is almost always transient. Electrolyte supplements may be necessary until the patient's fluid balance is restored.

CONCLUSION

We have tried to explain extracerebral tumors in enough depth to allow the nurse some basis in understanding the pathology of tumors as well as the symptoms one might expect to see. Information regarding the diagnostic measures is important in assisting in the neurologic work-up as well as providing some validity to the explanations you may be communicating to patients. The same is true regarding the description of the various treatments employed for patients with extracerebral tumors. The combined information in Sections I and II should give the intensive care nurse a clear definition of postoperative care of patients undergoing neurosurgery. You realize by this time the degree of responsibility designated to the qualified intensive care nurse. The nursing profession is obliged to consider you in high esteem.

BIBLIOGRAPHY

"Anxiety, Recognition and Intervention," A Programmed Text, *American Journal of Nursing*, 65 (No. 9):130–152, September 1965.

Beeson, Paul B., and Walsh McDermott, eds., *Textbook of Medicine*, Vol. 1, 14th ed., Philadelphia: W. B. Saunders Co., 1975.

Elliot, Carolyn St. John, "Radiation Therapy: How You Can Help," *Nursing 76,* September, pp. 34–41.

Elliott, Frank A., *Clinical Neurology*, Philadelphia: W. B. Saunders Co., 1971.

Ezrin, Calvin, "The Pituitary Gland," *Clinical Symposia*, Summit, New Jersey: CIBA Pharmaceutical Co., 1963.

Kintzel, Ray Corman, ed., *Advanced Concepts in Clinical Nursing*, 2nd ed., Philadelphia: J. B. Lippincott Co., 1977.

Luckman, Joan, and Karen Sorensen, *Medical-Surgical Nursing: A Psychophysiologic Approach*, Philadelphia: W. B. Saunders Co., 1974.

Read, Sharon, "Clinical Care in Hypophysectomy," *Nursing Clinics of North America,* 9 (No. 4): 647–654, December 1974.

Robbins, Stanley L., *Pathologic Basis of Disease*, Philadelphia: W. B. Saunders Co., 1974.

Rubin, Philip, *Clinical Oncology for Medical Students and Physicians, A Multidisciplinary Approach*, 4th ed., The American Cancer Society, 1974.

Shafer, Kathleen, et al., *Medical-Surgical Nursing*, St. Louis: The C. V. Mosby Co., 1975.

Wheeler, Priscilla, "Care of a Patient with a Cerebellar Tumor," *American Journal of Nursing*, February 1977, pp. 263–266.

Youmans, Julian R., ed., *Neurological Surgery*, Philadelphia: W. B. Saunders Co., 1973.

9
NEUROLOGIC AND INFECTIOUS DISORDERS

INTRODUCTION

Many neurologic and infectious disorders could be reviewed in depth, and the discussion certainly would benefit the nursing care provided the patients involved. The critical care nurse, however, may be exposed to only a selected few of these patients, whose difficulty with their problems requires admission to the unit. Or, perhaps the neurologic disease is a secondary diagnosis, and in these circumstances the nurse needs to be familiar with the condition.

The chapter has been divided into two sections: Section I, discussing neurologic diseases including parkinsonism, myasthenia gravis, and epilepsy; Section II, discussing infectious diseases including meningitis, encephalitis, brain abscess, poliomyelitis, and Guillain-Barré syndrome.

SECTION I: NEUROLOGIC DISEASES

Parkinsonism

Perspective. The major manifestations of Parkinson's disease were first described by James Parkinson. It has been known as Parkinson's disease, paralysis agitans, and shaking palsy. The etiology of the primary disease remains unknown, but secondary symptoms of the disease may be associated with, or a complication of, epidemic encephalitis, carbon monoxide poisoning, phenothiazine intoxication, vascular disorders, neurosyphilis, and head trauma. The word "parkinsonism" will be used here in describing the disorder regardless of the cause, which may further classify symptoms as primary or secondary.

Parkinsonism is the most frequently encountered disease of the extrapyramidal system and represents a ranking cause of debility from neurologic disease. It is considered to be the second most common neurologic ailment in the United States with an incidence of about one million cases and an estimated fifty thousand new cases reported each year. The onset of parkinsonism is usually between the ages of 50 and 65 years of age; it is known to be a slowly progressive disease of late adult life. It recognizes no sex or racial barriers, and no evidence exists to indicate a familial or heredity factor. The progression of the disease is relentless over a period of two or three decades, shortening life expectancy, with the cause of death usually being bronchopneumonia or urinary tract infection.

Parkinsonism is usually attributed to degeneration within the nuclear masses of the extrapyramidal system. The essential lesion is found in the substantia nigra, where groups of pigmented cells disappear. The cells and tracts of the striate bodies, globus pallidus, and substantia nigra all show a deficiency of the neural transmitter substance striatal dopamine.

Clinical manifestations. Parkinsonism is characterized by tremors, akinesia, and rigidity. It may begin insidiously with any one of these three cardinal symptoms alone or in combination. Tremors may go unnoticed by the patient or those around him for some time. Commonly the initial symptoms are tremors of the hands, involving the fingers in a pill-rolling motion, which may be followed by akinesia (a slowing of movements) until the patient's appearance becomes one of peculiar stillness. Ultimately, the face assumes a masklike appearance with a fixed unblinking stare. Movements become slow and do not flow smoothly one into another, creating delays. The patient may be unable to carry out routine daily activities. Rigidity involving muscles of all the extremities may occur. Stiff neck and a shuffling, short-stepped gait with loss of swinging of the arms may develop. It becomes increasingly difficult for the patient to maintain an erect posture; he is inclined to fall forward. As rigidity affects the facial muscles, dysarthria, monotonous voice tones, and drooling result. Parkinsonism involves an inevitable progression of symptoms, which may vary in rate of appearance and disabling effects.

Diagnostic measures. The diagnosis of parkinsonism is based on the symptomatology presented, particularly if tremors are present, and exploration of causes associated with other problems contributing to the development of extrapyramidal system symptoms. Cerebrospinal fluid analysis is usually normal; sometimes there are abnormal EEG tracings. Neurologic findings include lack of facial expression; rhythmical resting tremors of the distal limb segments, accented by suspension, decreased by active motion, and eliminated during sleep; muscular rigidity; akinesia; and postural abnormalities.

Treatment modalities. The treatment of parkinsonism is symptomatic, supportive, and palliative throughout the patient's remaining life. It includes psychotherapeutic measures, specific medications, physical therapy, and occasionally surgical intervention.

Psychotherapeutic measures are appropriate inasmuch as the symptoms of the disease are markedly influenced by psychic factors. The patient's overall attitude largely affects the degree to which the disability hinders his activity.

The drugs that are employed in the treatment of parkinsonism are either dopaminergic (levodopa and amantadine hydrochloride) or anticholinergic (benztropine mesylate and benzhexol hydrochloride) in nature. The dopaminergic and cholinergic mechanisms are thought to be antagonistic. Dopamine, a precursor of norepinephrine with its adrenergic (inhibiting) effect, is in reduced concentration in patients with parkinsonism. The symptoms of the disease reflect a dominance of the cholinergic (excitatory) mechanism, which is innervated by acetylcholine. The drugs administered either enhance the dopaminergic mechanism or block the cholinergic mechanism in an attempt to correct the imbalance between these two antagonists. Specific drugs are discussed in detail in Chapter 11.

Physical therapy measures, such as heat and massage, may alleviate muscle cramping and contractures causing pain. Postural exercises and gait training are important in the prevention of falls and injury to the patient.

Occasionally surgical intervention is the mode of treatment for parkinsonism. The integrity of certain neural pathways is essential for the production of symptoms. These pathways are surgically interrupted, using stereotactic procedures producing lesions in the ventrolateral nucleus of the thalamus. Candidates for the surgery are selected on the basis of age, the manifestation of unilateral symptoms that constitute a substantial handicap, and unresponsiveness to drug therapy.

Nursing objectives.   The critical care nurse may encounter parkinsonism in the following instances: the patient with parkinsonism who is admitted to the unit with a life-threatening problem that is unrelated to his parkinsonism diagnosis; the patient in parkinsonian crisis; or the patient suffering from a complication of parkinsonism.

The nursing goals for any patient admitted with a secondary diagnosis of parkinsonism are integrated to deal with the acute problem as well as those problems presented as a result of his disease.

The major threat to the parkinsonism patient's respiratory system is aspiration pneumonia. The patient may have dysphagia when muscle rigidity becomes advanced. Exercise caution at mealtime and proceed with feedings using common sense. The food served may have to be adjusted in quantity and consistency. Allow enough time for meals, never rushing the patient. If in your judgment a suction apparatus becomes necessary, place one at the bedside with a large bore suction catheter, such as a tonsil suction for emergency use.

Validate and administer all antiparkinsonism medications the patient has been taking. The sudden withdrawal of drugs is inadvisable and may precipitate parkinsonian crisis.

Nutrition may be a problem. If the patient has difficulty eating, he may suffer from weight loss and, of course, loss of energy. Weigh him daily, and as previously explained adjust his therapeutic diet including ample fluids to avoid constipation.

The psychological climate assumes increased importance with the parkinsonism patient. Lassitude tends to foster dependence. It becomes so much easier for these patients to allow someone else to do things for them; this is particularly true in the critical care unit where acute illness favors dependence automatically. Consider the patient's primary diagnosis; be aware of the emotional attitude prevalent in patients with parkinsonism; sustain as much independence as possible.

All efforts should be made to have the patient continue in a physical therapy program. If this is not possible, use preventive measures in the unit and encourage self-activity. If the patient must assume bed rest, prevent postural deformities; employ the usual techniques directed toward the complications of immobility.

Parkinsonian crisis. This emergency situation may develop as a result of undue psychological or physiological stress, or the abrupt withdrawal of antiparkinsonism medications. The clinical manifestations are: sudden exacerbation of tremor, rigidity, and dyskinesia; acute anxiety; diaphoresis; tachycardia and hyperpnea. Reinstate the patient on his antiparkinsonism drug regimen; if symptomatology is severe, administer IV sodium phenobarbital as directed. Cardiovascular and respiratory monitoring are usually indicated. Reduce environmental stress when possible by placing the patient in a quiet, semidarkened room. Assess the patient frequently until the crisis has subsided.

Complications of Parkinsonism. The most frequent complication encountered in these patients is aspiration pneumonia. Treatment is based on the maintenance of adequate ventilation, including respiratory toilet, and the administration of antibiotics and adjunctive steroid therapy as prescribed.

Myasthenia Gravis

Perspective. Myasthenia gravis is a neuromuscular disorder characterized by abnormal fatigability of muscles. The prevalence is estimated at approximately 33 people per one million population, with an annual incidence of 2 to 5 per million. New cases are reported as occurring with about the same frequency as systemic lupus erythematosis.[1] The disease occurs in any age group, but frequently it is reported in people between 20 and 30 years old. In young adults it is more common in females than in males. There is no evidence to conclude there are heredity factors.

[1]Beeson, Paul B., and Walsh McDermott, eds., *Textbook of Medicine*, 14th ed., Philadelphia: W. B. Saunders Co., 1975, p. 802.

The course of myasthenia gravis includes periods of remission, exacerbation, and improvement after the administration of anticholinesterase drugs. The muscle weakness and fatigability are thought to be caused by impaired neuromuscular transmission at the myoneural junction. Normally acetylcholine is released, transmitting the impulse at the motor end plate, following which the neurotransmitter is rapidly hydrolyzed by the enzyme cholinesterase. It has been postulated that the abnormal transmission defect is a result of: the diminished secretion and release of acetylcholine; the excessive secretion and release of cholinesterase; or an abnormal response of the end plate to acetylcholine. The anticholinesterase drugs used in treating myasthenic patients with resultant relief of symptoms increase the effective concentration of acetylcholine.

The cause of myasthenia gravis is not known, though it is thought to be an autoimmune disease, since multiple skeletal autoantibodies have been found in patient serum. Hyperthyroidism, thymomas, systemic lupus erythematosis, and rheumatoid arthritis occur more commonly in patients with myasthenia gravis. Many believe thymoma or thymic hyperplasia in particular is associated with the disease.

Clinical Manifestations. The symptoms of myasthenia gravis are related to muscle weakness and fatigability. Muscle strength diminishes with increased activity and seems to be restored with rest. The patient experiences periods of remission and exacerbation. The presenting symptom is usually weakness of the extraocular muscles producing ptosis or diplopia, which becomes more pronounced late in the day. All muscular functions including speech and swallowing become more compromised after prolonged activity. The patient often has a high-pitched, nasal voice, and a snarling nasal smile ("myasthenic smile"). Any somatic musculature may be affected.

Diagnostic Measures. A diagnosis of myasthenia gravis is based on a history, a pattern of muscle weakness and fatigability, and the patient's response to anticholinesterase drug therapy. Neostigmine and edrophonium chloride are used and should produce brief relief of symptoms in the myasthenic patient. The development of muscle fatigue may be investigated by performing electromyography.

Treatment Modalities. The medical management of patients with myasthenia gravis is based on the administration of anticholinesterase drugs. Adjunctive drug therapy with glucocorticoids and immunosuppressive agents is being evaluated.

The surgical management may include a thymectomy. Some neurologic centers perform a thymectomy on all patients under 60 years of age who are disabled by myasthenia gravis and are otherwise in good general health.

Thymectomy may not benefit patients in whom a thymoma has been established.

Nursing objectives. In the critical care unit nursing goals for the myasthenic patient include: patient teaching and understanding of his disease; management of surgical intervention; management of myasthenic crisis; and phychological support in helping the patient to adjust to his limitations.

Patient teaching. The patient as well as his family should be well acquainted with the disease process, the pharmacologic therapy, and the clinical manifestations of myasthenic crisis. The patient must be able to recognize the degree of his muscle fatigability and respond accordingly with rest. The family may observe increased weakness during special time periods and should reschedule activities based on the patient's strength. The patient and family need to be thoroughly familiar with the action of the drugs and the symptoms of adverse effects and to understand the importance of seeking medical attention when crisis is pending. Preventive measures, including some nutritional ones, and the maintenance of good general health should be encouraged.

Surgical management. If at all possible the critical care nurse should be in a position to assess the patient scheduled for a thymectomy prior to the procedure. The performance of an open thoracotomy as well as the possibility of postoperative myasthenic or cholinergic crisis may bring the patient to the unit for 24 to 72 hours after surgery. The patient often enters the unit intubated (unable to communicate), making assessment somewhat more difficult unless the nurse has evaluated the patient prior to surgery. Confirm the administration of all preoperative and postoperative drugs with the physician. Be prepared to assess and intervene if the patient develops symptoms of crisis.

Management of crisis. A crisis may occur as a result of an overdose of anticholinesterase drugs (cholinergic crisis) or from an exacerbation of the myasthenic involvement, requiring additional anticholinesterase drugs (myasthenic crisis). The most important aspect of detecting crisis in a myasthenic patient is prior assessment. The critical care nurse gathers information by speaking with the patient and identifying how quickly muscle fatigue occurs as he talks. Listen attentively to the patient who has had the disease over a period of time. He can usually describe the onset of crisis in the early stages. The patient may present with sudden onset of difficulty or inability to swallow, dyspnea with muscle weakness, nasal flaring, and other signs of respiratory distress. *Any* increase in muscle fatigability, respiratory distress, or quantity of secretions must forewarn the nurse of pending crisis. Neostigmine should be readily available, as well as equipment for respiratory assistance. In differentiating crisis, edrophonium chloride (Tensilon, an anticholinesterase) is used, since its maximum duration of action is 5 to 10 minutes. If there is marked improvement in the patient's clinical status after intravenous injection of Tensilon, the crisis is myasthenic in nature, caused by an exacerbation of symptoms of the disease and a need for more medication. If the patient's condition deteriorates with the administration of Tensilon, it is cholinergic in nature, from an overdose of anticholinesterase drugs; pralidoxine, a cholinesterase reactivator, may be given along with atropine to counteract the muscle weakness occurring with overdose of anticholinesterase drugs. The nurse must be knowledgeable about myasthenic pharmacology in order to observe "standing orders" in the unit in the event of crisis.

Psychological support.   The adjustment to myasthenia gravis may be a difficult one for the patient. Frustrations occur that are often overwhelming. The patient may not be able to accomplish physical tasks *when* he wants to, if at all. He suffers periods of remission and exacerbation. During crisis the patient becomes frightened and needs the reassurance that the nurse, with all of the respiratory equipment necessary to sustain life, is near, and that *life will be preserved.* Considerable work needs to be done with the family to deal with all of the emotional upsets and to resolve problems that occur as a result of the patient's physical incapabilities.

Epilepsy

Perspective.   The word epilepsy comes from the Greek *epilēpsia*, whose roots meant "to take or to seize." A *seizure* is a *symptom* of abnormal and excessive neuronal discharge in different parts of the brain. When a seizure involves musculoskeletal contractions, it is termed a convulsion. Seizures may occur as a symptom of a lesion of the brain which produces an irritable focus (such as a tumor, trauma, or infection), cerebral ischemia (cerebrovascular disease), or metabolic disturbances (such as electrolyte disturbances, low serum glucose level, acid–base imbalance, drug toxicity, or withdrawal). *Epilepsy* refers to *recurrent* seizures when there is *no* extracerebral *neurologic cause* for their appearance and is often termed "seizure disorder" or idiopathic epilepsy. The symptom of seizures then, in this instance, is not secondary to any other disease process. This section is devoted to a discussion of epilepsy with a description of seizure symptoms.

Epilepsy is estimated to occur in about 0.5 to 1.0% of the United States population.[2] There are no sex barriers for the disease, but it is felt that genetic

[2]Beeson, Paul, and Walsh McDermott, ed., *Textbook of Medicine*, 14th ed., Philadelphia: W. B. Saunders Co., 1975, p. 723.

factors do create a predisposition to epilepsy. The onset of seizures is usually before age 20 years. A person developing symptoms later in life strongly suggests other brain pathology.

Classification and Clinical Manifestations of Seizures.   Seizures are irritative phenomena characterized by abnormal synchronous activation of groups of cerebral neurons. These irritative phenomena manifest themselves in various clinical patterns, which primarily depend upon the normal function of the originally activated groups of neurons, the anatomical relationship of such neurons to other functional areas of the brain, and the facility and speed with which the discharge is propagated within the nervous system. Seizures are classified by a variety of clinical and EEG criteria. For our purposes they will be divided into two broad groups: generalized seizures and focal seizures.

Generalized seizures.   These seizures are thought to originate from deep within the central brain and rapidly propagate to the cerebral cortex, creating general activation of cerebral neurons.

(a) Grand Mal Seizures: This major seizure is often hallmarked by an aura. The aura may be dissimilar in individuals; some describe an odd epigastric sensation, memory phenomena, peculiar gustatory or olfactory sensations, or motor dysfunction such as spasm of a limb or turning of the eyes or head. The patient usually loses consciousness soon after his aura appears. Following loss of consciousness, the skeletal muscles undergo strong *tonic* (rigid and extended) contractions, often accompanied by the appearance of dyspnea and cyanosis. A few seconds later the patient develops severe generalized *clonic* (alternate contraction and relaxation) convulsive movements, which become less frequent as the attack persists. The patient often froths at the mouth, loses bowel and bladder control, bites his tongue, and may develop bruises and contusions. Following the clonic phase, the patient usually is in a state of flaccid-like coma during which time the pupils are dilated, corneal and deep tendon reflexes are lost, and he develops a Babinski response. Upon recovering the patient is usually confused, disoriented, and fatigued, and he will often fall into a deep sleep. This is referred to as the postictal state. The patient usually has amnesia for the seizure with the exception of recollection of the aura.

(b) Petit Mal Seizure: This minor seizure is manifested by myoclonic or akinetic episodes with a brief absence of memory (blank spells). There may be momentary loss of consciousness, but it is often so fleeting that the patient and even his associates are unaware of it. Classically, petit mal seizures are characterized by a sudden vacant expression, the cessation of motor activity, and loss of muscle tone. The patient's consciousness and mental and physical activity abruptly return. The patient may have as many as a hundred petit mal seizures per day, which may coexist with grand mal seizures.

Focal seizures.   A focal seizure is an abnormal discharge in a localized part of the cortex. It may be limited to one limb or area of the body and may be motor (clonic movements) or sensory (tingling or unusual sensation).

(a) Jacksonian Seizure: This is an example of a focal motor seizure during which there is no loss of consciousness. It commonly starts in one part of a limb such as the thumb or great toe and occurs as a localized clonic spasm. It usually spreads in a more or less orderly fashion. When the seizure spreads to the other side of the body and becomes generalized, the patient is apt to lose consciousness. The seizure may also remain confined to the site of origin and wax and wane in intensity.

(b) Psychomotor Seizures: In this category of focal seizures we include those attacks which do not conform to the classical criteria of seizures previously discussed. Psychomotor seizures are characterized by automatisms (patterned, purposeful movements), incoherent speech, turning of the head and eyes, smacking of the lips, twisting and writhing movements of the extremities, clouding of consciousness, and amnesia. Patients sometimes experience déjà vu, the feeling of reliving a scene of the past or a sense of vague familiarity while in a strange environment.

Status epilepticus.   Status epilepticus represents the rapid, repetitive recurrence of any type of seizure without recovery between attacks. The term is usually used to refer to attacks of generalized epilepsy. During status epilepticus the patient remains unconscious and is in continuous seizures with tonic and clonic fluctuations, incontinence, severely disturbed breathing, high fever, excessive diaphoresis, and elevation of the blood pressure. The state may last for hours or days and requires emergency treatment because of the possible danger of cerebral damage from ischemic hypoxia. The patient may also suffer cardiac and renal failure. The onset of status epilepticus is usually abrupt and frequently due to rapid withdrawal of or shift in medication.

Diagnostic Measures:

Medical history.   The patient's medical history usually provides a detailed description of the attacks, which helps to establish the existence of recurrent seizures. Episodes of altered consciousness should be explored. Special attention should be given to details of the aura and to any phenomenon that might provide localizing significance. A family history may reveal genetically determined cerebral disorders and/or other neurologic abnormalities. The general medical history may reveal evidence of other bodily systems disease pertinent to the development of seizures.

Clinical examination.   The majority of patients with seizures do not exhibit any significant physiologic or neurologic abnormalities upon physical examination. The only evidence of a seizure may be bruises about the body received when the patient lost consciousness and fell, or a bitten tongue.

Laboratory findings. Cerebrospinal fluid change is the only abnormality likely to be found. There may be a slight increase in cerebrospinal fluid protein and the white blood cell count. Skull and chest roentgenograms are done on all patients and may reveal maldevelopment, abnormal calcifications, pineal shift, or signs of increased intracranial pressure. The chest film may reveal pulmonary infection or tumor. Contrast media may be used to demonstrate the intracranial contents. Radioactive isotope brain scanning and CAT scans are useful and help to locate the site of focal lesions. The EEG is probably the most valuable tool in diagnosing epilepsy. Abnormal electrical brain activity is recorded, which may be used adjunctly in diagnosing the condition; a small percentage of patients with grand mal seizures have normal EEG tracings.

Treatment Modalities:

Medical therapy. There are literally hundreds of anticonvulsant drugs available today. None is capable of achieving total seizure control in all patients, but optimal results can usually be obtained for most patients with various drug combinations. The more popular and successful of these drugs are found in Chapter 11.

Surgical therapy. Patients who suffer from seizures may have a surgically remediable brain lesion such as a tumor. Surgical intervention for removal of an area of abnormal discharge is appropriate for only a selected few patients. These patients, who usually have intractable seizures after an intensive medical regimen, are often the ones with focal motor or psychomotor seizures. The surgery enjoys very limited success.

Nursing Objectives:

The nursing care for the patient with seizures in the critical care unit centers around the following: maintenance of adequate ventilation; maintenance of a safe environment; observation of seizures and subsequent reporting; provision of prescribed drug therapy; and attention placed on the psychosocial aspects of epilepsy.

Maintenance of adequate ventilation. It is imperative that an oral airway be placed in the patient's mouth during a seizure, prior to the development of tonic or clonic movements. After such activity has occurred, it is nearly impossible to insert such a device without damaging the teeth. The patient who requires massive amounts of anticonvulsant drugs may also require oral or nasal endotracheal intubation and assisted ventilation. A firm bite-block must be utilized with the oral endotracheal tube to prevent the patient from occluding (biting) the tube during seizure activity. The patient's cardiovascular and respiratory status must be carefully monitored to prevent or discover hypoxia and its related complications, which may increase the frequency of seizures.

Maintenance of a safe environment. The patient's bed must be padded along side rails and headboards to prevent physical injury to him during seizure activity. Side rails must be up and secure at all times.

Observation and reporting of seizures. The nurse is responsible for observing and reporting the following:

1. The duration of the seizure; the time it begins and ends; the time consumed in the tonic, clonic, flaccid, and postictal phases.
2. The presence of and description of an aura.
3. The patient's level of consciousness. This should be determined and changes in the level noted.
4. The motor activity during the episode, including where the activity begins and what parts of the body become involved. Note any deviation of eyes or tongue.
5. The presence or absence of bowel or bladder incontinence.
6. The patient's response to the seizure.
7. The patient's response to drug therapy.
8. The frequency and number of seizures.

Provision of prescribed drug therapy. Medications must be readily available and the critical care nurse thoroughly familiar with their pharmacokinetics. Medication schedules must be adhered to and the patient assessed for adverse effects.

Psychosocial aspects of epilepsy. The patient and family need to be educated about the disease and its symptoms. A thorough explanation of actions to be taken during a seizure is necessary. As with all pharmacologic regimens, the patient and family need information about the drugs, how to schedule them, what adverse reactions there are, and when to seek medical attention.

In many cases of epilepsy, there are concurrent personality problems that require psychological management. The achievement of a psychological adjustment depends on the patient's age, family, and social stratum. The family must understand it is most beneficial to the patient to adapt in a normal home and school setting.

Society's response to the epileptic is changing, becoming broader in its view of the diagnosis of epilepsy. Most patients are now granted a driver's license if seizures are under control. Employment opportunities are restrictive if the occupation involves situations in which the epileptic or others may be injured if a seizure occurs. All states have repealed laws prohibiting epileptics from marrying. If the epilepsy seems to be genetically related, genetic counseling is advisable before decisions are made by the couple regarding children. Public education is expanding, and outmoded beliefs are being replaced by a more rational perspective, relieving the patient of the social stigma once attached to his condition.

SECTION II: INFECTIOUS DISEASES

Infections of the central nervous system constitute a medical emergency; they dictate the immediate institution of diagnostic steps to establish the causative agent and immediate treatment to preserve life and minimize serious neurologic sequelae. The central nervous system infectious diseases presented here include meningitis, encephalitis, brain abscess, poliomyelitis, and Guillain-Barré syndrome.

Meningitis

Meningococcal Meningitis

Pathology.   Meningococcal meningitis is also known as cerebrospinal fever or epidemic cerebrospinal meningitis. It is caused by the gram-negative diplococcus *Neisseria meningitidis*. The infection usually occurs sporadically and in localized or widespread epidemics. Infants and children, especially under 15 years of age, are most commonly affected. For unknown reasons military recruits are especially vulnerable. The incidence of cases and carriers is predominantly male. The range of the incubation period is 1 to 10 days and the portal of entry is the upper respiratory tract, transmission occurring from direct or intimate contact, air-borne droplets, or articles contaminated by infected respiratory secretions. Mouth-to-mouth resuscitation has resulted in several cases.

The organism multiplying in the bloodstream produces a fulminating septicemia, the development of a rash, and subsequent meningeal invasion, resulting in capillary endothelial damage, inflammation of vessel walls, and subsequent necrosis and thrombosis. Focal hemorrhages occur into cutaneous, subcutaneous, submucosal, and synovial tissues. For unknown reasons meningococcal infections are innocuous in some people and overwhelming in others.

Clinical manifestations. The striking manifestation of meningococcal meningitis is the rash. It appears soon after onset of other symptoms, varies in severity, and each lesion measures 1 or 2 millimeters to 1 centimeter or more in diameter. The lesions are pink or reddish-blue and actually purpuric in the severest form. Light pink macules appear before petechiae, purpura, or ecchymoses. The rash usually appears first on the wrists and ankles and may result in superficial or deep ulcerations, ultimately requiring grafting. The lesions fade to a rusty brown color in three to four days, although new crops may appear.

Signs of sepsis usually occur with the rash, including shaking chills, low blood pressure, rapid quiet respiration, and overwhelming bacteremia.

Inflammation of the meninges produces pain in the neck and back with forward flexion of the head, stiff neck, retraction of the head, opisthotonus, Kernig's and Brudzinski's signs, hyperesthesia, hyperirritability, and exaggerated reflexes. Unequal reflexes may be present. The increasing intracranial pressure may lead to headache, generalized convulsions, nausea, vomiting, dilated or irregular pupils, papilledema, elevated blood pressure, and Cheyne-Stokes respiration. The patient may become depressed and finally stuporous or comatose. The course is extremely variable, but greatly influenced by therapy. Death or severe neurologic sequelae usually occur in untreated cases.

Diagnostic measures. The cerebrospinal fluid is under increased pressure and may vary from clear to frankly purulent. A gram stain reveals diplococci, and the white blood count is elevated, consisting mostly of neutrophils. The total protein is increased and sugar reduced. The meningococci may be cultured from cerebrospinal fluid. In addition, a complete blood count and posterior nasopharyngeal and blood cultures should be obtained. Blood coagulation analysis should be performed to determine the presence of coagulopathy.

Treatment modalities. Antibiotic therapy is used for the treatment of meningococcal meningitis. Sulfonamides, penicillins, and aminoglycosides are the primary drugs of choice. Most of these drugs are used IV in massive doses.

Nursing objectives. Nursing objectives center around the medial regimen. A CVP or PA catheter is usually inserted, since patients tend to become dehydrated. The CVP, PAWP, and urinary output must be kept at adequate levels to ensure proper hydration. If coagulopathy occurs, it is treated by the usual measures. Vasopressors may be required to maintain an adequate blood pressure. If signs of adrenal collapse appear, steroids must be used. Stress ulcers frequently occur; gastrointestinal bleeding must be watched for carefully and routinely. Dyspnea or respiratory distress requires standard treatment. Increased intracranial pressure or cerebral edema may require urea or mannitol. Symptomatic or supportive treatment is offered by the nurse for all patients. The patient will require sedation to assure adequate rest, although it should not interfere with nursing assessment. Antiemetics or nasogastric suction is used for persistent nausea and vomiting. Strict isolation is required for only 24 to 48 hours after initiation of appropriate therapy. The patient must have vital signs monitored closely so that circulatory collapse, shock, gastrointestinal bleeding, adrenal failure, and respiratory distress may be treated early. Frequent neurologic assessment is required to detect signs of increasing intracranial pressure or the recurrence of infection which will require further treatment. Meticulous attention to the skin lesions may prevent secondary infection and/or breakdown.

The family's often intense fear of the disease spreading must be understood. It is recommended that intervention rather than prevention be the therapy for families. If symptoms appear, they should, of course, be treated immediately.

Some authorities recommend observation of nasopharyngeal cultures from those staff members caring for the patient. Positive cultures from the nursing personnel require treatment. Prophylactic medication for staff members is not necessary. Those critical care nurses who are not in good health or especially those with upper respiratory system infections should not care for the patient.

Meningococcal meningitis is a medical emergency requiring prompt attention. The critical care nurse must realize that no other microbe may kill more quickly. In addition, the patient is often left with serious neurologic deficits such as deafness, cranial nerve paralysis, mental deficiencies, and even blindness or hydrocephalus.

The diagnosis itself often generates fearful hysteria within the hospital. In addition to caring for the patient, the nurse must use discretion when discussing the disease with others, abide by the principles of ethical conduct, and refrain from comments to people who are not involved in the unit or care of the patient. For those who need information and are disturbed by the diagnosis, some explanation of the preventive measures being taken to avoid transmission is extremely important.

Bacterial Meningitis

Pathology. The most common causes of bacterial meningitis are *Diplococcus pneumoniae*, *Neisseria meningitidis*, *Hemophilus influenzae*, *Staphylococcus aureus*, and *Escherichia coli*. Meningeal infections with pseudomonas have been reported following lumbar puncture and spinal anesthesia, and after the establishment of shunting procedures to relieve hydrocephalus. The route of infection is not always so clearly defined. The incidence of bacterial meningitis is difficult to determine, since the meningococcal type is the only one reportable.

Clinical manifestations.   The mode of onset varies; some patients complain of headache, fever, and stiff neck associated with otitis, rhinitis, or other infections one to seven days prior to the onset of the full meningitis syndrome. Others rapidly develop headache and confusion, without antecedent respiratory infection. Other symptoms include backache, photophobia, and generalized myalgia. Patients almost always demonstrate signs of meningeal irritation, especially stiff neck and Kernig's and Brudzinski's signs. Skin lesions are rare. Although intracranial pressure is usually elevated, papilledema is rare. The level of consciousness varies from confusion and mild lethargy to coma. Signs of neurologic damage appear in approximately 50% of the cases and include cranial nerve pareses, fixed pupils, and Babinski responses. Complications of bacterial meningitis include coagulopathy, temporal lobe and cerebellar tonsillar herniation, endocarditis, purulent arthritis, subdural effusions, and of course the aforementioned neurologic residua.

Diagnostic measures.   The diagnosis of bacterial meningitis should be considered in all patients with a history of upper respiratory tract infections interrupted by nausea and vomiting, headache, lethargy, confusion, or stiff neck.

The cerebrospinal fluid pressure is usually elevated, the gross appearance varying from slight turbidity to gross purulence. Gram stains usually identify the offending organism. The hallmark of bacterial meningitis is a low cerebrospinal fluid sugar, which distinguishes it from viral meningitis. Protein content is usually elevated, and cultures are positive.

Treatment modalities.   The mainstay of therapy is antibiotics. These should be administered parenterally at the earliest possible moment. When gram stain reveals the organism, specific treatment may be instituted from the beginning. Otherwise, either IV Gentamycin or penicillin is usually the initial drug of choice.

Encephalitis

Pathology.   Encephalitis is defined as an inflammation of the brain. It may be classified according to the cause, although signs and symptoms, diagnosis, treatment, and nursing objectives are the same for all forms. The four general forms and their causes are:

1. Viral encephalitis: the principle cause of viral encephalitis is arboviruses, which are arthropod-borne viruses. Forms include California encephalitis,

Eastern or equine encephalitis, St. Louis encephalitis, Venezuelan encephalitis, and Western or equine encephalitis. The most common vector is the mosquito. All forms are found in the United States except Venezuelan encephalitis. The equine varieties often produce encephalitis in horses at the same time that they are infecting humans. Many other viruses may produce the disease. Herpes simplex produces an encephalitis with masslike lesions in the temporal lobes. The rabies virus invariably produces encephalitis. Other causes are the mumps and polio viruses.

2. Encephalitis that accompanies exanthematous disease of childhood: this form of encephalitis often occurs in the course of measles, infectious mononucleosis, and rubella.

3. Encephalitis associated with vaccines: encephalitis may present following the use of certain vaccinations, especially those for smallpox, rabies, and pertussis.

4. Toxic encephalitis due to drugs or poisons: this form may present, but is usually indistinguishable from other forms.

Clinical manifestations.   The symptoms are usually fever, general malaise, sore throat, nausea and vomiting, lethargy, stiff neck, and convulsions. The patient usually displays signs of meningeal irritation, tremors, signs of upper motor neuron lesion (exaggerated deep tendon reflexes, spastic paralysis, and Babinski's), and cranial nerve paresis. The level of consciousness may progress rapidly from stupor to coma.

Diagnostic measures.   Cerebrospinal fluid is usually elevated and protein count increased. The glucose content is normal. The virus is rarely isolated from the fluid.

Other laboratory tests may include isolation of the virus from blood and serologic tests of blood, which may be diagnostic in some cases.

Treatment modalities.   Specific treatment is not available for most forms of encephalitis. However, a variety of treatment measures and procedures may contribute significantly to a successful outcome. These measures include reduction of increased intracranial pressure by osmotic diuretics, control of convulsions, maintenance of airway, administration of oxygen, and attention to nutrition during comatose states.

Nursing objectives.   The nursing care is based on the treatment measures instituted. The nurse must be alert for the development of complications, which include bronchopneumonia, urinary retention and infection, mental deterioration, parkinsonism, and epilepsy. The family needs support, especially when neurologic deficits become apparent.

Brain Abscess

Pathology. Cerebral abscess or brain abscess represents a suppurative process of brain substance that results from the extension of adjacent infective foci or hematogenous spread. The incidence of brain abscess is approximately 7 per 1000 neurosurgical procedures.[3] In general it is seen approximately one-fifth as frequently as bacterial meningitis in large hospitals. Most brain abscesses are a consequence of an adjacent primary infection, particularly of the middle ear, mastoid, paranasal sinuses, or face, scalp, or skull. Other causes include craniotomy wound infections, lung abscess, acute bacterial endocarditis, and skin infections. Sometimes an underlying cause cannot be identified. A wide variety of organisms may produce a brain abscess; a careful attempt must be made to isolate the causative organism.

Clinical manifestations. The history of a brain abscess usually consists of an acute or subacute febrile illness accompanied by headache and localizing neurologic symptoms. Headache is the most frequent initial symptom and may develop suddenly or insidiously. It is usually not a localizing headache. The focal signs that occur totally depend on the location of the abscess within the brain. Increased intracranial pressure may occur and be manifested by nausea and vomiting, drowsiness, confusion, cranial nerve paresis, and stupor. Papilledema may occur late and is not a common finding.

Diagnostic measures. Preliminary X-rays of chest, skull, sinuses, and mastoids should be obtained. The next step is usually radioisotope brain scanning, or CAT scanning, which is abnormal in most cases. Once the abscess is localized, cerebral angiography may be beneficial. The EEG is also utilized for localization.

Cerebrospinal fluid analysis is usually done when meningitis is suspected, but it is done cautiously when a space-occupying lesion is suspected. The pressure is elevated, and cells may or may not be elevated. The sugar is within normal limits unless suppurative meningitis is also present. The protein content is usually elevated.

Treatment modalities. Prompt antibiotic treatment is crucial. Osmotic diuretics may be used to decrease intracranial pressure. Surgery is required after cerebral edema is under control. The surgery consists of initial aspiration of the abscess cavity with excision of the abscess if possible. Of course, the method employed depends on the site of the abscess.

Nursing objectives. Nursing management centers around general neurologic or post-craniotomy care with special attention directed toward recog-

[3]Beeson, Paul B., and Walsh McDermott, eds., *Textbook of Medicine*, 14th ed., Philadelphia: W. B. Saunders Co., 1975, p. 672.

nition of further abscess. Residual neurologic damage, especially seizures, is common and managed the same way as seizures from other causes.

Poliomyelitis

Pathology. Acute poliomyelitis is a highly contagious disease caused by one of three viral strains that attack the motor cells of the anterior horn of the spinal cord. It varies widely in severity; some patients exhibit infection, while others develop overwhelming paralytic illness and death. Since the advent of effective vaccines, polio has become virtually nonexistent in this country. Occasionally minor outbreaks occur in nonimmunized children. It must be emphasized that continued vaccination in all populations remains paramount. Because of the virtual elimination of polio the disease will be presented only briefly.

Clinical manifestations. Poliomyelitis usually presents with a prodromal phase of illness consisting of a history of malaise, low grade fever, coryza, and mild gastrointestinal disturbances. The incubation period is about three weeks. As the illness progresses, muscle weakness, stiff neck, and nausea and vomiting are seen. The patient may develop a lower motor neuron lesion with flaccid paralysis, diminished deep tendon reflexes, and muscle wasting. When paralysis complicates polio, it takes one of two forms: spinal poliomyelitis or bulbar poliomyelitis. Spinal polio results in weakness of the muscles supplied by spinal nerves; the bulbar form results in weakness of the muscles supplied by the cranial nerves, as well as signs of encephalitis. Respiratory paralysis may complicate bulbar polio.

Diagnostic measures. There will be changes in cerebrospinal fluid such as increased protein content and increased white blood cell count. Primary diagnosis is based on the recovery of the virus from throat washings, stool, and blood.

Treatment modalities. All intervention is supportive and oriented toward the prevention of complications. Special attention should be given to the detection of cranial nerve paralysis, difficulty in swallowing, and weakness of respiratory muscles. The patient must receive extensive rehabilitative therapy; active exercise is to be avoided in the febrile stage.

Nursing objectives. Primarily the nursing goals are aimed at prevention of complications and deformities. Because of the low incidence of the disease in this country, poliomyelitis no longer constitutes a major health problem. Although infants are routinely immunized, adults no longer are. The community, nevertheless, continues to need education about immunization programs. The vaccine is easily administered, safe, and effective. The emphasis for the critical care nurse must then be on public education and caring for those unfortunate people crippled from vast epidemics prior to 1955.

Guillain-Barré Syndrome

Pathology. Guillain-Barré syndrome is also called Landry-Guillain-Barré syndrome, Guillain-Barré-Strohl syndrome, acute polyneuritis, acute inflammatory polyradiculoneuropathy, or French polio. The cause is unknown, but it usually occurs as a postinfectious process. The disease is thought to be a hypersensitivity or autoimmune response to nerves leading to a mononuclear inflammatory reaction and subsequent demyelination. Patients frequently develop the disease one to two weeks after a mild upper respiratory infection or gastroenteritis. It also occurs after the administration of certain vaccinations such as that for influenza.

Clinical Manifestations. A few days (7 to 10) following a mild infection the patient develops lower extremity weakness. This extends within a few more days to the upper extremities and the face. Facial diplegia and dysphagia may be present. Weakness of the trunk and extremity muscles may be severe, and total flaccid paralysis (including the respiratory muscles) may occur, necessitating assisted ventilatory management in the critical care unit. Sensory changes are not common, but muscle pain and tenderness and nerve sensitivity to pressure are almost always present. When sensory changes do occur, they usually are manifested as paresthesias of the toes and fingers ("stocking and glove"). Progression of these symptoms may cease at any point in the course.

The prognosis for recovery from paralysis is generally good. Death is usually from respiratory or vasomotor failure or complications of same.

Diagnostic measures. A cerebrospinal fluid examination usually reveals "albuminocytologic dissociation" with total protein content as high as several hundred grams per hundred milliliters with few or no white cells. Since the albumin content is elevated and the cell count normal, it is said to be dissociated.

Treatment modalities. Although adrenal corticosteroids have been widely used, there are no controlled studies to demonstrate their value.

Nursing objectives. The most important aspect of treatment is skilled nursing care in the critical care unit to manage respiratory difficulties. Since the patient is often in flaccid paralysis for months, patience and communications skills are imperative. When the patient is apneic and flaccid, he must always have two alarm systems functioning on the respirator to warn of mechanical problems. In addition, it is the author's belief that these patients must *never* be left unattended. Physical therapy prevents further bodily complications and must be initiated early in the phase of the illness.

CONCLUSION

Neurologic and infectious disorders of the central nervous system occur with sufficient frequency that the critical care nurse is obliged to have a thorough understanding of their pathology. Oftentimes intervention varies, and nursing measures vary accordingly. There are no absolutes, but certain standard nursing actions are expected. The expectations are growing increasingly more compelx, and the profession recognizes this growth. Nursing practice is expanding and hopefully gaining a significant positive correlation between consumer expectation and nursing practice.

BIBLIOGRAPHY

Beeson, Paul B., and Walsh McDermott, eds., *Textbook of Medicine*, 14th ed., Philadelphia: W. B. Saunders Co., 1975.

Bruya, Margaret, and Rose Bolin, "Epilepsy: A Controllable Disease," *American Journal of Nursing*, March 1976, pp. 388–397.

Elliott, Frank A., *Clinical Neurology*, Philadelphia: W. B. Saunders Co., 1971.

Luckman, Joan, and Karen Sorensen, *Medical-Surgical Nursing: A Psychophysiologic Approach*, Philadelphia: W. B. Saunders Co., 1974.

Moidel, Harriet, et al., eds., *Nursing Care of the Patient With Medical-Surgical Disorders*, 2nd ed., New York: McGraw-Hill Co., 1977.

Shaffer, Kathleen, et al., *Medical Surgical Nursing*, St. Louis: The C. V. Mosby Co., 1975.

10
NEUROVASCULAR
DISORDERS

INTRODUCTION

It has been estimated that there are approximately two million people living today with neurologic manifestations of cerebrovascular disease. In all varieties of stroke there are perhaps 200,000 deaths in the United States annually, making it the third leading cause of death. At least 500,000 Americans suffer a new, acute cerebrovascular attack each year. Recurrent strokes are common in all types of cerebrovascular disease, the recurrence carrying a higher rate of mortality. However, the overall problem is even more imposing than the statistics indicate. Survivors are inflicted with a high degree of disability and dependence, necessitating admission to medical care facilities and the assistance offered by social service departments and other supportive agencies.

Stroke-Prone Profile

The Council of Cerebrovascular Disease of the American Heart Association has drawn up a tentative Stroke-Prone Profile along with recommendations as to its interpretation and use. This guide classifies those patients prone to stroke syndromes. The profile is as follows:

1. Transient ischemic attacks; previous cerebral infarction.
2. Hypertension.
3. Cardiac abnormalities: EKG abnormalities—left ventricular hypertrophy, myocardial infarction, cardiac dysrhythmias, particularly atrial fibrillation, cardiac enlargement on X-ray—particularly if accompanied by EKG criteria of LVH, congestive heart failure.
4. Clinical evidence of atherosclerosis, angina, myocardial infarction, intermittent claudication, arterial bruits—especially carotid, absent pulses.
5. Diabetes mellitus, any evidence of impaired glucose tolerance.
6. Elevated blood lipids—cholesterol, beta lipoprotein and possibly endogenous triglyceride and pre-beta lipoprotein.

There is no doubt that the profile can be used to effectively identify susceptible persons and that treating one or more of the noted risk factors may help prevent a catastrophic stroke, or modify its course significantly.[1]

CEREBRAL ISCHEMIA AND INFARCTION

Cerebral infarction means cerebral necrosis from ischemia that produces swelling and the disintegration of neural cells. Cerebral thrombosis and cerebral emboli produce such ischemia. Cerebral infarction is twice as frequent in males as females, with the peak age at 60 to 68 years, incidence rising in a positive correlation with age.

Cerebral ischemia is caused by generalized or localized prolonged reduction of blood flow to the brain. Many factors contribute to occlusive vascular disease, including:

1. Atherosclerotic disease of the intracranial and extracranial arteries.
2. Cerebral arterial spasm after subarachnoid hemorrhage.
3. Cerebral arterial vasoconstriction associated with migraines.
4. Cerebral emboli from rheumatic heart disease, myocardial infarction, atrial fibrillation, subacute bacterial endocarditis.
5. Cerebral thrombosis adjacent to an area of intracerebral hemorrhage.
6. Cerebral thrombosis due to arteritis from collagen disease or bacterial arteritis.
7. Cerebral thrombosis from polycythemia or ischemia from severe anemia.
8. Dissecting aortic arch aneurysm.
9. Generalized cerebral hypoxia from cardiopulmonary insufficiency, pulmonary emobli, or carbon monoxide poisoning.
10. Reduced cerebral blood flow from severe hypotension or arrhythmias.

Pathology

It must be remembered that the brain is dependent on its oxygen supply and that the cerebrum contains no reserve of oxygen that will sustain its metabolism when perfusion is lacking. The EEG actually reflects changes within approximately 15 seconds following general or local oxygen deprivation. After 3 to 10 minutes of oxygen deprivation there is extensive and irreversible neural damage. Cerebral edema usually accompanies cerebral infarction, and may be severe enough to cause tentorial herniation. The cerebral edema also causes changes in the space relationships in the cranial

[1]Kannel, W. B., quoted by C. H. Millikan, "The Stroke-Prone Profile," *Current Concepts of Cerebrovascular Disease–Stroke*, Scientific Publication of the American Heart Association, 4:17–20, (September, October 1969).

vault, which further impair blood flow and cerebrospinal fluid flow and increase the cerebral ischemia.

Cerebral infarction is usually caused by simultaneous changes in several of the following factors:

1. Status of the arterial system from the heart to the brain.
2. Status of the venous system draining the brain.
3. The efficiency of the heart as a pump.
4. The character of the blood; viscosity and oxygen-carrying capacity.

Any alteration in these factors may produce cerebral ischemia or infarction. Perhaps the most common type is the alteration of the arterial system between the heart and the brain by the development of atherosclerosis, which is the condition resulting from the collection of fatty plaques on the intima of large and medium-size arteries. These lesions may lead to the development of a thrombus within the lumen, creating stenosis and reducing blood flow, progressing in size and causing vessel occlusion, or fragmenting and producing an embolus.

Cerebral infarction may occur without atherosclerosis, as by an extracerebral embolus occluding the arteries. Such emboli are commonly produced by the heart from atrial fibrillation, rheumatic heart disease, or mitral stenosis. The mural thrombi following an acute myocardial infarction may produce cerebral emboli, which may also be a product of subacute bacterial endocarditis and long bone fractures (fatty emboli).

Cerebral infarction may also result from thrombosis of a cerebral venous sinus, especially the superior sagittal sinus. Extensive thrombotic occlusion of cortical veins may also occur. Dehydration, head injury, intracerebral hemorrhage, polycythemia, leukemia, infection, and the puerperal state may all cause cerebral venous thrombosis. Infections in the eye, face, or nose may produce cavernous sinus thrombosis.

Cardiac disease in itself is an important causative factor in cerebral infarction in patients with atherosclerosis. Hypotension and hypertension are excellent examples of cardiac disease contributing to cerebral infarction. Hypotension such as that following a myocardial infarction may produce cerebral ischemia, especially when the lumen of the affected vessel is embarrassed by atherosclerosis. Such ischemia may also be produced by cardiac arrhythmias and Stokes-Adams attacks. Hypertension may evoke and increase cerebrovascular resistance, and if this is coupled with stenosed vessels, a significant reduction in cerebral blood flow may result. Hypertension may actually cause vasoconstriction in small cerebral vessels, which in turn produces ischemia or infarction.

Another factor related to cerebral infarction may be medications. Cerebral infarction occurring in young females of childbearing age may be related to the use of oral contraceptives. This relationship has been traced to the estrogen content of the medication, which may alter blood coagulation capabilities. Females with high blood pressure and migraines apparently show greater susceptibility to cerebral infarction when using oral contraceptives.

Clinical Manifestations of Stroke Syndrome

There are several clinical states that indicate some degree of ischemia and infarction. These profiles of stroke syndrome will be discussed: transient ischemic attack, stroke-in-evolution, completed stroke, internal carotid artery occlusion, vertebrobasilar infarction, and cerebral venous sinus thrombosis.

Transient ischemic attack. Transient ischemic atack (TIA) is sometimes called incipient stroke and is defined as transient episodes of neurologic dysfunction caused by cerebrovascular disease. The attacks are produced by cerebral ischemia of mild duration with dysfunction lasting 5 to 30 minutes; there is a return to preattack status with no permanent brain damage. Episodes that last longer signify infarction or some other pathological process. The symptoms of TIA vary, depending upon the area of the brain deprived of blood and carotid artery or vertebrobasilar involvement. Symptoms of carotid artery involvement include: transient contralateral weakness of distal musculature, progressing in an ascending fashion to involve the entire extremity and perhaps the entire side of the body; and sensory symptoms of tingling in the contralateral body parts. Dominant cerebral hemisphere ischemia may produce aphasia. Occipital lobe ischemia may produce transient visual field defects. When vertebrobasilar insufficiency occurs, the following symptoms result: vertigo (the most common symptom), diplopia, dysarthria, dysphagia, dysphonia, tinnitus, unilateral distal musculature weakness, and tingling. Although patients have neurologic deficits during the episodes, the results of a neurologic examination between attacks are normal. Transient ischemic attacks may occur at any interval: daily, weekly, or monthly. The patient may suffer from these attacks for years before there is insult from a cerebral infarction; patients may have a series of TIA lasting only hours before complete occlusion produces cerebral infarction. Nearly 75% of patients with complete strokes have a history of previous episodes of ischemic attacks.[2] The significance of TIA is the implication of cerebrovascular disease and the potential danger of cerebral infarction.

Stroke-in-evolution. This is sometimes referred to as an impending stroke, a progressive stroke, or an evolving stroke. The term refers to

[2]Fields, William, "Aortocranial Occlusive Vascular Disease (Stroke)," *CIBA Clinical Symposia*, Vol. 26, No. 4, 1974, p. 20.

increasing neurologic dysfunction caused by cerebral ischemia. Stroke-in-evolution is characterized by the gradual onset of paralysis and sensory impairment over a period of minutes or up to one or two days. The symptoms may appear as a series of steplike changes or a steady progressive deterioration. The patient may present with a mild weakness, which becomes more severe and involved in time. Otherwise the symptoms are the same as those of a completed stroke.

Completed stroke. The completed stroke is defined as the clinical picture seen in patients who cease to exhibit any further neurologic deterioration. Cerebral infarctions produced by emboli, atherosclerosis, or thrombosis are distinguished by clinical presentation, the pattern of onset suggesting the cause. Cerebral embolus usually produces an abrupt onset of symptoms, with headache preceding other neurologic symptoms by several hours. In the patient with cerebral infarction caused by atherosclerosis and thrombosis, symptoms appear more slowly, the patient showing signs of stroke-in-evolution. The attack may have been preceded by a series of transient ischemic attacks. Headache usually precedes atherosclerotic infarction also, usually mild in nature and localized to the side of the infarction. Consciousness may be reduced at the onset of infarction, but is usually not lost until severe insult occurs to the dominant cerebral hemisphere. Focal or generalized seizures may occur in the course of the acute or convalescent phase of infarction. A serious consequence of dominant cerebral hemisphere ischemia is dysphasia, occurring in varying degrees of severity from mild deficit of expression to aphonic mutism. Such dysphasia is usually a combination of expressive and receptive aphasia.

Internal carotid artery occlusion. The carotid bifurcation (the division of the common carotid artery into the internal carotid artery and the external carotid artery) is the site most often involved by atherosclerosis, particularly stenosis near the origin of the internal carotid artery. The symptoms of internal carotid artery occlusion are intermittent visual impairment or blindness, ipsilateral to the occlusion (from retinal artery insufficiency) and contralateral hemiparesis with sensory loss. These symptoms are usually preceded by transient ischemic attacks. In the paretic extremity, hyperactive deep tendon reflexes and Babinski's become evident, as well as increased muscle tone with marked spasticity and early contracture. Sensory impairment is usually manifested by an abnormality in position sense, vibratory sense, two-point discrimination, and tactile perception of shape or texture.

Vertebrobasilar infarction. Occlusion of a branch of the basilar or posterior cerebral arteries may produce dysfunction of the brain stem, the cerebellar hemispheres, or the occipital lobes of the cerebral hemispheres. The extent of the infarct determines whether the symptoms are unilateral or bilateral. Unilateral symptoms usually consist of ipsilateral third cranial nerve palsy with contralateral hemiparesis (Weber's syndrome or crossed motor paralysis) and ipsilateral third cranial nerve palsy with ipsilateral disturbance in gait or coordination (Nothnagel's syndrome). The bilateral symptoms may include loss of consciousness, quadriparesis, impairment of vertical eye movements, and midposition and fixed, or dilated and fixed, pupils. The nonpurposeful, flail-like, involuntary movements that may occur in an arm or leg are called hemiballismus. Midbrain infarction may also produce akinetic mutism or coma vigil. This state produces an unusual appearance in the patient; he appears almost awake, although unable to communicate in any fashion.

Cerebral venous sinus thrombosis. This is usually a result of local infection. Regardless of which sinus is involved, the patient usually has some evidence of sepsis with fever, malaise, headache, and an elevated white blood count. Cerebral venous sinus thrombosis is a likely cause of postpartum cerebral infarction. The symptoms are headache, delirium, drowsiness, diplopia, seizures, and signs of increasing intracranial pressure. When thrombosis occurs to the cavernous sinus, it is usually caused by sinus or paranasal skin infection. The symptoms of cavernous sinus thrombosis are proptosis, orbital chemosis, edema, pain around the eye, papilledema, retinal hemorrhage, and fever.

Diagnostic Measures

The physical examination should include a systems review for cerebrovascular disease and other disorders such as cardiac problems and diabetes mellitus. The status of the peripheral pulses should be described. They should be palpated bilaterally because if they are absent, decreased, or different in side-to-side comparison, that is suggestive of atherosclerotic lesions in the peripheral circulation and should make one suspect the possibility of cerebrovascular disease. In addition to vital signs the examiner should auscultate the right and left carotid arteries and the eyes for the detection of a bruit, which may suggest stenosis of the internal carotid artery.

Laboratory tests should include complete blood count, urinalysis, and determination of glucose, cholesterol, and triglyceride levels.

A lumbar puncture is done cautiously to prevent tentorial or foraminal herniation in patients with suspected expanding lesions.

X-rays are examined for evidence of fracture, pineal shift, or suggestion of chronic increased cranial pressure.

An electroencephalogram is helpful to the physician for differential diagnosis when there are abnormal tracings.

An electrocardiogram should be done to rule out acute myocardial infarction, atrial fibrillation, or other arrhythmias. It should be noted that cerebral infarction may produce T wave and ST segment abnormalities unrelated to cardiac disease.

Brain scanning usually shows a high area of uptake of contrast media in the infarcted areas, although this finding cannot be distinguished from the findings of a tumor.

Special procedures.   There are procedures specific for the diagnosis of cerebrovascular disease. The noninvasive techniques are ophthalmodynamometry, thermography, and ultrasonography.

Ophthalmodynamometry (ODM) is a procedure in which an instrument measures retinal artery pressure for side-to-side comparison (Fig. 10-1). If the pressure in the internal carotid artery is diminished, the arterial pressure in the ophthalmic artery may be reduced. The retinal artery may also be observed through an ophthalmoscope while the intraocular pressure is simultaneously increased by external pressure. Skill and judgment must be exercised while performing the procedure; it does have its limitations.

Facial thermography is a procedure that measures the skin temperature photographically. The supraorbital area of the forehead is supplied by branches of the internal carotid artery. If the skin temperature is reduced (temperature changes with blood flow), that is an indication of internal carotid artery occlusion.

Ultrasonography measures blood flow in the supraorbital region. It is a highly successful technique used to determine internal carotid artery occlusion.

Angiography is an invasive technique used for differential diagnosis and has been found to be *the most accurate technique in demonstrating site, extent, and incidence of arterial occlusion.* Also, important knowledge is obtained that is used to understand the role of collateral circulation.

Treatment Modalities and Nursing Goals

The primary goal for the patient in the intensive care unit suffering cerebrovascular insufficiency is the maintenance of an adequate airway and ventilation. Neurologic assessment is important in determining the development of cerebral edema or further cerebral infarction. The first few days are important, and the patient is kept flat in bed to assist cerebral perfusion. He is allowed to rest, and the environment is kept as quiet as possible. When the patient regains consciousness, he may be unable to communicate as he gradually becomes aware of the residual effects of infarction. At this time he will need a great deal of support, and every effort should be made to anticipate his needs to avoid frustration. The maintenance of a fluid and electrolyte balance, caloric intake, and elimination all deserve the usual consideration.

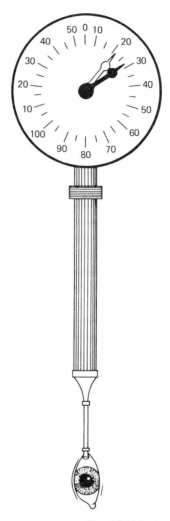

Fig. 10-1. Ophthalmodynamometer (ODM). The ODM is shown being used on the eye to measure retinal artery pressure.

Medical regimen.   Many neurologists consider anticoagulant therapy the treatment of choice in cerebrovascular insufficiency. Primarily, it is used to prevent the formation of emboli and to correct progressive stroke. The nursing administration of these drugs requires an understanding of their pharmacokinetics as well as patient teaching regarding precautions used when the body's coagulation mechanism is altered. Cerebrovasodilators are used to increase collateral circulation, thereby improving cerebral perfusion. If cerebral edema occurs, osmotic diuretics or steroids may be used, although many authorities believe these agents are not as useful in the presence of cerebral infarction; careful nursing care alone may suffice to carry the patient through such episodes.

Surgical regimen.   The precipitating factor in cerebrovascular disease is atherosclerosis. Somehow normal circulation to the brain must be restored and limitations placed on the progression of the underlying disease. The surgical procedures employed for these purposes are endarterectomy, patch-graft angioplasty, and a bypass graft procedure. Selection criteria for surgical candidates have been established and include, naturally, the location of the lesion. Surgical procedures may prove effective in certain patients in removing occlusive lesions, emboli, and in the restoration of cerebral blood flow.

Conclusion

Rehabilitative programs are usually begun for patients with cerebrovascular infarction as soon as possible when their neurologic findings have stabilized, usually within 12 to 24 hours. The goal is to retrain the patient to use his remaining capabilities for maximum effectiveness. These programs include sitting, standing, and other techniques for increasing mobility. It is the responsibility of the health care team to begin such a program in the critical care unit and provide for continuity of the program when the patient is moved to the floor.

Many critical care units are actively engaged in discussion of whether or not to allow stroke patients admission to the unit. The policies of many units include a list of conditions both eligible and ineligible for admission; often stroke appears on the latter list. The rationale in support of ineligibility is the fact that many stroke patients are moribund on admission or shortly thereafter, many physicians feel they are not candidates for CPR, and little can be done to improve their neurologic status. The rationale in support of eligibility is the prevention of complications and the restoration of physiologic function. The critical care setting may easily prevent further neurologic damage in a rehabilitatable patient by simply preventing pneumonia with its attendant risk of hypoxia and carbon dioxide narcosis. It is the authors' belief that admission policies should be reexamined and acute stroke patients be admitted. We agree that circumstances must be individually explored and decisions based on not only the condition of the patient but also the situation peculiar to each unit. There is no doubt that nurses should be active participants in this decision-making process.

INTRACRANIAL HEMORRHAGE

Nontraumatic intracranial hemorrhage is a serious cerebrovascular illness that carries a high mortality rate. The causes of hemorrhage are numerous, but the clinical pictures quite similar. Intracranial hemorrhage may be caused by the rupture of an arterial aneurysm, an arteriovenous anomaly, hypertensive vascular disease, or intracerebral tumor hemorrhage. The pathology of each of these conditions will be discussed.

Pathology

Arterial aneurysm. An arterial aneurysm is a sac formed by the dilatation of the wall of an artery and filled with blood. The cause of the condition is uncertain, but believed to be a combination of congenital and acquired factors. An important congenital factor is the maldevelopment of the media (middle muscle layer) of the vessel at an arterial bifurcation where the muscular coat is incomplete. The importance of age and acquired factors is demonstrated by the rarity of aneurysms in infants and children; their common occurrence is in adults. Hypertension and atherosclerosis may be acquired factors that contribute to the development of aneurysms. Aneurysms may occur singularly or in combination. A single aneurysm may range in size from 0.5 to 1.5 centimeters in diameter. They may become extremely large (greater than 3 centimeters in diameter) and are then called giant aneurysms. These aneurysms are likely to compress cerebral substance and/or the cranial nerves. Not all aneurysms bleed; some are found incidentally on postmortem examination. The relationship of exertion and trauma to rupture is disputed. For the most part aneurysms rupture while the patient is at rest or engaged in minimal activity. Arterial aneurysms that are found in cerebral vasculature occur as saccular (berry), fusiform, mycotic, or dissecting aneurysms.

Saccular aneurysms. Saccular or berry aneurysms are small, round, berry-shaped dilatations usually found at arterial bifurcations at or near the circle of Willis. They arise from the internal carotid artery, posterior communicating artery, middle cerebral artery, anterior communicating artery, or anterior cerebral artery. The most common site of involvement is the point of junction of the posterior communicating artery and the internal carotid artery. They may be microscopic or large enough to act as a tumor. They appear to expand progressively with time and produce symptoms when they rupture.

Fusiform aneurysms. Fusiform aneurysms are spindle-shaped dilatations on an artery due to atherosclerosis. They are most commonly found on the basilar artery and carotid artery in the cavernous sinus. They are commonly large enough to cause compression of the cranial nerves or the brain, but rarely hemorrhage.

Mycotic aneurysms. These aneurysms are produced by septic emboli usually associated with bacterial endocarditis. The wall of the artery is weakened from within by a small infective embolus. After the embolus lodges, a necrotic vasculitis is produced with resultant thinning and dilatation of the vessel wall. Mycotic aneurysms may eventually rupture. They tend to occur at multiple sites and are the only aneurysm found distally in the smaller branches of the middle cerebral artery.

Dissecting aneurysms. These aneurysms are rare, but have been seen in association with saccular aneurysms. A cavity is formed by blood that has been forced between the layers of the arterial wall.

Arteriovenous Anomalies. Arteriovenous anomalies are called arteriovenous fistulas, arteriovenous malformations, and cavernous angiomas. They are congenital malformations that appear as tangled, interconnected networks of vessels in which arterial blood communicates directly with venous blood without intervening capillaries. These arteriovenous anomalies gradually enlarge, since they offer a path of less resistance to blood flow than the normal capillary bed. Consequently, the arteries must dilate to bring more blood to the lesion, and veins must dilate to carry more blood away. The vessels themselves tend to be malformed so that some structurally resemble arteries and others veins. These malformed vessels have friable walls and are carrying arterial blood under high pressure, contrary to their structural capability; therefore, they rupture, producing a subarachnoid hemorrhage or an intracerebral hemorrhage or both.

Hypertensive Vascular Disease. Hypertension produces thickening and degeneration of cerebral arterioles. Red blood cells can be found free in the perivascular space around the involved vessels, and microaneurysms are common. The degeneration usually gives way eventually to necrosis and rupture. The rupture and subsequent hemorrhage may occur anywhere in the brain, but it is most common in the cerebrum. Small branches of the middle cerebral artery penetrating the region of the basal ganglia are the most susceptible. These lesions produce intracerebral hemorrhage.

Intracerebral Tumor Hemorrhage. Intracerebral hemorrhage may occur from primary or metastatic tumors. It is most common in rapidly growing, heavily vascularized tumors. Hemorrhage is most commonly seen in patients with glioblastoma multiforme and metastatic bronchogenic carcinoma.

Clinical Manifestations

The clinical manifestations of intracranial hemorrhage are associated with the symptoms produced by a subarachnoid hemorrhage (bleeding into the subarachnoid space) or an intracerebral hemorrhage (bleeding into the substance of the brain itself).

Subarachnoid hemorrhage. An understanding of the pathophysiology of subarachnoid hemorrhage will clarify the presence of signs and symptoms. When blood is suddenly released (ruptured aneurysm) into the subarachnoid space, several deleterious events occur. The sudden high pressure jet stream (arterial blood) tends to raise intracranial pressure and act as a concussion, or it may cause rapid brain displacement. The blood is a noxious and irritating agent, particularly when the hemolytic process begins. The blood irritates the blood vessel, the meninges, and the brain itself, producing a sterile meningitis in hours. This meningitis is a source of serious problems in itself, since it produces subjective discomfort, systemic toxicity, and eventually meningeal scarring which can impede cerebrospinal fluid absorption. The blood also irritates the underlying brain ' tissue and provokes adverse descending autonomic impulses, which produce hypertension and cardiac arrhythmias. Vascular spasm and vessel wall edema also follow a subarachnoid hemorrhage and produce cerebral ischemia and infarction.

The most common initial symptom following a subarachnoid hemorrhage is a *sudden violent headache*, described as excruciating, bursting, or explosive. Some patients actually hear a burst or snap inside the head. Although it usually remains severe, the headache may later subside to a dull throbbing ache. It is usually a generalized headache and is frequently accompanied by severe neck and back pain.

Other symptoms include dizziness, vertigo, nausea, vomiting, drowsiness, sweating, and chills. The majority of patients show some alteration in consciousness. This may range from a mild disturbance with confusion to a severe disturbance with no response to painful stimuli.

Meningeal irritation often produces irritability, photophobia, hyperesthesia, nuchal rigidity, opisthotonus, and Kernig's and Brudzinski's signs.

Hypothalamic regulatory mechanisms may be altered, producing vomiting, sweating, increased serum glucose levels, glycosuria, and proteinuria.

Neural tissue is often compressed by the hematoma, producing focal neurologic signs. The nature of symptoms is, of course, determined by the area of involvement. Such symptoms may include paralysis or paresis, speech disorders, seizures, and visual alterations such as diplopia and even loss of vision.

Retinal hemorrhage of the subhyaloid type is characteristic of subarachnoid hemorrhage. It is a large, prominent hemorrhage seen at the side of the optic disc. The hemorrhage is caused by subarachnoid blood being forced along the optic nerve sheath with sufficient vigor to occlude the retinal vein and subsequently traverse the intervaginal spaces around the optic nerve.

Papilledema from increased intracranial pressure is seen in only a minority of patients. It may develop quickly or over a period of days.

The patient's condition *after* the rupture of an aneurysm has important prognostic value. The most commonly used grading system for patients with subarachnoid hemorrhage involves five levels, the lower grades indicating a more favorable prognosis, the higher grades connoting a less favorable prognosis.

Grade I   Minimal bleeding: The patient is alert and with minimal neurologic deficit and minimal signs of meningeal irritation.

Grade II   Mild bleeding: The patient is alert and with minimal neurologic deficit and increased signs of meningeal irritation.

Grade III   Moderate bleeding: The patient is drowsy or confused, with or without neurologic deficit.

Grade IV   Moderate bleeding: The patient is stuporous, with or without neurologic deficit.

Grade V   Severe bleeding: The patient is deeply comatose, decerebrate, and moribund.

Intracerebral hemorrhage.   When intracranial hemorrhage occurs into the brain, the onset of symptoms is usually abrupt; initially the patient may have a headache, nausea, and vomiting. Loss of consciousness or neurologic deficit may precede initial symptoms by several hours, a result of the abrupt increase in intracranial pressure. The neurologic deficit that follows is often hemiplegia or hemisensory defects caused by the disruption or the distortion of the main cerebral motor and sensory pathways. Loss of consciousness may occur within minutes and probably indicates either a large hemorrhage or an intraventricular bleed. There is often a progressive decline of consciousness leading to coma, decortication, and decerebration, the symptoms of tentorial herniation and brain stem compression. The presence of bloody cerebrospinal fluid on a lumbar puncture may be the only sign distinguishing intracranial hemorrhage from cerebral infarction.

Diagnostic Measures

Cerebrospinal fluid examination can usually be done safely on patients with intracranial hemorrhage, though it should be employed with caution when there is evidence of impaired consciousness or a progressive decline in awareness, indicative of brain stem compression. In subarachnoid hemorrhage the cerebrospinal fluid is invariably bloody; in intracerebral hemorrhage it is frequently bloody. If an intracerebral hemorrhage has occurred and cerebrospinal fluid is examined 1 to 24 hours after the bleed, the red blood cell count is constant in sequential samples. If the fluid is bloody as a result of a traumatic puncture, the pink or yellow discoloration on centrifuged cerebrospinal fluid (caused by oxyhemoglobin and degradation of oxyhemoglobin to bilirubin, respectively) is absent; in addition the red blood cell count on sequential samples will decrease. The white blood cell count in intracerebral hemorrhage is usually high in proportion to the red blood cell count, and the protein content is usually elevated in the presence of blood. Elevation of cerebrospinal fluid pressures is proportionate to the degree of bleeding.

Arteriograms are successful in distinguishing the cause of an intracranial bleed. They are used early in the diagnostic work-up and will be helpful in determining whether the existing problem can be surgically corrected. Skull X-rays do not usually reveal any significant evidence for diagnosis unless the hematoma produces a pineal shift.

An electroencephalogram may reveal enough information to clarify the diagnosis, but cannot distinguish with any certainty between hemorrhage, thrombosis, or embolus.

Brain scanning will usually show only giant aneurysms, while CAT scans will show aneurysms greater than 9 millimeters in diameter. The CAT scan may also outline the area of clot, infarction, and edema, differentiating parenchymatous, subdural, and intraventricular hemorrhage from edema and infarction.

Air contrast studies play a diminishing role in the investigation of patients with intracranial hemorrhage.

Treatment Modalities and Nursing Goals

Medical therapy. Medical therapy is singularly used in patients with an intracranial hemorrhage when the arteriogram reveals the lesion to be surgically inaccessible, when the patient is classified as Grade III, IV, or V and is not improving, when multiple aneurysms exist, or when the patient refuses surgery. The goals of medical therapy in the treatment of intracranial hemorrhage are designed to preserve life, minimize the residual neurologic deficits of the patient, and prevent recurrence of the hemorrhage. The specific treatment is directed toward the cause of the hemorrhage. The objectives include the prevention and control of increased intracranial pressure, the promotion of cerebrovascular perfusion, and the prevention of complications.

Prevention and control of increased intracranial pressure. The patient should be ministered to in a quiet, restful atmosphere. Absolute bed rest is essential; every effort must be made to provide comfort means. Diminish as many stresses as possible such as coughing, straining, and so forth, which tend to elevate intracranial pressure. Attend as well to the psychological needs of the patient, alleviating anxiety whenever possible. Narcotics are avoided, but sedatives may be administered as well as other measures to relieve the patient's headache. Minimize the effects of hyperthermia, if they exist, decreasing the metabolic needs of the brain tissue. Treat seizures, if indicated, with routine nursing measures and the drugs prescribed. If continuous ventricular drainage is used to relieve pressure, the nurse has certain responsibilities in setting it up and measuring, recording, and maintaining sterility. Above all, frequent neurologic assessment is essential in recognizing increasing intracranial pressure. Any dramatic change in the patient's neurologic status may require immediate surgical intervention.

Promotion of cerebrovascular perfusion. The patient's blood pressure must remain under control. Hypotension brings ill effects to cerebral tissue; hypertension brings disaster to already insulted cerebral vessels. Antihypertensive drugs may be administered if radical pressure reduction is necessary. Monitor the patient's blood pressure frequently and observe for symptoms of abnormal perfusion. The prevention of vasospasm is important. Adequate blood oxygenation must be maintained. The patient's respiratory status must be assessed and blood gases monitored at intervals to detect hypoxia.

Prevention of complications. Cerebral edema must be controlled in the hemorrhage patient; the process involves swelling of brain tissue, creating increased volume. Adequate respiratory status (competent airway and assisted ventilation if necessary) will preclude or reduce hypoxia, which contributes to edema. Osmotic diuretics (urea or mannitol) are used to reduce cerebral hydration by promoting diuresis. Fluid maintenance is under close surveillance with CVP lines inserted; replacement is often with sodium-restricted fluids. Steroids (dexamethasone) are used in treating cerebral edema effectively, but the action of the drugs in this instance is not clearly understood. Again a prime nursing responsibility is patient assessment to detect the presence of any alteration in the patient's status and to be prepared for any method employed to correct the problem.

Another area requiring attention is the prevention of recurrence of the hemorrhage. Intervention in this regard is interrelated with controlling hypertension, vasospasm, cerebral edema, and so on. Antifibrinolytic agents (aminocaproic acid) may be used, as well as antihypertensive drug therapy. Prevent stress, promote rest and comfort, assess frequently, and be prepared for immediate surgical intervention if a bleed recurs.

Surgical therapy. Surgery is the preferred mode of treatment for intracranial hemorrhage. The optimum time for surgical intervention is debatable. Early surgery carries a higher mortality and morbidity rate, by increasing vasospasm, edema, and poor perfusion, than surgery delayed 7 to 14 days after hemorrhage; however, this time frame still presents a dilemma, since rebleed and death may occur in the interim. Some surgeons prefer to operate on Grade I or II category patients within the first few days after hemorrhage in the hope of eliminating the often fatal rebleeding. These surgeons feel that the rebleeding associated with the delay will balance the somewhat higher mortality rate of early surgery. Because of the surgical incidence of vasospasm and infarction, most surgeons prefer to operate 5 to 7 days after hemorrhage. Meanwhile the patient is maintained for as long as possible on a medical regimen until these risks are reduced.

Surgical therapy involves the surgical evacuation of the hemorrhage and the restoration of normal cerebral perfusion. As with ischemia and infarction, surgical procedures may include endarterectomy, angioplasty, and grafting. Two other techniques for the treatment of intracranial hemorrhage will be discussed: surgical obliteration of an aneurysm and carotid artery occlusion for the prevention of bleed recurrence.

Obliteration of aneurysm. A temporal, frontotemporal, or suboccipital craniotomy is performed to expose the aneurysm. A surgical microscope providing three to four times magnification is generally used. This microtechnique allows the surgery to be performed through a smaller cranial opening and minimizes the need for brain retraction. It also permits the surgeon more accurate identification of the anatomy of the aneurysm and the surrounding area. When the aneurysm is located, a noncrushing-type clip with a spring mechanism is employed to allow removal and repositioning (Fig. 10-2). The aneurysm is then resected. If resection is not feasible, coagulation may be used to reduce its size, or the aneurysm may be encased with surgical gauze or plastic. The wound is closed, and the patient is returned to the intensive care unit. The nursing measures are based on the principles previously outlined in accord with the surgical approach, being either supratentorial or infratentorial.

Carotid artery occlusion. The ligation of the carotid artery may be performed on selected patients with intracranial hemorrhage from aneurysms (giant aneurysms and those in the cavernous sinus), arteriovenous anomalies, and hypertensive vascular disease. This technique is less common since the development of microsurgery. When carotid ligation is indicated, it is usually performed on the internal carotid artery. A gradual occlusion of the artery over a period of two or seven days is performed by using an adjustable clamp which allows gradations of closure; in common use are the Selverstone and Crutchfield clamps. Permanent ligation of the carotid artery reduces blood flow and lowers the pressure in the aneurysm, reducing the threat of rupture. The clamp is positioned on the carotid artery in surgery through a stab wound

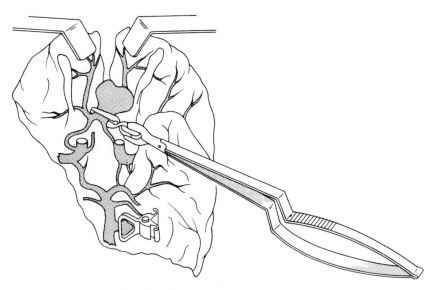

Fig. 10-2. Surgical treatment of aneurysms. Two types of noncrushing clips are applied to aneurysms off the basilar artery (below) and on the anterior cerebral artery (above). The aneurysms are magnified in this picture for adequate visualization.

(Fig. 10-3). On the day after surgery the clamp is adjusted daily until the artery is occluded. Postoperatively the patient is kept at absolute bed rest in the intensive care unit under close surveillance until clamp closure is complete. Vital signs are observed and recorded every 30 minutes and the strength in each hand is tested at 5-minute intervals for 8 hours following clamp adjustment.

The critical care nurse must be totally familiar with the operation of the clamp; if neurologic deficits from cerebral ischemia occur after clamp adjustment, the clamp must be released immediately; some surgeons prefer to do this themselves. Retinal artery pressure may be measured with an ophthalmodynamometer during the occlusion proceeding to determine the presence of thrombosis. In adjusting the clamp, it is preferable to effect a systolic or diastolic ipsilateral retinal artery pressure drop of 10%. If retinal artery pressure is equal bilaterally, thrombosis of carotid vessels has presumably not occurred. If the retinal artery pressure on the side of the ligation remains significantly decreased after full opening of the clamp and the patient's condition shows no change, the common carotid or internal carotid artery or both are probably thrombosed. This requires immediate surgical exploration of the neck vessels. When the common carotid artery has been totally occluded for longer than one hour, when ischemic neurologic complications arise, many surgeons will reopen the neck incision to ensure

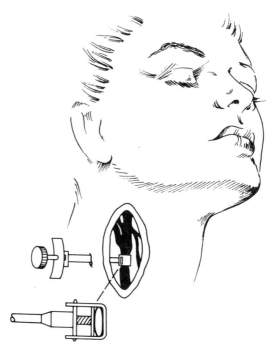

Fig. 10-3. Carotid occlusion. A Crutchfield clamp shown in place for occlusion of the common carotid artery.

that there are no clots in the carotid vessels *prior* to opening the clamp. This procedure has the disadvantage of not obliterating the offending aneurysm and may be associated with late rebleeding. Some surgeons employ the use of an IV vasopressor to moderately elevate systemic blood pressure for two to three days during closure of the clamp. This may increase perfusion of the brain and lessen the incidence and degree of cerebral ischemia. The use of a vasopressor is best monitored by installing an indwelling arterial catheter attached to a transducer to provide continuous blood pressure monitoring.

Conclusion

The diagnostic and technical advances introduced in the last decade dealing with intracranial hemorrhage have led to a better understanding of the nature, origin, location, and repair of aneurysms and arteriovenous anomalies. Subsequently the critical care nurse has reduced postoperative morbidity and mortality through the use of refined technical skills and professional management of patient care.

The patient with an intracranial hemorrhage will require all of the nursing skills available to prevent further core body system complications. Rehabilitative nursing begins in the intensive care unit, and arrangements must be made for the continuity of care when he is transferred to the ward. Physical and psychological adjustment to limitations may be a long-term process for the patient as well as the family. The patient may be in the unit only a short time, but every consideration must be given to his present life and his future life.

BIBLIOGRAPHY

Beeson, Paul B., and Walsh McDermott, eds., *Textbook of Medicine*, 14th ed., Philadelphia: W. B. Saunders Co., 1975.

Elliott, Frank A., *Clinical Neurology*, 2nd ed., Philadelphia: W. B. Saunders Co., 1971.

Fields, William, "Aortocranial Occlusive Vascular Disease (Stroke)," *CIBA Clinical Symposia*, Vol. 26, No. 4, 1974.

Hudak, Carolyn, et al., *Critical Care Nursing*, 2nd ed., Philadelphia: J. B. Lippincott Co., 1977.

Kannel, W. B., quoted by C. H. Millikan, "The Stroke-Prone Profile," *Current Concepts of Cerebrovascular Disease-Stroke*, Scientific Publication of the American Heart Association, 4:17–20, (September, October 1969).

Luckman, Joan, and Karen Sorensen, *Medical-Surgical Nursing*, Philadelphia: W. B. Saunders Co., 1974.

Shafer, Kathleen, et al., *Medical-Surgical Nursing*, 6th ed., St. Louis: The C. V. Mosby Co., 1975.

Youmans, Julian R., ed., *Neurological Surgery*, Vol I, Philadelphia: W. B. Saunders Co., 1973.

11
PHARMACOLOGY

ANTICONVULSANTS

BARBITURATES

Phenobarbital, Phenobarbital Sodium
Barbipil, Barbita, Luminal, Eskabarb

ACTIONS AND USES: Phenobarbital is the most widely used anticonvulsant in treating major motor, psychomotor, and other focal seizures. It may be used as primary therapy, but more commonly it is added when diphenylhydantoin has not completely controlled the patient's seizures. The pharmacodynamics of phenobarbital remain unclear; it may effectively suppress the seizure without altering abnormal brain waves. It is considered one of the safest anticonvulsant drugs.

PREPARATION AND DOSAGE: Phenobarbital PO: adult 120–200 mg daily at h.s.; pediatric 1–6 mg/kg.
Phenobarbital sodium IM, IV (slowly) for status epilepticus: adult 200–320 mg; pediatric 3–5 mg/kg.

ADVERSE EFFECTS AND NURSING CONSIDERATIONS: Drowsiness is the most common, though transient, side effect of phenobarbital. A paradoxical effect of hyperactivity may be seen in children. Ataxia may occur and usually requires a reduction in dosage. Skin eruptions and megaloblastic anemia are uncommon effects. When it is used in pregnancy, a clotting defect may occur in the newborn. Barbiturates may not be used to treat acute intermittent porphyria, since they are metabolized in the liver. In patients with epilepsy abrupt withdrawal may produce seizures. It is unlikely that drug dependency or drug inebriation will occur with the usual dose given for epilepsy. Respiratory depression may occur from parenteral use of phenobarbital, but this should not preclude the use of a full anticonvulsant dose, since fractional doses may produce paradoxical drug-induced depression with continued status epilepticus.

Mephobarbital
Mebaral

ACTIONS AND USES: Mephobarbital is metabolized in the body to phenobarbital, and the two have similar properties and uses. However, larger doses of mephobarbital are given than of phenobarbital.

PREPARATION AND DOSAGE: PO: adult 200 mg h.s. and 600 mg daily in divided doses; pediatric under 5 years of age 16–32 mg 3–4 times daily; over 5 years of age 32–64 mg 3–4 times daily.

Metharbital
Gemonil

ACTION AND USES: The properties and uses of metharbital are similar to those of phenobarbital, but it is less potent on a weight basis, making dosage adjustment necessary.

PREPARATION AND DOSAGE: PO: adult initially 100 mg h.s. to 300 mg daily in divided doses, which may be increased to 600–800 mg daily if required; pediatric 5–15 mg/kg in divided doses.

Primidone
Mysoline

ACTIONS AND USES: Although primidone is not a barbiturate, it is considered with this group because of its close chemical relationship to the group and because it is partially metabolized in the body to phenobarbital. In epilepsy it is used for patients who do not initially respond to a phenobarbital-hydantoin regimen. It may be used specifically for psychomotor epilepsy.

PREPARATION AND DOSAGE: PO: adult 250 mg daily h.s. to 2 g daily in divided doses; pediatric: children younger than 8 years old one-half of the adult dose.

ADVERSE EFFECTS AND NURSING CONSIDERATIONS: The side effects and contraindications for primidone are the same as for phenobarbital. In addition primidone may produce pronounced sedation. This symptom often diminishes with gradual dose increase in continued administration.

HYDANTOINS

Phenytoin Sodium
Dilantin sodium

ACTIONS AND USES: Phenytoin sodium is probably the most useful drug for major motor, psychomotor, and other focal epilepsies. It is often used in combination with phenobarbital, especially when one or the other drug is ineffective. Phenytoin exerts selective action on the cerebral cortex without drastic alteration in the sensory areas. Although an anticonvulsant, it is not a hypnotic. Phenytoin is not indicated in petit mal or most minor motor seizures, since it does not improve them and often increases their frequency. Although it does not cure the mental deterioration found in some epileptics, it does not produce such marked deterioration either. It is commonly prescribed after cerebral neurosurgical procedures and for severe head injury patients to prevent convulsive disorders. It may be used parenterally to treat status epilepticus, but it is not as effective as phenobarbital or diazepam. Phenytoin has the advantage of producing little or no sedation in usual doses.

PREPARATION AND DOSAGE: Phenytoin PO: must be individualized according to patient response, adult initially 300 mg daily; children 3–8 mg/kg daily.
Phenytoin has a long half-life; thus single doses are as effective as divided ones.
Phenytoin sodium IV for status epilepticus: adults 150–250 mg infused, not to exceed 50 mg per minute; pediatric dose is calculated according to body surface area.

ADVERSE EFFECTS AND NURSING CONSIDERATIONS: Phenytoin produces a higher incidence of toxic reactions than phenobarbital. Less serious effects include apathy, nervousness, dizziness, ataxia, blurred vision, hyperplasia of the gums (especially in the youth), and hirsutism. Other reactions include tremor, excitement, hallucinations, psychosis, nausea, and vomiting. Skin rash, exfoliative dermatitis, fever, or dyspnea may also develop in patients particularly sensitive to phenytoin. Serious toxic effects include hepatitis, blood dyscrasias, periarteritis nodosa, and lupus erythematosis. Since it is an alkaline preparation, it may produce gastric irritation. Its high alkalinity contraindicates IM injection when the IV route is possible. If it is administered too rapidly IV, dangerous hypotension may occur. Subcutaneous and perivascular injections are definitely avoided.

DRUG INTERACTIONS:

Drugs That Potentiate Phenytoin	*Drugs That Inhibit Phenytoin*
Aspirin	Alcohol
Phenylbutazone	Antihistamines
Chloramphenicol	Barbiturates
Cycloserine	Glutethimide
Isoniazid	Sedatives
Estrogens	Hypnotics
Griseofulvin	
Chlordiazepoxide	
Sulfonamides	
Anticoagulants	

Phenytoin Potentiates	*Phenytoin Inhibits*
Antihypertensives	Corticosteroids
Folic acid antagonists	Digitalis
Methotrexate	
Propanalol	
Quinidine	
Tubocurare	

Mephenytoin
Mesantoin

ACTIONS AND USES: Mephenytoin is effective in major motor, psychomotor, and other focal epilepsies. Its toxicity, however, is greater than that of phenytoin; therefore it should be reserved for use in patients who prove refractory to other drug therapy.

PREPARATION AND DOSAGE: PO: adult initially 50–100 mg daily with weekly increases by the same amount until maintenance dose is reached, 200–600 mg in 3–4 divided doses; pediatric initially the same as adult, maintenance 100–400 mg, depending on the age of the child and the severity of the seizure disorder.

ADVERSE EFFECTS AND NURSING CONSIDERATIONS: Unlike phenytoin, mephenytoin does produce sedation. There are fewer side effects; however, more serious life-threatening complications may arise. These include severe skin eruptions; blood dyscrasias such as aplastic anemia, leukopenia, agranulocytosis, thrombocytopenia, megaloblastic anemia; hepatitis; systemic lupus erythematosis; and lymphadenopathy which resembles lymphomas. In addition, a toxic synergism between trimethadione or paramethadione and mephenytoin exists.

Ethotoin
Peganone

ACTIONS AND USES: Ethotoin is moderately effective in grand mal seizures and slightly effective in psychomotor epilepsy. It is usually ineffective when used alone.

PREPARATION AND DOSAGE: PO: adult initially 1 g daily in divided doses and for maintenance 2-3 g in 4-6 divided doses; pediatric initially 750 mg daily and maintenance 500 mg to 1 g in divided doses.

ADVERSE EFFECTS AND NURSING CONSIDERATIONS: Although toxic effects resemble those of phenytoin, the incidence of their occurring is much lower. The drug then is less toxic, but is also less effective.

MISCELLANEOUS ANTICONVULSANTS

Carbamazepine
Tegretol

ACTIONS AND USES: Carbamazepine is a tricyclic compound that is chemically related to imipramine. Although introduced for the treatment of trigeminal neuralgia, it has anticonvulsive properties comparable to those of phenobarbital, phenytoin, or primidone. Carbamazepine is not effective in treating petit mal or minor motor epilepsy. It does produce a psychotropic effect, which may increase alertness and promote mood elevation in epileptics.

PREPARATION AND DOSAGE: PO trigeminal neuralgia adult: 100 mg b.i.d. increased by increments of 100 mg q 12 hrs until pain is relieved; usual range is 200 mg to 1.2 g daily; administer with meals. PO seizure control adult: 100 mg t.i.d.; pediatric under 6 years old 100 mg daily, 6-12 years old 100 mg b.i.d. The dose may be increased by increments of 100 mg each week. The average effective daily dose is 1 g.

ADVERSE EFFECTS AND NURSING CONSIDERATIONS: A small percentage of the patients receiving carbamazepine experience adverse reactions. Most symptoms subside spontaneously or after dosage is reduced. The most common reactions are neurologic in origin and include dizziness, drowsiness, ataxia, confusion, fatigue, blurred vision, headache, diplopia, oculomotor dysfunction, dysphasias, abnormal involuntary movement, peripheral neuritis, paresthesias, depression with agitation, talkativeness, nystagmus, and tinnitus. Digestive disorders include nausea and vomiting, gastric distress, abdominal pain, diarrhea, constipation, anorexia, dryness of the mouth, and stomatitis. Dermatologic reactions of all varieties occur in few patients. Hematopoietic reactions that include transitory leukopenia, eosinophilia, leukocytosis, purpura, aplastic anemia, and thrombocytopenia occur rarely. Fatalities have been reported. Patients should discontinue the drug and notify their physician if signs of hematologic toxicity occur. These signs include fever, sore throat, stomatitis, easy bruising, appearance of petechiae, or purpura. The patient should also have blood and platelet counts performed during therapy. Other miscellaneous reactions to carbamazepine include cardiovascular symptoms, aggravation of hypertension, hypotension, syncope, edema, aggravation of ischemic heart disease, congestive heart failure, and recurrence of thrombophlebitis, as well as urinary frequency or retention, elevated BUN, impotence, cholestatic and hepatocellular jaundice, fever and chills, lymphadenopathy, myalgia, arthralgia, leg cramps, and conjunctivitis. Carbamazepine should be used cautiously in patients with cardiovascular, liver, renal, or urinary tract disease, or in patients with increased intraocular pressure, and patients receiving MAO inhibitors or tricyclic antidepressants.

Diazepam
Valium

ACTIONS AND USES: Diazepam was introduced as an antianxiety agent, but has important anticonvulsive properties. It is a benzodiazepine derivative. This drug is extremely valuable when used parenterally for the treatment of status epilepticus and is regarded by many as the drug of choice. It may also be useful when given orally for refractory myoclonic seizures.

PREPARATION AND DOSAGE: IV (slowly) for status epilepticus: adult 5-10 mg; pediatric 2-5 mg.

ADVERSE EFFECTS AND NURSING CONSIDERATIONS: The most common adverse effects of oral diazepam are drowsiness, dizziness, fatigue, and ataxia, somnolence, nystagmus, and muscle weakness. Paradoxical stimulation may occur. Parenteral administration for status epilepticus requires astute nursing observation for respiratory depression, hypotension, and cardiac arrest. These effects are more likely to occur in the elderly. Respiratory depression may be reversed by naloxone hydrochloride (Narcan). When diazepam is given IM, it is absorbed slowly, erratically, and incompletely. When administered PO, it is rapidly and completely absorbed, reaching peak blood levels in about 2 hours. Therefore, the drug should be given IV or PO. After a single PO or IV dose the effects may seem to wane rapidly, due to rapid tissue distribution. Furthermore, it is metabolized slowly with a half-life of 20–50 hours. Repeated dosage leads to a cumulative effect. Diazepam cannot be mixed or diluted with other solutions or drugs. It must not be added to intravenous solutions and must be given directly IV. Extreme caution must be exercised to avoid extravasation or intra-arterial administration. When it is used IV, the patient must be closely monitored to detect respiratory depression, apnea, hypotension, or cardiac arrest.

Paraldehyde
Paral and Paraldehyde

ACTIONS AND USES: Paraldehyde is an effective drug for status epilepticus. It may be given orally, rectally, IM, or diluted IV, and is a rapid-acting sedative-hypnotic. Although it is primarily metabolized by the liver, a small amount is excreted through the lungs, giving a characteristic pungent odor to the breath of the patient.

PREPARATION AND DOSAGE: IV or IM for status epilepticus: suggested doses vary and manufacturers' recommendations are vague; approximately 0.15 ml/kg seems to be a reasonable dose.

ADVERSE EFFECTS AND NURSING CONSIDERATIONS: Gastric irritation may occur after oral administration of paraldehyde. Intragluteal injection is irritating but relatively safe; it should be reserved for emergencies only. IV administration produces severe coughing, which may cause pulmonary hemorrhage; for this reason paraldehyde should be diluted with sodium chloride injection and administered by drop infusion slowly. Fatalities have occurred with IV use. Rectal administration makes dosage difficult to control, but may be employed in children. Bronchopulmonary disease is a relative contraindication for use of the drug. Sedation usually occurs and is intensified and prolonged in patients with liver damage.

SPECIAL PRECAUTIONS:

1. Paraldehyde may react with plastic equipment.
2. Give it slowly IV; dilute with sodium chloride injection. Administer by slow IV drip.
3. Avoid extravasation when giving the drug IV.
4. Avoid giving paraldehyde near peripheral nerves if giving IM, and give intragluteally, since it may be irritating.
5. If severe coughing occurs, discontinue the infusion.
6. Observe for severe sedation or respiratory depression.
7. Use only freshly prepared solution.

ANTIFIBRINOLYTIC AGENTS

Aminocaproic Acid
Amicar

ACTIONS AND USES: Aminocaproic acid is an agent that inhibits plasmin (fibrinolysin) and prevents the formation of excessive plasmin responsible for the destruction of fibrin, fibrinogen, and other important clotting components. Aminocaproic acid inhibits the dissolution of clots. It is well absorbed orally or IV, is excreted rapidly in the urine, and provides peak plasma levels in approximately 2 hours. The major use of this drug is to control hemorrhage occurring with cardiopulmonary bypass, portocaval shunt, thoracic surgery, and obstetrical complications. Recently, aminocaproic acid has become a popular drug in the medical management of subarachnoid hemorrhage and other neurovascular diseases. It has been used in an attempt to control local hemorrhage not related to abnormal fibrinolytic activity. Its primary neurologic role is in the treatment of bleeding secondary to aneurysm. The rationale for this is that hemostasis of weeping and leaking aneurysms will occur. Furthermore, if such leaking has already stopped, inhibition of normal local fibrinolytic activity should increase the persistence of a physiologic seal and reduce the incidence of rebleeds.

PREPARATION AND DOSAGE: PO or IV (slowly): initially 5 g; doses of 1 g are then given at hourly intervals. When given IV, sodium chloride injection, 5% D/W, or Ringers may be used to dilute the drug. The injection of undiluted aminocaproic acid or the rapid infusion of this drug is not recommended.

ADVERSE EFFECTS AND NURSING CONSIDERATIONS: Adverse effects include pruritis, erythema, rash, hypotension, dyspepsia, nausea, vomiting, diarrhea, conjunctival erythema, and nasal congestion. Aminocaproic acid is contraindicated in the presence of depletion coagulation disorders and may potentiate fatal thrombotic disorders. For this reason frequent laboratory tests should be performed to evaluate the patient's hemostatic mechanisms and prevent the development of a hypercoagulable state. Since aminocaproic acid is totally excreted in the urine, it should be used in smaller doses in patients with renal disease or oliguria.

ANTIHYPERTENSIVE AGENTS

Severe high blood pressure may occur as a complication of neurologic disease and often presents an emergency situation. Table 11-1 reviews the major drugs used in the treatment of hypertension, and any one of them may be used in the neurologic patient. It is usually advisable to lower the patient's blood pressure

Table 11-1. Major Antihypertensive Drugs

Diuretics	Thiazides (benzothiazides)
	Chlorothiazide (Diuril)
	Hydrochlorothiazide (HydroDiuril)
	Methyclothiazide (Enduron)
	Ethacrynate NA (NA Edecrin)
	Furosemide (Lasix)
	Potassium-sparing agents
	Spironolactone (Aldactone)
	Triamterene (Dyrenium)
	Methyclothiazide (Enduron)
	Polythiazide (Renese)
	Trichlormethiazide (Naqua)
	Chlorthalidone (Hygroton)
Agents that depress the activity of sympathetic nervous system at the postganglionic site	Rauwolfia alkaloids
	Reserpine (Serpasil)
	Methyldopa (Aldomet)
	Guanethidine (Ismelin)
	Propanolol (Inderal)
Drugs that act directly on vascular smooth muscle	Hydralazine (Apresoline)
	Sodium nitroprusside (Nipride)
	Diazoxide (Hyperstat)
Ganglionic blocking agents	Mecamylamine (Inversine)
	Trimethaphan (Arfonad)
	Pentolinium (Ansolysen)

rapidly, and for this reason certain rapid-acting drugs are employed: diazoxide, sodium nitroprusside, and trimethaphan camsylate, which will be presented in this discussion. For further information the critical care nurse is referred to either the formulary or a reference such as *AMA Drug Evaluations*.

Diazoxide
Hyperstat

ACTIONS AND USES: Diazoxide is a thiazide derivative that is a nondiuretic agent. It acts directly on vascular smooth muscle, affecting only arterioles and causing peripheral vasodilatation. Diazoxide does not affect capacitance vessels and in fact increases cardiac output. When given rapidly IV, it produces an immediate fall in blood pressure in 1 to 5 minutes. The pretreatment blood pressure usually returns within 24 hours. Major advantages are: there is a rapid onset of action; it does not require continuous infusion; it does not require careful titration of dosage; it does not usually produce excessive hypotension; it has no sedative effect, and thus allows careful evaluation of the patient's mental status; and drug resistance does not occur if it is given concomitantly with a diuretic.

PREPARATION AND DOSAGE: IV adult: 300 mg or 5 mg/kg; pediatric 5 mg/kg. The drug must be injected rapidly (within 30 seconds), thus ensuring a maximum response. Slow injection may be ineffective, probably because diazoxide is rapidly bound to plasma protein. The hypotensive effect appears to depend on a high initial concentration of the drug in its free form. The injection may be repeated in ½-hour to 24-hour intervals, depending on the patient's blood pressure.

ADVERSE EFFECTS AND NURSING CONSIDERATIONS: Sodium retention, water retention, and hyperglycemia are the major side effects of diazoxide therapy. When an adequate dose of an effective diuretic is given, fluid overload is prevented, and the antihypertensive effect of diazoxide enhanced. A potent rapid-acting diuretic such as furosemide (Lasix) is usually given concurrently. The hyperglycemic effect of diazoxide is usually transient and can be controlled when necessary by oral hypoglycemic agents or insulin. The degree of hyperglycemia is increased by the concurrent use of thiazide diuretics and furosemide. Therefore, serum glucose levels should be measured frequently, especially in diabetic patients and patients requiring repeated doses of diazoxide. Orthostatic hypotension may occur when patients are treated with diazoxide and furosemide. For this reason the patient's blood pressure should be closely monitored for 8 to 10 hours following combined therapy, and the patient should avoid the upright position. Diazoxide occasionally causes gastrointestinal disturbances such as nausea, vomiting, and anorexia. It may also produce headache, flushing, and supraventricular tachycardia. Hypersensitivity reactions include rash, leukopenia, and fever, but these are uncommon. Extravasation should be avoided, since it produces local pain, although tissue sloughing has not been reported. Other adverse effects have been reported in patients on long-term oral use of diazoxide.

Sodium Nitroprusside
Nipride

ACTIONS AND USES: Sodium nitroprusside is an extremely potent peripheral vasodilator, acting directly on vascular smooth muscle. It is preferred by many physicians when other agents have proved ineffective. It has a rapid onset of action, 1–2 minutes, but requires continuous infusion to maintain its hypotensive effect.

PREPARATION AND DOSAGE: IV: 3 mcg/kg/min is the average dose if the patient is not receiving any other antihypertensive drug. The dose is adjusted (not to exceed 8 mcg/kg/min) by the desired effect based on the pretreatment blood pressure and the use of concurrent antihypertensive drugs. If the blood pressure has not been reduced at the higher rate of infusion in 10 minutes, the drug should be discontinued.

ADVERSE EFFECTS AND NURSING CONSIDERATIONS: Precise measurements of the IV flow rate and continuous blood pressure monitoring are both essential for safe administration of sodium nitroprusside. The rapid reduction of blood pressure may cause apprehension, headache, restlessness, dizziness, nausea, diaphoresis, palpitations, and abdominal pain. The symptoms have been found to disappear with a slowing of the infusion rate or the temporary discontinuance of the IV; symptoms do not recur when the infusion begins again at a slower rate.

SPECIAL PRECAUTIONS:

1. Prepare IV administration of sodium nitroprusside in a solution of 5% D/W.
2. Do not add any preservative or other drug to the solution.
3. If prepared in advance the infusion solution should be protected from heat, light, and moisture.
4. Administer prepared drug in solution within 4 hours.
5. The solution is light brown; if it is any other color, discard it.
6. Protect infusion during administration by wrapping the IV bottle in aluminum foil or some opaque material.

Trimethaphan Camsylate
Arfonad

ACTIONS AND USES: Trimethaphan camsylate is a short-acting ganglionic blocking agent administered IV only. In addition, it has a direct vasodilating effect, which increases the patient's hypotensive response. A continuous infusion is necessary to maintain an antihypertensive effect. Patients may become refractory to trimethaphan camsylate after 48 hours of therapy. This drug is frequently employed in neurosurgery to produce some degree of hemostasis in capillary beds, arterioles, and venules. It prevents excessive bleeding and increases visualization and exposure of the surgical field.

PREPARATION AND DOSAGE: Continuous IV infusion 1.0 mg/ml in 5% D/W.

ADVERSE EFFECTS AND NURSING CONSIDERATIONS: Trimethaphan camsylate may cause urinary retention, orthostatic hypotension, anorexia, nausea, vomiting, dryness of the mouth, mydriasis, and cycloplegia. It may precipitate an anginal episode in the patient with angina pectoris. Respiratory depression and tachycardia may also occur.

SPECIAL PRECAUTIONS: An indwelling arterial line should be employed to facilitate blood pressure monitoring for the patient on trimethaphan camsylate. The blood pressure must be observed every 5 minutes. The patient may be placed supine to increase the hypotensive response. In addition the critical care nurse must observe closely for respiratory depression, especially if the patient has been receiving a muscle relaxant. Cardiac monitoring will provide a means of recognizing the potential complication of tachycardia.

ANTIPARKINSONISM AGENTS

Levodopa
Bendopa, Dopar, L-dopa, Levopa

ACTIONS AND USES: Levodopa is the most widely used and the most effective drug available for the symptomatic treatment of parkinsonism. It is a precursor of dopamine, a neurotransmitter that seems to be deficient in patients suffering from this disease. The majority of patients when treated with levodopa have a reduction of akinesia and rigidity. Tremors may increase in severity during the initial phase of therapy and later improve. The patient usually shows improvement in balance, posture, gait, speech, and handwriting. Drooling and oculogyric crises are usually reduced. Intellectual function may be improved and mood elevation achieved.

PREPARATION AND DOSAGE: The dose of levodopa is carefully adjusted to the individual patient and the severity of symptoms. The drug is available in 250 and 500 mg capsules and tablets for oral administration with meals. The dose is not to exceed 8 g daily.

ADVERSE EFFECTS AND NURSING CONSIDERATION: There are numerous adverse effects associated with levodopa therapy, which may be considered by bodily systems. Gastrointestinal effects include nausea, vomiting, anorexia, constipation, diarrhea, and bleeding. Cardiovascular symptoms include arrhythmias, orthostatic hypotension, palpitations, hypertension, and phlebitis. Musculoskeletal effects include a wide variety of symptoms ranging from involuntary muscular movements to opisthotonus. Psychological side effects include anxiety, confusion, depression, hallucinations, paranoia, and even suicidal tendencies. Neurologic side effects include ataxia, convulsions, headaches, tremors, weakness, and numbness. Most side effects are dose-related and disappear following dosage reduction. Neurologic and psychologic effects are more persistent.

SPECIAL PRECAUTIONS: Levodopa must be administered carefully when a patient has almost any physiologic disorder of organic basis. It is not recommended for use in children under 12 years of age, pregnant women, or nursing mothers.

1. Advise the patient and family of the action, side effects, and symptoms that should provoke medical attention.
2. Explain drug interactions and particularly have the patient refrain from taking vitamins containing vitamin B_6, which rapidly reverses levodopa effect.
3. Instruct the patient to adjust his schedule of activities slowly, in accordance with the best effects of the drug.
4. Question the physician regarding drug withdrawal and reinstatement orders.
5. Be certain the patient and family understand the prescribed dosage (not to exceed 8 g daily), the dosage schedule, and the expected effects of the drug.

DRUG INTERACTIONS:

1. MAO inhibitors increase the adrenergic effect of levodopa.
2. Sympathomimetic drugs also increase the adrenergic effect of levodopa.
3. Any antihypertensive or antianxiety drug that blocks adrenergic receptors decreases the effect of levodopa.
4. Pyridoxine reverses the effect of levodopa.

Amantadine Hydrochloride
Symmetrel

ACTIONS AND USES: Amantadine hydrochloride is an antiviral agent that produces moderate reduction of parkinsonian symptoms. Although the method of action is not understood, it is believed to be related to the release of dopamine as well as other catecholamines from neuronal sites. Amantadine hydrochloride is considerably less effective than levodopa, although it does produce more rapid clinical improvement initially and has fewer untoward reactions. Its primary use is in patients who cannot tolerate large doses of levodopa.

PREPARATION AND DOSAGE: Oral administration for idiopathic or postencephalitic parkinsonism for adults is initially 100 mg daily after breakfast for 5 to 7 days. If adverse reactions do not appear and symptoms are not under control, the dose may be increased to up to 200 mg per day.

ADVERSE EFFECTS AND NURSING CONSIDERATIONS: The primary adverse effect of amantadine hydrochloride is livedo reticularis. This is a peripheral vascular condition characterized by a discoloration of the skin due to passive congestion, which appears as a reddish-blue, net like mottling of the skin in the extremities. It disappears after the drug is discontinued. Edema of the ankles, apparently from increased capillary permeability, may also occur. Other symptoms include dizziness, nervousness, the inability to concentrate, ataxia, slurred speech, insomnia, lethargy, blurred vision, dryness of the mouth, gastrointestinal upset, and rash. The peripheral and central adverse effects of the anticholinergic drugs are increased by amantadine hydrochloride. Combined therapy has produced psychotic reactions in some people.

CENTRAL-ACTING ANTICHOLINERGIC AGENTS

Generic Name	Trade Name
TRIHEXYPHENIDYL	Artane, Tremin
BIPERIDEN	Akineton
CYCRIMINE	Pagitane
PROCYCLIDINE	Kemadrin
DIPHENHYDRAMINE	Benadryl
CHLORPHENOXAMINE	Phenoxene
ORPHENADRINE	Norflex
BENZTROPINE	Cogentin
ETHOPROPAZINE	Parsidol

ACTIONS AND USES: These agents are used as adjuncts to levodopa therapy or as the sole drug in patients who cannot tolerate levodopa. Their effect seems to be related to their central cholinergic blocking action. In fact, those anticholinergic agents that do not readily cross the blood-brain barrier, such as quaternary ammonium compounds, have no effect on the symptoms of parkinsonism. The anticholinergic drugs are considered to be less effective than levodopa for treating parkinsonism; however, they do produce slight to moderate improvement of symptoms with some improvement in functional capabilities. Unfortunately, their usefulness is limited by side effects, which often preclude the administration of a therapeutic dose, and their tendency to be less effective with continued use.

PREPARATION AND DOSAGE: The dosage of the individual anticholinergic agent should be referred to prior to administration.

ADVERSE EFFECTS AND NURSING CONSIDERATIONS: Some degree of toxicity will usually appear with all of the anticholinergic drugs when a therapeutic dose is employed. The most common adverse effects include dryness of the mouth, mydriasis, cycloplegia, tachycardia, constipation, urinary retention, and psychic disturbances. Because the anticholinergic drugs have a mydriatic effect, they may precipitate acute glaucoma. These drugs, however, may be used safely in the open-angle glaucomatous patient on miotic drug therapy. Patients who suffer from prostatic hypertrophy must be closely observed for urinary retention. In addition those patients with gastrointestinal disorders must be observed for signs of intestinal obstruction. The most common psychic disturbances are impairment of recent memory, mild confusion, insomnia, and restlessness. More serious disturbances such as agitation, disorientation, delirium, paranoid reaction, and hallucinations may occur, especially in the elderly. Large doses of anticholinergic drugs have produced marked elevation in body temperature, especially in children, which may be life-threatening.

ANTICHOLINESTERASE DRUGS

ACTIONS AND USES: The agents used to treat myasthenia gravis are the reversible anticholinesterase compounds. These drugs are thought to alleviate symptoms by inhibiting cholinesterase (the enzyme that destroys acetylcholine), producing an increase in acetylcholine at the motor end plate. The drugs most effective in accomplishing this are: the quaternary ammonium compounds neostigmine bromide, ambenonium chloride, and pyridostigmine bromide; and edrophonium chloride. Exacerbations of myasthenia gravis commonly progress to the more acute symptomatology of myasthenic crisis. As pointed out on p. 214, the manifestations of myasthenic crisis and cholinergic crisis are similar, so that it is often difficult clinically to gain a differential diagnosis. Some authorities prefer a pharmacologic test as a diagnostic aid. This test is performed in a critical care unit where facilities for endotracheal intubation and respiratory support are available for the patient. Usually a small IV dose (1–2 mg) of a short-acting cholinesterase inhibitor, edrophonium chloride, will produce a brief remission of myasthenic crisis and an exacerbation of a cholinergic crisis. If an overdose of the anticholinesterase drug is suspected (cholinergic crisis), 500 mg of pralidoxime is given slowly IV. Pralidoxime is a cholinesterase reactivator, which may temporarily increase muscle strength in cholinergic crisis. This drug is given very cautiously, since it may convert a cholinergic crisis to a myasthenic crisis. When neostigmine bromide is used IV or IM to treat exacerbations of myasthenia gravis, atropine may be used as a supplemental agent to control the side effects of anticholinesterase drugs on the secretory glands, heart, and gastrointestinal smooth muscle.

Neostigmine Bromide ⎫ **ORAL**
Prostigmine Bromide ⎭

Neostigmine Methylsulfate ⎫ **IM or IV**
Prostigmine Methylsulfate ⎭

ACTIONS AND USES: Neostigmine bromide is a quaternary ammonium compound that inhibits cholinesterase, the enzyme which destroys acetylcholine. The effect is an increase in the concentration of acetylcholine at the motor end plate.

PREPARATION AND DOSAGE: Neostigmine bromide PO for myasthenia gravis: adult 15–45 mg q 2–4 hrs; pediatric 7.5–15 mg 3–4 times daily. Neostigmine methylsulfate IM or IV for diagnosis of myasthenia gravis: 0.22–0.31 mg/kg in conjunction with atropine 0.011–0.016 mg/kg IM for control of side effects; pediatric 0.025 mg/kg in conjunction with atropine 0.011 mg/kg, SC for control of side effects.
Neostigmine methylsulfate IM or IV for treating exacerbations of myasthenia gravis: adult 0.5–2 mg q 1–3 hrs in conjunction with atropine 0.2–0.6 mg IM q 3–6 hrs; pediatrics 0.1–0.2 mg q.i.d. SC in conjunction with atropine 0.01 mg/kg SC q 1–8 hrs.

ADVERSE EFFECTS AND NURSING CONSIDERATIONS: Neostigmine may produce miosis, hyperhidrosis, hypersalivation, gastrointestinal distress, and bradycardia. Although atropine may be used to treat these side effects, it must be kept in mind that a sudden increase in adverse symptoms is often the first sign of overdose, which may be masked by the atropine. Anticholinesterase drugs are contraindicated in the presence of mechanical obstruction of the intestinal or urinary tract.

SPECIAL PRECAUTIONS: When signs of overdose appear (cholinergic crisis), neostigmine should be temporarily discontinued and 1–2 mg of atropine given IV. Respirations must be supported as indicated. Pralidoxime may be given slowly and cautiously to reverse respiratory arrest and improve muscle strength. A dose of 50 mg IV is administered every minute (not to exceed 1 g) until symptoms of overdose subside. Pralidoxime may convert cholinergic crisis to myasthenic crisis.

Ambenonium Chloride
Mytelase Chloride

ACTION AND USES: Ambenonium chloride is an oral anticholinesterase drug used to treat myasthenia gravis. It produces fewer side effects than neostigmine and may possess a longer duration of action. It may be used for patients who are unable to tolerate neostigmine bromide because of a bromide ion sensitivity.

PREPARATION AND DOSAGE: The dose is regulated by the patient's response and the severity of the disease. PO: adult maintenance 10-30 mg q 3-4 hrs; pediatric maintenance 1.5 mg/kg in 24 hrs in 3-4 divided doses.

ADVERSE EFFECTS AND NURSING CONSIDERATIONS: The adverse effects and contraindications for ambenonium chloride are the same as those for neostigmine bromide.

Pyridostigmine Bromide
Mestinon

ACTION AND USES: Pyridostigmine is an anticholinergic agent used orally to treat myasthenia gravis. Like ambenonium chloride, it produces fewer side effects than neostigmine and has a longer duration of action.

PREPARATION AND DOSAGE: Pyridostigmine bromide is available in a syrup, which is useful if the patient is unable to swallow or for one with a nasogastric tube. Pyridostigmine bromide PO: adult 60-300 mg q 4 hrs; pediatric 7 mg/kg q 24 hrs in divided doses.

ADVERSE EFFECTS AND NURSING CONSIDERATIONS: The adverse effects and contraindications for the use of pyridostigmine bromide are the same as for neostigmine.

Edrophonium Chloride
Tensilon

ACTIONS AND USES: Edrophonium chloride is a drug used to diagnose myasthenia gravis and for differential diagnosis of myasthenic crisis and cholinergic crisis. It is a short-acting cholinesterase inhibitor whose effects are felt but briefly. When it is administered IV, muscle strength increases within 1-3 minutes in myasthenic patients.

PREPARATION AND DOSAGE: Edrophonium chloride for diagnosis of myasthenia gravis: adult IV 2 mg injected within 15-30 seconds; if there is no response in 45 seconds, an additional 8 mg IV may be used. In patients over 50 years old, 0.4 mg of atropine SC 10 minutes prior to the test may be given to prevent bradycardia and hypotension. Pediatric 0.2 mg/kg with 1/5 of this dose given within 1 minute; if there is no response, administer remainder of the dose. Edrophonium chloride for differential diagnosis of crisis: adult IV 1-2 mg.

ADVERSE EFFECTS AMD NURSING CONSIDERATIONS: The adverse effects of edrophonium chloride are the same as for all anticholinesterase agents. In patients with myasthenic crisis a small dose IV should produce remission of symptoms. If the patient is in cholinergic crisis, it will further weaken him. Therefore, the drug should be used under these circumstances in a critical care setting with facilities available for intubation and assisted ventilation.

MISCELLANEOUS DRUGS

ANTI-INFLAMMATORY DRUGS

Dexamethasone Sodium Phosphate
Decadron Phosphate, Hexadrol Phosphate

ACTIONS AND USES: Dexamethasone is a synethetic glucocorticoid used parenterally for the treatment of cerebral edema. The edema may be in association with brain tumor, head injury, subarachnoid hemorrhage, irradiation, or other causes. The drug is a potent anti-inflammatory agent, but its direct effect on the cerebrovasculature is poorly understood. For this reason it is used on a short-term basis.

PREPARATION AND DOSAGE: Initially 6-10 mg IV followed by 4-6 mg IM or IV q 6 hrs until maximum improvement results, generally within 2-4 days.

ADVERSE EFFECTS AND NURSING CONSIDERATIONS: Since all glucocorticoids cause a thinning of the gastric mucosa, the risk of gastrointestinal bleeding in patients with active ulcers or gastrointestinal bleeding with the development of stress ulcers must be emphasized. Most neurosurgeons recommend concommitant, prophylactic use of antacids and routine examination of nasogastric aspirate and stools for occult blood.

OSMOTIC DIURETICS

Urea
Ureaphil, Urevert

ACTIONS AND USES: Urea is an osmotic diuretic given IV for the temporary reduction of intracranial or cerebrospinal pressure in the control of cerebral edema. Urea appears in the glomerular filtrate, remains in the tubular fluid, and limits the reabsorption of sodium. The effect of urea persists for 3–10 hours.

PREPARATION AND DOSAGE: The usual dose of urea is an IV administration of a 30% solution in 5 or 10% D/W or 10% invert sugar. To prepare 135 ml of a 30% solution of urea, mix the contents of one 40 g vial with 105 ml of diluent. Each ml then provides 300 mg of urea. Adult dose: 1–1.5 g (3.3–5 ml of 30% solution) per kg; pediatric 0.5–1.5 g/kg.

ADVERSE EFFECTS AND NURSING CONSIDERATIONS: Headache, nausea, vomiting, syncope, disorientation, and transient agitation may occur during the infusion of urea. Hyponatremia and hypokalemia may occur, and signs such as muscle weakness and lethargy must be observed for. If urea is allowed to extravasate, local reactions ranging from irritation to necrosis may occur. Phlebitis and thrombosis may occur along the infusion site. Urea must not be used in veins of the legs, as superficial and deep leg thrombosis may occur. Urea must be used cautiously in patients with cardiac, hepatic, or renal disease. It is contraindicated in patients with severely impaired renal function or liver failure. It should not be used on patients with elevated BUN or creatinine levels. In the presence of a space-occupying lesion, urea may increase the bleeding, resulting in cerebellar tonsillar herniation.

SPECIAL PRECAUTIONS: To avoid hemolysis, do not exceed a rate of infusion greater than 4 ml/min of a 30% solution. A prepared solution may be stored no longer than 48 hours in the refrigerator. Urea may never be mixed with blood in a transfusion.

Mannitol
Osmitrol

ACTIONS AND USES: Mannitol has the same effect as urea, but a larger volume is required to produce the same response. Mannitol is less irritating than urea, is less likely to cause thrombophlebitis, and does not cause tissue necrosis following accidental extravasation.

PREPARATION AND DOSAGE: IV administration of 15% mannitol in water, 150–500 ml over 1 hour until the patient's clinical signs improve. This may be repeated if necessary.

ADVERSE EFFECTS AND NURSING CONSIDERATIONS: These are uncommon when recommended doses are not exceeded. Symptoms may include headache, nausea, chills, thirst, dizziness, and chest pain. Signs of water intoxication have occurred only when the dosage has exceeded 200 g/8 hrs. Transient pulmonary congestion may occur.

SPECIAL PRECAUTIONS: Administer slowly to prevent overexpansion of the intravascular space. Avoid extravasation. In severely ill patients, fluid and electrolyte balance, urine volume, and vital signs must be carefully monitored. Hypertonic solutions of mannitol should not be mixed with blood transfusions, as crenation and agglutination of red blood cells may occur.

BIBLIOGRAPHY

AMA Drug Evaluations, 2nd ed., prepared by the AMA Department of Drugs, Acton, Massachusetts: Publishing Sciences Group, Inc., 1973.

Bergersen, Betty S., *Pharmacology In Nursing*, 13th ed., St. Louis: The C. V. Mosby Co., 1976.

Falconer, Mary W., et al., *Current Drug Handbook, 1976-1978*, Philadelphia: W. B. Saunders Co., 1976.

Loebl, Suzanne, et al., *The Nurse's Drug Handbook*, New York: John Wiley and Sons, Inc., 1977.

Rodman, Morton J., and Dorothy W. Smith, *Pharmacology and Drug Therapy in Nursing*, Philadelphia: J. B. Lippincott Co., 1968.

12
TEST AND REVIEW

I *Admission Situation:* 1100 hrs Friday. Patient is a 27-year-old female admitted to ICU at 1100 hrs on a Friday, following a fall from the top of a ladder. She landed on the back of her head.

Admitting diagnosis: Head injury with concussion; no skull fracture. VS: B/P 128/70, HR 88, R 24, T 98.

Neuro exam on admission: Patient is lethargic, but otherwise the neuro exam is grossly normal.

Problem Situation: 1300 hrs Friday.

Subjective: Pt. complains of increased headache over last 2 hrs. She states the headache is not localized and is now moderately severe. She also states that her head is sore. Denies nausea, vomiting, or other symptoms.

Objective: II–XII cranial nerves intact. Level of consciousness is lethargic; no restlessness; well oriented; no aphasia; cognitive thought intact. DTR's symmetrical; no pathological reflexes. Motion and coordination intact. B/P 132/68, HR 84, R 24, T 98.4. Breath sounds clear, ventilation adequate. Color pink, warm, and dry.

Assessment:

Plan:

II *Admission Situation:* 0200 hrs Wednesday. Patient admitted to ICU at 0200 hrs following motor vehicle accident at 0010 hrs. Pt. was unconscious approx. 20 min, has retrograde amnesia. Skull films in E.D. revealed frontal and cribiform plate fractures. No other apparent injuries. Initial exam in ICU unchanged from that in ED. Neuro: II–XII C.N. intact; II, III, IV, VI difficult to check because of severe periorbital ecchymosis and edema. Level of consciousness lethargic; answers a few questions with confused answers. Is not aware of situation, time, or place.

Moves all extremities without apparent paresis or paralysis.

DTR's symmetrical, no pathological reflexes.

Cardiac: NSR by ECG at 74. Heart tones loud at apex without murmurs, gallops, or rubs. No neck vein distention. Peripheral pulses symmetrical. Color pink, warm, and dry.

Respiratory: Chest clear to P and A. 0200 PaO_2 96, $PaCO_2$ 42, pH 7.43, resp. freq. 18.

GI/GU: no active bowel tones. No n/v. Foley in place to straight-drain; urine clear 180 cc out with sp. gr. 1.016.

Musculoskeletal: intact other than skull fracture; C-spine films negative.

Orders: IV of 1000 Ringer's lactate over 10 hrs

      TXM for hold

      Decadron 4 mg q 6 hrs IV

      Neuro checks every 30 min

Problem Situation: 0300 hrs Wednesday.

Subjective: Pt. complains of a "runny" nose; denies prior cold symptoms. Complains of slight nausea, no vomiting.

Objective: Pink serous exudate from both nares. Patient swallowing frequently. All other systems unchanged.

Assessment:

Plan:

III *Admission Situation*: Refer to patient admission situation II.

    Problem Situation: 0600 hrs, day of admission.

    Subjective: N/A.

    Objective: Resp. freq. increased to 32/min. Respirations shallow. Stertorous noise during inspiration.

    Auscultation: multiple loud rhonchi over large airways; BS equal; color: pale lips and nailbeds cyanotic. Skin warm and dry. B/P 146/76, HR 72.

    Neuro: Increased lethargy and restlessness; otherwise same as 0200 hrs.

    Assessment:

Plan:

_____

IV *Problem Situation*: Refer to patient admission situation II.
Time is now 1100 hrs.
Subjective: N/A.
Objective: Neuro: Right pupil dilated and fixed
Left Babinski
Jackknife spasticity in left arm
Left hemiparesis
Stuporous
Asymmetrical increase in DTR's in left arm/leg

Assessment:

Plan:

_____

V *Admission Situation*: A 17-year-old male high school student presents with a 3-week history of sinusitis, postnasal drip, persistent low
grade fever, and malaise. All symptoms followed a blow to the frontal
area by a basketball. He was treated in an outlying community
doctor's office with low dose oral penicillin. Despite treatment, the
pt.'s symptoms became increasingly more severe. He experienced a 10-
kg weight loss due to persistent nausea and vomiting. On the day of
admission the patient awakened with total motor aphasia and urinary
incontinence. This prompted the parents to bring the pt. to an urban
neuro center. Initial admission data (1500 hrs): Appears extremely ill,
emaciated, restless.
Neuro: lethargic, restless, seems oriented when presented with yes-no
questions.
Total motor aphasia
C.N.'s intact
Bilateral Babinski's
Left ankle clonus
Brudzinski's and Kernig's signs
Nuchal rigidity
Motion, coordination intact

Other systems:
 Purulent, malodorous nasal discharge.
 Continuous vomiting
 Poor skin turgor, eyeballs soft
 Color pale, profuse diaphoresis
 B/P 96/60, HR 122, T 104.6
 Resp. freq. 38
Ancillary data:
 C-spine, skull films normal
 PA/lat. chest film normal
 CBC Hgb 19
   Hct 54
   WBC 32,000 with marked increase in mature and immature
    polymorphonuclear cells.
   Platelets adequate
 CSF by LP revealed grossly purulent fluid with many WBC's and
  normal pressures.

Assessment:
 1. Brain abscess with meningitis
 2. Urinary incontinence very bothersome and embarrassing to pt.
 3. Poor nutritional status
 4. Fever
 5. Communication difficult

Plan: Develop a plan for each area cited above. Include alternates.

VI *Admission Situation*: A 63-year-old female is admitted to ICU after
 a motor vehicle accident.
 E.D. 1400 hrs: Respiratory system: intact; chest film normal.
 Cardiovascular system: intact with B/P 128/70, HR 78, resp. 26.
 Neuro: Pt was unconscious for approximately 1 hr and has retrograde
 amnesia. No skull or C-spine fractures.
  Stuporous
  CN's intact
  No paresis/paralysis
  Bilateral Babinski's
 Musculosketetal: left compound, comminuted femoral fracture.
 Steinman pin to Thomas splint with traction. Other systems intact.

IV with Ringer's lactate.
Problem Situation: ICU at 1645 hrs.
Subjective: N/A.
Objective: B/P 98/60, HR 112, resp. 26.
All systems unchanged except VS; skin cool, moist.

Assessment:

Plan:

VII *Admission Situation*: Refer to patient admission situation VI.
Problem Situation: Time now 2000 hrs.
Subjective: N/A.
Objective: Pt. regains consciousness. Neurologically intact except patient states she is totally blind.

Assessment:

Plan:

VIII *Admission Situation*: A 47-year-old female was assaulted with a hammer at 2230 hrs. The one blow to the head produced brief, transient loss of consciousness. No other injuries.
Skull films in Emergency Department reveal nondepressed closed right temporal fracture.
Initial neuro: intact.
Admitted to ICU 0030 hrs.
Physical exam including neuro unremarkable.
Problem Situation: 1030 hrs next morning.
Subjective: C/O severe nonlocalized headache.
Objective: Neuro: Right pupil fixed and larger than left. No consensual response in left eye. Otherwise intact.

Assessment:

Plan: Set priorities for plan.

IX *Situation*: A 20-year-old male army recruit in ICU for 4 days with acute fulminant purpuric meningococcal meningitis. For duration of stay the pt. has been comatose with decorticate motor response and is opisthotonic. Intubated and on MA-1 for apnea.
1700 hrs.:
Subjective: N/A.
Objective: Develops repeating grand mal seizures 40 sec duration; followed by flaccid paralysis, then seizure repeats. Is on anti-seizure medication. Bites off endotracheal tube during each seizure.

Assessment:

Plan:

X *Situation*: A 52-year-old male myasthenic pt. (for several years) admitted to ICU with diagnosis of pending crisis, unknown etiology. Myasthenic symptoms have increased over last week.
Subjective: N/A.
Objective: On 3 occasions his wife has visited him in ICU. It has been noted that when she leaves he has an increase in weakness, increase in inability to swallow, and increase in inability to handle secretions. In addition, his wife has offered that they are contemplating divorce.

Assessment:

Plan:

XI *Situation*: A 36-year-old married female with children is in ICU following a supratentorial craniotomy for tumor excision of a glioblastoma multiforme. She is on her 6th postop day and has done very well. Her neurosurgeon discussed her diagnosis with her yesterday. The only medication she is on is dexamethasone.

Subjective: C/O hallucinations.

Objective: Neuro check grossly normal, although pt. is irritable. She is now disoriented and confused, and freely hallucinating.

Assessment:

Plan:

XII *Situation*: A postop supratentorial craniotomy pt. is doing well following removal of a meningioma. He is 52 years old. It is 11 hrs since he returned from surgery. Neuro checks are every hour.

Subjective: N/A.

Objective: Neuro: Level of consciousness has declined in 1 hr from alert to stuporous. He has become restless. Otherwise normal. Resp: Adequate ventilation. All other systems normal.

Assessment:

Plan:

XIII *Situation*: A 24-year-old male is admitted to ICU from OR at 2300 hrs. He sustained a .38 caliber gunshot wound in the posterior neck just lateral to the area of C-4. He was brought to ED 2 hrs following the injury, at which time he was found to be quadriplegic. He was taken to OR for debridement.

At 0800 hrs the next day:

Subjective: C/O lightheadedness, dizziness.

Objective: B/P down (from 116/60) to 98/48. HR (from 82) to 58. Pale, moist. Cyanotic lips and nailbeds.

Resp: Shallow at 12 min.

Neuro: unchanged.

Assessment:

Plan:

XIV *Situation*: A 44-year-old female is admitted to ICU for observation following a subarachnoid hemorrhage. On admission she is alert, oriented; C.N.'s intact; motion, coordination intact; DTR's symmetrical; has a Brudzinski's sign, Kernig's sign, and nuchal rigidity. She has been stable for 3 days.
Third day:
Subjective: C/O severe nonlocalizing headache of sudden onset.
Objective: Neuro: only change is decrease in level of consciousness from alert to stuporous.

Assessment:

Plan:

XV *Situation*: A 27-year-old female is on the med-surg ward 6 hrs following the transsphenoidal removal of a small pituitary chromophobe adenoma. She developed severe polyuria (895 ml in 1 hr) with a specific gravity of 1.001 and also dropped her B/P from a normotensive state to 94/60. Her HR increased to 120. Because of these developments, the neurosurgeon is transferring the pt. to ICU.

Plan: What are you prepared for? How will you anticipate her arrival?

XVI *Situation*: A 16-year-old male is suspected of having an A-V anomaly. He will be going for an angiogram and a brain scan, about both of which he is very anxious.

How can you prepare him?
How can you involve his family?

XVII *Situation*: An 18-year-old male is on the neuro ward 8 weeks following a C-6 fracture. He is quadriplegic. The head nurse is approached by a student nurse who is concerned about the pt. The s.n. finds the pt. extremely agitated, anxious; he states that feeling must be returning because he is having severe flexor muscle spasms in both legs.

Plan: How should this problem be dealt with?

XVIII *Situation*: A 9-year-old female is in ICU 9 hrs following an infratentorial craniotomy for partial excision of a medulloblastoma. She has been stable since surgery, although she has remained stuporous.
Subjective: N/A.
Objective: *Sudden onset* of Cheyne-Stokes respirations with 30-sec apneic periods every 2 min, pupils dilated, and fixed, bilateral decerebration.

Assessment:

Plan:

IXX *Situation*: 14-year-old female who, following a dive into shallow water (2300 hrs), is admitted through ED to ICU. C-6 fracture by X-ray; C-6 quadriplegia. Admitted to ICU at 0200 hrs.
Subjective: N/A.
Objective: At 0230 on admission to ICU, on admission physical her bladder is percussed at the umbilicus.

Assessment:

Plan:

XX *Situation*: A 43-year-old female is admitted to ICU with idiopathic epilepsy and possible status epilepticus. If she has seizures, what would be important to observe, report, and record?

DISCUSSION

I *Assessment*: Pt.'s headache is probably due to concussion.
Plan:
1. Observe neuro signs every 30 min for possibility of developing intracranial bleed or cerebral edema.
2. Give pain medication if ordered.
3. Notify neurosurgeon if any further deterioration.

II *Assessment*: Probable CSF rhinorrhea. Nausea from swallowing CSF.
Plan:
1. Place pink serous exudate on a 4 × 4 gauze. If clear fluid haloes around pink, CSF leak is probable.
2. Notify neurosurgeon if suspicion confirmed and discuss alleviation of nausea.
3. Elevate HOB 45°.
4. Instruct pt. not to blow nose; tell him why and what is happening.
5. Do not suction nose or insert tubes.
6. Have pt. spit out CSF exudate so he won't swallow it.
7. Administer antiemetic if ordered.
8. Monitor ability to handle CSF drainage with decreased level of consciousness.

III *Assessment*: Respiratory insufficiency and/or failure, probably due to decrease in level of consciousness affecting ability to handle secretions.
Plan:
1. Arterial blood gases.
2. Try to cough and deep-breathe pt.

    3. Notify neurosurgeon.
    4. Elevate HOB 45° and position pt. in lateral semi-Fowler's.
    5. Monitor respiratory status every 30 min.

IV *Assessment*: Probable subdural hematoma (may be epidural) with subsequent tentorial herniation onto III C.N. (right) and pressure on upper motor neuron in brain stem.
  Plan:
    1. Notify neurosurgeon immediately.
    2. Call OR or appropriate person (i.e., nsg. supervisor) to prepare for pending surgical decompression.
    3. Prepare twist drill tray and necessary equipment.
    4. Type and crossmatch (10 min) for 2–4 units whole blood.
    5. Notify family; obtain phone permission with two witnesses.
    6. Call appropriate clergy or have operator do same.
    7. Shave scalp, retaining hair.
    8. Prepare to intubate pt.
    9. Monitor EKG and neuro status until neurosurgeon arrives.

V 1. Brain abscess/meningitis: Be ready for surgical decompression. Darken room. Keep quiet. Give medications as directed. Observe for further neuro sequelae.
    2. Urinary incontinence: Try Texas condom or other means before resorting to Foley. Pt.'s resistance is extremely poor, and any indwelling device must be considered cautiously.
    3. Nutritional status: Try feeding pt. several small feedings/day. Encourage fluids and use pt.'s favored food and drinks. Discuss hyperalimentation—both parenteral and PO; weigh daily.
    4. Fever: Avoid hypothermia blankets to avoid breakdown of skin on bony prominences (from pt.'s severe emaciation). Try tepid water sponges and/or alcohol sponges.
    5. Communication: Offer pt. paper and pencil on clipboard, or offer slate board for communication. Have parents stay with pt. as much as possible. Assign consistent staffing pattern to pt.

VI *Assessment*: Pt is probably hypovolemic and suffering blood loss from fractured femur.
  Plan:
    1. Notify appropriate physician.
    2. Increase rate of IV infusion until orders received.
    3. Type and crossmatch.
    4. CBC for Hct and Hgb stat.
    5. Monitor VS every 15 min.

VII *Assessment*: Possible occipital cortical bruise causing cortical blindness.

Plan:

 1. Notify neurosurgeon.
 2. *Stay with pt.* and try to offer psychological support to reduce
    anxiety and fear. The tremendous shock may be overwhelming
    for the patient, and having someone in physical contact with
    verbal empathic responses may be helpful.

VIII *Assessment*: Possible epidural hematoma (more likely than subdural).

Plan:

 1. Notify neurosurgeon.
 2. Prepare twist drill tray or call OR according to neurosurgeon's
    preference.
 3. Type and crossmatch (10 min) for 2–4 units whole blood.
 4. Notify family; obtain phone permission with two witnesses.
 5. Call appropriate clergy.
 6. Shave scalp, retaining hair.
 7. Prepare to intubate pt.
 8. Monitor EKG, neuro status until neurosurgeon arrives.

IX *Assessment*: Trismus of jaw causing pt. to bite off endotracheal tube.

Plan: When pt. is flaccid, insert solid bite-block and oral plastic
airway, and secure ETT. This should alleviate problem.

X *Assessment*: The psychological environment of the marriage may be
affecting the patient's physical condition.

Plan: The conflict may be influencing the impending crisis and may
further interfere with the patient's recovery. Initially the nurse may be
able to discover the basis of the problem and validate some existing
feelings between the husband and wife. Interviewing techniques and
communication skills become invaluable. Perhaps temporarily the
wife should not visit—at least this would be one alternative. If the situation is intense, certainly a referral to a specialist in counseling,
mental health, etc., would be appropriate. The "hurting family" needs
support, an opportunity to discuss problems on a feeling level, and
often some guidance in problem solving.

XI *Assessment*: The patient's psychological disorganization is probably
related to the shock and stress of becoming aware of her prognosis.

Plan: Initially the patient may need protection from herself or her
environment. The doctor may prescribe psychotropic drugs. The

patient and her family may need assistance in dealing with death and dying. Nursing intervention is based on fostering cohesion of the family unit and exploring and combating despair. Utilize family strengths in support of the patient. There will be many hurdles for the patient and family to overcome; the reality of bereavement must be approached slowly and gently. The nurse must CARE.

XII *Assessment*: Patient is probably developing cerebral edema.
   Plan:
   1. Notify neurosurgeon.
   2. Observe pt. closely, as he may develop brain stem compression with subsequent respiratory embarrassment.
   3. Prepare urea or mannitol for administration (whichever physician prefers).
   4. Note time of last dose of dexamethasone.

XIII *Assessment*: GSW probably produced ischemic cord damage, which is possibly now increasing, converting the C-4 quadriplegia to C-3 quadriplegia. This is producing autonomic response and respiratory embarrassment.
   Plan:
   1. Arterial blood gases.
   2. Bag pt.
   3. Administer low flow O_2.
   4. Notify neurosurgeon.

XIV *Assessment*: Possible rebleed.
   Plan:
   1. Notify neurosurgeon.
   2. Monitor neuro signs frequently (every 30 min).

XV What are your prepared for?
   The patient has probably developed diabetes insipidus; the polyuria has depleted her blood volume, producing hypovolemia.
   How will you anticipate her arrival?
   1. Prepare pitressin for administration.
   2. Have IV tray ready with plasmanate and Ringer's lactate readily available.
   3. Take urometer and hydrometer to bedside.
   4. Have equipment ready to obtain serum electrolytes.

XVI Preparation of the patient: Generally a boy of this age would understand an explanation of the procedure. Information can often relieve the anxiety of the unknown. One interesting approach might be to have him draw the anatomy he is familiar with; or if he is knowledgeable about machinery, tools, etc., he might be able to discuss the X-ray and other equipment. If you can get an idea of what he does understand, then you can proceed from that point on to what he needs to know about the diagnostic techniques. It is surprising how anxiety diminishes when you allow the patient to use the energy generated by stress in talking, drawing, and so on.

Preparation of the family: The family needs a comprehensive understanding of the procedure to be done along with a description of the risks involved. If the relationship is supportive, the family may become involved in providing strength and encouragement for the boy.

XVII How should this problem be dealt with?
1. Explain mechanism of spinal shock, recovery, and spinal automatisms to the student.
2. Explain the importance of the pt.'s understanding to prevent false encouragement.
3. Discuss different methods of communicating this to the pt.

XVIII *Assessment*: Probable brain stem herniation from cerebral edema.
Plan:
1. Place HOB flat.
2. Call anesthesia to intubate pt; call respiratory therapy for MA-1.
3. Notify neurosurgeon immediately.
4. Prepare urea or mannitol (whichever neurosurgeon prefers).
5. Call clergy.
6. Notify family.

IXX *Assessment*: Urinary retention from spinal shock. Patient should have been catheterized in ED. This step is extremely important to facilitate future bladder training.
Plan:
1. Foley to straight drain.
2. Drain 800 cc urine every 30 minutes until bladder is empty.

XX Observation and reporting of seizures: The nurse is responsible for observing and reporting the following:
1. The duration of the seizure; the time it begins and ends; the time consumed in the tonic, clonic, flaccid, and postictal phases.
2. The presence of and description of aura.
3. The patient's level of consciousness; it should be determined and changes in the level noted.

4. The motor activity during the episode, including where the activity begins and what parts of the body become involved. Note any deviation of eyes or tongue.
5. The presence or absence of bowel or bladder incontinence.
6. The patient's response to the seizure.
7. The patient's response to drug therapy.
8. The frequency and number of seizures.

INDEX

Page numbers in italics are either tables or illustrations.